Chronic Disease Management:
A New Paradigm for Care

PATRICK J MCEVOY

FRCGP

General Medical Practitioner

Londonderry

Foreword by

PROFESSOR MIKE PRINGLE

President

Royal College of General Practitioners

Radcliffe Publishing

London • New York

Radcliffe Publishing Ltd
St Mark's House
Shepherdess Walk
London N1 7BQ
United Kingdom

www.radcliffehealth.com

British Library Cataloguing in Publication Data

A catalogue record for this book is available from the British Library.

ISBN-13: 978 190891 156 8

The paper used for the text pages of this book
is FSC® certified. FSC (The Forest Stewardship
Council®) is an international network to promote
responsible management of the world's forests.

Typeset by Darkriver Design, Auckland, New Zealand
Manufacturing managed by 21six

Contents

Foreword

In the next 20 years, the Department of Health in England expects the number of those aged over 80 years to double and the number of people with a long-term condition to increase by 3 million. The same trends apply in all developed countries. While there is nothing we can do to alter these facts, there is much we can do to address the way we conceive of and manage chronic disease.

As this book sets out, health systems have been trying to squeeze the management of chronic disease into an acute care mould. Furthermore, it is perverse that chronic disease represents so much loss of quality of life for patients, so much work for primary care teams, so much resource use in our hospitals, yet we do not place proportionate weight on understanding, training for and planning chronic care. Long-term conditions along with multi-morbidity will be the priority challenge for this century in all health systems, and we need fresh thinking and new tools to confront this challenge.

Our major resource is, of course, those with chronic diseases themselves. They are the experts on their experience of the illness and care pathway, on their expectations and on the trade-offs that they will find acceptable. At the same time, health professionals are the custodians of scientific information and service resources. The best decision-making comes when the consultation is a meeting of the two experts, both striving from different perspectives to achieve the same overall goals of effective care and maximum well-being along the continuing path of illness and disability.

For those who aspire to achieve optimal outcomes, this book is their invaluable guide. It presents an evidence-based, generic profile of chronic disease as well as putting a recognisable face on the main players – the patients, their carers, the clinicians, all involved in training and the health system. Three key elements emerge: (1) a generic paradigm of chronic disease, (2) a trajectory-based model of clinical management and (3) a curriculum for chronic care. These have universal application. Dr McEvoy, who has written extensively on medical education, presents us with a timely analysis of current issues in chronic disease as well as a unique teaching and learning resource.

Professor Mike Pringle
President
Royal College of General Practitioners
March 2014

About the author

Patrick J McEvoy was born in Larne, Northern Ireland, in 1947 and was educated at St MacNissi's College and The Queen's University of Belfast. He graduated in medicine in 1971 and was made Fellow of the Royal College of General Practitioners in 1994. From 2000 to 2002 he was Provost, Royal College of General Practitioners Northern Ireland.

Following hospital posts in Belfast and Kenya, he worked in general practices in Belfast before taking up partnership at The Aberfoyle Medical Practice, Derry, in 1978. He was also Honorary Lecturer at the Faculty of Medicine, The Queen's University of Belfast, 1998–2012; Trainer and Programme Director with the Northern Ireland Medical and Dental Training Agency, 1982–2008; and Chair of the Association of Course Organisers, 2005.

He is the author of the UK training manual for GP postgraduate programme directors, *Educating the Future GP: The Course Organisers' Handbook* (1993; 2nd edition 1998), published by Radcliffe Medical Press.

Between 1994 and 2006 he undertook medical educational consultancies in Slovakia, Romania and Egypt.

He is married to Hazel, who is a counsellor, and they have four children and five grandchildren. His interests include music, choral singing, poetry, history, countryside walks and leisurely swimming.

Acknowledgements

I gratefully acknowledge the supportive assistance of my wife, Dr Hazel McEvoy, for her constant encouragement, suggestions, logistic support and her forbearance during my absence while writing; my sons Mark, for IT support and suggestions, and John, for aspects of healthcare in the United States; my daughters Siobhan, for insights into multidisciplinary work, and Frances, for comments on mental health. In the development of the book, Dr Paul Sackin provided invaluable formative guidance at all stages. Dr Kathleen Dunne, Professor Hugh McGavock and Professor Philip Reilly helped greatly by reading and commenting on the full text. Thanks are also due to all my former medical colleagues at The Aberfoyle Medical Practice, who willingly agreed to read and comment on various chapters; special thanks to Shane Cunning for computer assistance. The staff at Radcliffe Publishing have been unfailingly supportive in the production of this book. I am grateful to the late Dr Peter Fallon, and to all who taught me medicine. I also owe a debt of gratitude to all my trainees, from whom I have learned so much.

The Association of Course Organisers, sadly no longer in existence, was the collective voice of programme directors for general practice training in the UK from 1985 until it was wound up in 2010. I owe a great deal to its founders and members over the years. Their supportive influence through annual conferences and other meetings made me, in as far as I am, a teacher and a writer. I wish to pay tribute here to the Association of Course Organisers and its fundamental contribution to GP training in these islands over 25 years, with gratitude for all of the people who contributed to its successes.

This book is dedicated to the memory of my brother, Professor James McEvoy, priest, philosopher and teacher; also to my grandchildren, Caedmon, Brigid, Theodore, Leo and Teagan, who for me represent all future beneficiaries of healthcare in the UK and USA.

Introduction: chronic disease, its natural history and ecology

The neglected epidemic of chronic disease.[1]

For long it has been my ambition to write about the natural history of a particular, common medical condition. Its name is chronic disease.

It is a complex condition whose myriad components are individually documented in extreme detail but whose composite story appears to be remarkably untold. As the poet Charles Kingsley observed, 'Odes to every zephyr; Ne'er a verse to thee'. My years spent as a clinical teacher and a reader of medical literature have failed to reveal much readily accessible work that holds between two covers the fascinating story of this complex entity, by contrast with the wealth of published information there exists on the innumerable individual conditions that comprise it. Aspects of it are familiar to everyone who lives with a significant long-term condition, whether as victim, family member, carer or therapist. Its life cycle reaches into every area of the health and social sciences. It is talked about increasingly in terms such as a global threat,[2] the healthcare challenge of the twenty-first century,[3] a tsunami of unquantifiable need,[4] an impending asteroid strike,[5] the overwhelming of our health services[6] …

A century and a half of scientific medicine has succeeded in identifying and describing the components of this class of disease, yet we appear to stand helpless in the face of the dimensions of the phenomenon as a whole and the growing threat that it poses. There is a large body of literature on the consequences of chronic disease from two opposite polarities: the macrocosm of the epidemiologists who, with health economists, chart the scale of its impact and, to a lesser extent, the intimacies of life for the victims in their quest for effective responses, self-help and support in the community. The middle ground is like a battlefield where squadrons of health and social care professionals struggle, confronting the various manifestations of the force that is chronic disease.

What seems to be lacking is a descriptive, quasi-journalistic account of the broad terrain, one that provides a comprehensible overview and tells the big story. Avoiding the temptation of lurid headlines and sensationalism, such a piece would fill in the backstory, interrogate the main constituents, zoom in on illustrative vignettes for human interest, and try to discern commonalities and patterns that make sense of apparent chaos and complexity. It might conclude with a composite picture, even if definitive solutions were beyond its grasp or remit.

This story is based on a hypothesis that I hope will become clear: that an identity can be constructed around chronic disease through discerning what truths underlie, and are shared by, chronic diseases in general. Such truths may be considered as operating at various levels, in sociology, epidemiology, therapeutics, clinical management and health policy, and pre-eminently in the experience of the patients and their carers.

To propose an analogy, all biology is based on four fundamental truths, the base pairs of amino acids. How these are arranged and interact builds further layers of reality through DNA and the field of molecular biology that is the foundation for all organisms, whatever their identity; these in turn are classifiable into innumerable species. Beyond this, an ecosystem can be described that contains the many species that coexist and interact with an environment.

With this imagery in mind, it may be seen that much of our everyday clinical knowledge is focused on what equates to the species level – that of the various individual diseases, when there are several other dimensions that are at least equally influential. This story, then, seeks to identify and address the truths that describe the genus and its ecosystem, how chronic diseases collectively impinge on the lives of people and society, and the implications of these for clinical professionals. Since every story has to have a narrator, its particular perspective is that of the general physician and his or her quest for effective partnership with people who are victims of chronic disease. These, in turn, may be likened to hosts whose lives have been blighted by long-term conditions, with their consequences in death, illness, disability and disruption of daily life.

Young professionals in early stages of career experience a syllabus of clinical training that leaves them overburdened with information and under-equipped with perspective. This imbalance is understandable. As lifelong learners, all professionals will recognise that they continue to share this syndrome to a degree. We have to know the nuts and bolts, but these need to be supplemented by the provision of cross-linkages to the pillars of knowledge in order to contextualise them. We are trained to be good at differentiation (and thus favour specialisation), but our capacities for integration are less well developed. The curriculum of learning for the general clinician, at whatever stage in professional life, is a strand that runs through this story. This is the educational task that needs to be undertaken, to place chronic disease in a philosophical context that makes sense in terms of the fundamental medical sciences and the array of repetitive clinical and administrative tasks that characterise professional life.

BUT, IS IT POSSIBLE TO GET EXCITED ABOUT CHRONIC DISEASE?

I suggest there are at least six good reasons why the study of chronic disease should grab our interest.

1. It poses a great and growing threat: to our patients' lives and lifestyles, to professional modes of practice, to our healthcare systems and the provision of social care, and to the economic well-being of nations.[7]
2. It accounts for up to 80% of the work of general medical practitioners, and it is increasing to the point where it threatens to displace acute care as the core function of general practice.[8]
3. General practitioners are considered to constitute the only division of the medical profession that is capable of mounting a coherent and comprehensive response to the needs of the victims of chronic diseases.[9]
4. It is a 'hot topic'; whether we know it or not, it is dominating the national agenda of healthcare and will increasingly affect all that we do as clinicians.
5. An understanding of chronic care is essential to making sense of everything we do in practice and draws upon everything we ever learned in training.
6. Chronic disease encompasses endless variety and reaches into every discipline that goes to make up the body of knowledge that is clinical medicine, yet it has not been taught or practised as a coherent discipline.

Therefore, chronic disease is like the elephant in the room that we have not been learning or talking about; we examine endlessly the consequences of its presence without reflecting much on its attributes.

It is clear that general practitioners cannot and do not function in isolation. They are surrounded and supported by a legion of co-workers within the practice, the community and the hospitals. Therefore, this story should be of interest to all involved in the provision of health and social care, whatever their particular discipline in the medical, nursing, social work and allied health professions. It is not confined to any one particular health system or country, for it is a universal story.

In telling the story it is necessary to avoid becoming bemired in detail or aspiring beyond what is realistic. Rather, the aim is to connect with human experience, to make sense of the forces that impinge on the plot, to provoke thought and to stimulate readers to imagine for themselves.

SUGGESTIONS FOR USING THIS BOOK

This account of chronic disease attempts to tell its story and, at the same time, fill in the substantial background information; there are textbook and reference elements, carved up into chapters that are more or less free-standing. Hence there will be a degree of repetition and summarising. Each chapter has an overview, conclusion and learning point questions that may be of use to teachers, and some curriculum thoughts, along with some signposted shortcuts to facilitate a 'speed-read' for time-poor professionals. The various scenarios are fictional; they do not represent any particular patient, colleague or trainee but are there to lighten the tone while conveying real issues and their context. If you, like me, can't wait to get through a book to find out 'who done it', you may wish to read the 'Chapter overview: executive summary' section in Chapter 1 and then jump straight to Chapter 7. The last two chapters are the closest approach to a how-to manual. While it is not exhaustively referenced (who needs exhaustion?), most assertions are substantiated. These point to a small core of major source works that are worthy of note for further reading.

SO, WHAT'S ON OFFER?

Storytelling is more about plot than punchline. No one has yet come up with the theory of everything that resolves the problems posed by chronic disease. Natural history and ecology are about cyclical systems, feedback loops, complexity and randomness. The descriptive sections that follow are an attempt to map this terrain. Whether we are doctors, nurses or patients the territory is the same. Although each has a separate journey to undertake, the various paths we navigate intersect frequently.

A chronic disease paradigm is described and proposed as an educational model that should also help practitioners to imagine beyond the particular to the general, to draw some conclusions, to work out some strategies for everyday use and to make sense of all the tedious and annoying bits of the day's work that are yet so essential. The text is evidence-based where possible, with definitions and lists, a good deal of opinion, some untamed trouble spots and, of course, fuzzy boundaries 'beyond which there be dragons and demons'.

It is my hope that this guide will be of value to students, trainees, practitioners, trainers and managers in a broad range of clinical disciplines (not confined to the UK and its National Health Service), and to all who follow the daunting but intriguing journey of lifelong learning about the Hippocratic triad: the doctor, the patient and the illness.

REFERENCES

1. Horton R. The neglected epidemic of chronic disease. *Lancet.* 2005; **366**(9496): 1514.
2. Strong K, Mathers C, Leeder S, *et al.* Preventing chronic diseases: how many lives can we save? *Lancet.* 2005; **366**(9496): 1578–82.
3. World Health Organization. *Global Report: innovative care for chronic conditions.* Geneva: WHO; 2002.
4. Dillner L. How services for long-term conditions could be reborn. *BMJ.* 2011; **342**: d1730.
5. Kane R, Priester R, Totten A. *Meeting the Challenges of Chronic Illness.* Baltimore, MD: Johns Hopkins University Press; 2005.
6. Department of Health. *Quality and Innovation Division.* London: DH; 2010.
7. Ibid.
8. Belfield G, Colin-Thomé. *Improving Chronic Disease Management.* Available at: www.natpact. info/uploads/ChronicDiseaseDHNote.pdf (accessed 8 April 2014).
9. Rothman AA, Wagner EH. Chronic disease management: what is the role of primary care? *Ann Intern Med.* 2003; **138**(3): 256–61.

CHAPTER 1

Chronic disease: what's so special about it?

Contents

CHAPTER OVERVIEW: EXECUTIVE SUMMARY

As president of the United States, Ronald Reagan is said to have required that a briefing on any subject, however important, should fit on one side of a page. Cynics remarked that sometimes he would want to skip the detail and get to the bottom line. This summary strays beyond the one page limit but there is a bottom line.

Chronic diseases have at least as many similarities with one another as they have differences. Who says so? For a start, the UK government, the US Centers for Disease Control and Prevention (CDC), European Union, the Organisation for Economic Co-operation and Development (OECD) and the World Health Organization (WHO). Patients and the alliances of long-term conditions sufferers also concur. Exploring these similarities will reveal an underlying profile that may be termed the 'chronic disease paradigm', and this will be examined in detail.

Chronic illness affects all age groups and is not simply a matter of ageing. It correlates with indices of poverty, and other social determinants of health, but affluence introduces hazards also – the so-called lifestyle disorders that merge into the territory of disease. It increases in prevalence worldwide with population growth, longevity and improved illness survival. Its economic impact is huge. This affects individuals and their families, health systems and the national wealth through rising costs of treatments and manpower, lost productivity and welfare dependency. It gives rise to an incalculable burden of distress. With improvements in treatments and support the victims live longer, but not necessarily healthier, lives.

Over their extended time span, chronic diseases are likely to intensify (progression), render the victim more susceptible to further disease (debilitation), accumulate (multi-morbidity), diversify (co-morbidity) and interfere with ability to function normally in society (disability), resulting in a perception of 'otherness' (stigma). They selectively afflict the disadvantaged and elderly (social antecedents of disease). For the patient, the treatment pathways are perplexing and hazardous due to complexity, multi-morbidity, polypharmacy and iatrogenic risk. Nevertheless, chronic diseases are amenable to preventive measures. A limited number of modifiable risk factors and lifestyle issues contribute to the bulk of chronic disease. These include hypertension, poor nutritional practices, hyperlipidaemia, obesity, addictions, trauma and physical inactivity.

Chronic diseases manifest observable stages in the course of their natural history, each of which is modifiable through medical and social interventions. This, the trajectory model, illuminates how chronic disease behaves. Stages in this trajectory include the premorbid or latent phase, leading to clinical onset, acute episode, relapse, plateau, progression, crisis, acceleration, palliative and terminal phases. Resources appropriate to each of these stages have to be identified and made available and accessible, taking into account coexisting conditions and patients' self-management capacities. Multidisciplinary, community-based teamwork is essential to meet the challenges that patients and families face through chronic illness and disability. Families and carers of those suffering chronic illness have an overarching contribution to make. The expert patient has a key role in helping others.

Primary healthcare is the clinical hub for chronic disease management. Complex systems of prevention and intervention, both clinical and social, have to be coordinated in order to achieve quality of care that is comprehensive, continuing and patient centred. These require the backup of diagnostic and therapeutic specialist services, along with robust healthcare policy and intersectoral action at government level. All physicians and allied health professionals could benefit from familiarity with a clear chronic disease paradigm in order to optimise their grasp of the issues, the efficacy of their interventions, to predict and modify the course of the disease, and its consequences. The knowledge, skills and attitudes implicit in managing chronic disease are largely generic, and this reflects the composite nature of the condition. They encompass the entire curriculum of training and continuing learning for primary care physicians. The principles of chronic disease should inform the training of all clinicians and be foundational to the undergraduate curricula. A chronic disease management paradigm will be presented as a curriculum construct.

A test of the humanity of a society is how it treats its chronic sick, and that is 'the bottom line'.

CHRONIC DISEASE MANAGEMENT IN A NUTSHELL

A generic view of chronic disease has been embraced by WHO over the 40 years since its seminal report, commonly known as the Alma-Ata Declaration.[1] A more recent WHO global report sums up its analysis thus:

> Chronic conditions … require ongoing management over a period of years or decades. Considered from this perspective, "chronic conditions" cover an enormously broad category of what could appear on the surface as disparate health concerns. However, persistent communicable (e.g. HIV/AIDS) and non-communicable diseases (e.g. cardiovascular disease, cancers and diabetes), certain mental disorders (e.g. depression and schizophrenia), and ongoing impairments of structure (e.g. amputations, blindness and joint disorders) while seemingly different, all fit within the chronic conditions category … [and] share fundamental themes.[2]

At a more intimate level, chronic disease resides at the home of the patient, profoundly affects the core social unit of immediate family and friends, and is most likely to receive treatment locally by a general practitioner (GP) in the low-tech, high-turnover setting of primary care in the community. Health systems that have a strong foundation of primary care have been shown to be more cost-effective and deliver better health outcomes than do alternative models of care.[3] High-quality primary medical care is capable of providing person-centred continuing care across the full spectrum of chronic disease. Between the global, epidemiological view of WHO on the one hand and the intimate personal experiences by patients on the other lies an extensive territory that may be characterised as chronic disease management.

The generic model of chronic disease, as embraced by WHO, is becoming familiar, having gained currency rapidly since the millennium. This is a useful landmark in contemporary history. It is easy to forget the existential angst that accompanied the approach of the year 2000. The foremost example was 'The Millennium Bug', which was supposed to risk the collapse of our global communications and control systems at midnight of the turn of the century. There was a global sigh of relief when the new day dawned without airliners crashing or thermonuclear war breaking out. Was this a masterpiece of prevention, a hugely successful business opportunity or the needless squandering of precious resources based on an unfounded myth or mistaken analysis? The years since 2000 have brought a number of pervasive anxieties that were not clearly foreseen, but whose roots go back long before that nodal point. Among these are climate change related to global warming, new kinds of transcultural conflicts and an economic bubble of unprecedented scale and consequence. We have to keep such examples in mind when evaluating other threats as they begin to gain currency. They tell us something about the difficulties of future-scoping, confronting uncertainty, the nature of risk, how much we are prepared to spend to avert a prophesy of doom, and how we would know if it worked. The chronic disease phenomenon might be less spectacular than any of these examples, but there is a growing realisation of its significance at both macro (national) and micro (domestic) levels. Unspectacular but insidious, it has been termed 'the healthcare challenge of the 21st century'.[4] It demands our attention, because consciousness-raising is the beginning of problem-solving, and the problems raised by chronic disease are far from being solved. A list of common-sense observations that relate to the chronic diseases may convey a sense of what chronic disease management means and begin to delineate the territory to be explored.

- Chronic diseases are amenable to prevention and treatment, but not usually to cure; they go on and on.
- They gather strength and accumulate complications with time (co-morbidity).
- Their extended duration allows other intercurrent illnesses to coincide and accumulate (multi-morbidity).
- Frequently they do not directly result in death, but commonly 'people die with rather than from chronic disease'.[5]
- The prevalence of chronic disease is not randomly distributed.[6] It clusters with poverty, deprivation, age and minority group status (social determinants of health, or social antecedents of disease).
- They constitute the fastest-growing cause of morbidity and mortality worldwide.
- Complexity is a feature of the health status and clinical pathway of those affected; multiple interventions, fragmented or absent treatment planning, polypharmacy and iatrogenic issues are salient features of their experience.
- Medical and social interventions are effective in prolonging life, but not necessarily healthy life.
- Many kinds of professional input are required simultaneously, sequentially or continually.
- Multidisciplinary (multi-professional, interdisciplinary) team-working requires coordination and management to achieve integration of care.

- Social interventions are necessary to support living with chronic and complex illness and disability.
- Social care is recognised as an unresolved, problematic area; public policy favours care in the community; the need for carers and care workers is increasing.
- The caring burden falls disproportionately on individuals and the immediate family circle.
- Family carers require specific support, since they themselves are likely to be vulnerable through age, illness and attrition. Psychological, emotional and relationship complications and social stress are intrinsic to the experience of carers in chronic disease and these need to be addressed.
- The responsibility of the patient for self-care has to be recognised, affirmed, nurtured, and facilitated – for example, through self-management programmes.
- The community resources of voluntary and self-help organisations, the third sector or non-governmental organisations play an important role in supporting patients and carers through chronic disease.
- Half of all those who live with disability live below the poverty line, according to reports from the OECD; financial support (social security systems) and welfare rights advice are vital supports for the chronic sick and those with disabilities.
- In addition to the costs of medical and social care, there is great economic cost to society through loss of work capacity and productivity.
- The lifelong nature of chronic disease and the resource implications that result emphasise the importance of prevention and health promotion.
- Effective prevention involves programmes of risk factor management, screening, case-finding, early diagnosis and intervention, monitoring, immunisation and other public health approaches; these are all achievable at the level of primary healthcare.
- Protocols and guidelines play an important part in decision support, formulating and implementing treatment plans, and delivering high-quality care that is effective and economically affordable.
- Evidence-based medicine, audit and reflective practice are among the drivers of a quality agenda; governance procedures further protect the interests of the citizen and society.
- Sophisticated use of information technology (IT) is essential in carrying out prevention, monitoring, clinical management, continuing care and quality assurance in chronic disease programmes.
- Management skills are necessary for the delivery of services in a coordinated and efficient manner; management is not an optional extra; commissioning of care services is an essential aspect of management.
- Research and development are required to address all levels of chronic care and

should not be subordinated to fundamental research in molecular biology and pathophysiology.

- Education and training, including continuing professional development (CPD), underpin the clinical effectiveness of the various professionals who deliver services for the long-term sick and disabled; curricula for clinical training for doctors, nurses and allied health professions should emphasise chronic care.
- The scale and implications of the chronic disease phenomenon are such that all professionals in health and social care should have an understanding of the principles of chronic illness care, based on a **chronic disease paradigm** and how this connects with all the contributing sectors, in order to make sense of the special contribution each makes to the overall story of chronic disease management. A universal, integrated paradigm of chronic disease management is shown in Figure 1.1. The four main conceptual areas cluster around that of the patient. I refer to them as 'complexes' because each one is a story in itself, like a 'dropdown menu', and these will be unpacked in the course of subsequent chapters (*see* Figure 1.1).

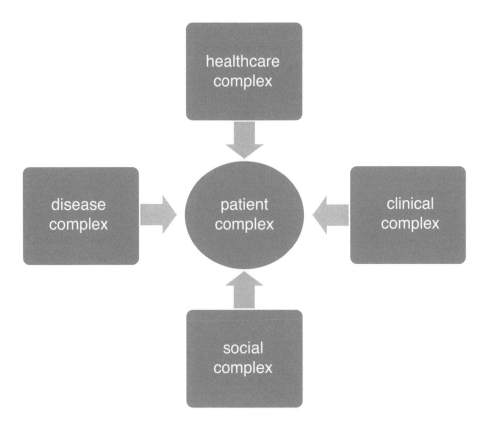

FIGURE 1.1 A simple integrated chronic disease management paradigm

ARE YOU INTERESTED IN CHRONIC DISEASE?

Unglamorous maybe, but perhaps you should be … especially if you are a patient, a carer, a physician in hospital or community practice, a nurse, a physiotherapist, a social worker, an occupational therapist, a manager who commissions or administers health services, a politician, a health economist, or are involved in training for these social roles or professions. Most people have an involvement in some chronic disease for personal, family or professional reasons. It seems that hardly anyone is free of disease or risk factors for any great length of time, and that is what the doctor–patient relationship in primary healthcare is about. Chronic disease impinges on the majority of the population, whether as victims, carers or professionals. All doctors are involved, but particularly those in general medical practice in the community.

But how many chronically ill people go through life with one disease? How many families are free to devote their energies to a single dependent person with an illness or disability? How many consultations in general practice are about one issue from beginning to end? Life is not like that, and even if diseases were to occur randomly, they would certainly not be evenly distributed. It is a common occurrence for individuals to harbour several unconnected but contemporaneous diseases or several distinct but interconnected ones.

These considerations validate the need for the general practitioner (GP). If a longitudinal model of medicine, defined by a focus on the course of this or that disease, were valid and sufficient, a system based firmly on specialist services would be desirable and appropriate. However, where individuals and families bear a heavy burden of several simultaneous disorders, it is necessary to shift the focus of attention from the disease to the patient and family. To do otherwise fragments resources and degrades the effectiveness of services involved, rendering them fragmentary. Clearly, however, both kinds of doctor are essential and play complementary roles. Specialists function at their best when managing episodes on the expectant pathway of defined pathology; the generalist addresses the experience of the individual patient, however diverse or long-lasting that experience might be.

As with any good fabric, it is the weft that binds together the strands of the warp upon the loom. Medical literature, mirrored by our professional formation, tends to focus on the longitudinal warp. A lot less consideration is given to the cross-linking, lateral strands. These, by the way, tend to dominate in the creation of the patterns within a fabric. As the horizontal weave of the generalist works its way across the vertical warp of the patho-physiological perspective, patterns or images emerge that are the themes that underlie all chronic disease. This vertical and horizontal integration is a mantra oft-encountered in chronic disease management, and just about as findable as the Holy Grail.

So what's the big idea?

The human life cycle is subject to ill health from cradle to grave, and its effects extend even beyond these limits! Nevertheless, people have little interest or concept about the science of what ails them. They want competent interventions that deal with their crises; solutions, assistance, a diagnosis, relief, support and holding relationships that enable them to live normally. Health and social care services have to be comprehensive enough to respond to any number of different diseases and combination of conditions, relying on a core of personnel and other resources, in ways that are economical in time, effort and cost, while ensuring quality of care. These must be multipurpose and flexible enough to accommodate the individual needs of patients. A generic model of chronic disease is, therefore, desirable as a theoretical framework on which to hang the components of a responsive service. Such a model is equally important as a matrix for learning and teaching about chronic illness and how health services might achieve congruence with the needs of people who live with long-term conditions.

So, having defined chronic disease as a generic force, we may proceed to reflect on its characteristics, its impact on those affected, and what knowledge and tools we already have and might develop in order to mount effective, consistent, long-term responses to the needs that arise.

HOW MANY CHRONIC DISEASES DO *YOU* HAVE?

How many chronic diseases do *you* have? None? Well, just pause a moment. Perhaps you have a history of asthma, psoriasis, an episode of depression, you have been a smoker, you have had recurring indigestion, migraine, joint pains or you have even relied on alcohol to see you through life's ups and downs? If none of these, perhaps you are very young or you have been extraordinarily fortunate in how you selected your parents.

Think, now, through your close family circle and what manifestations of chronic disease reside there. Count them up and double the number to get a rough estimate of your family prevalence. Of course, you immediately encounter questions such as how to define family circle, what threshold to use for counting disease, not to mention chronicity, and how much you know about your family history. Inviting you into a hypothetical family will avoid any distressing rumination or invasion of privacy. Suppose you have a brother who gets occasional seizures, a brother-in-law with type 2 diabetes, a sister who suffers anxiety; your father has a stent, your mother takes blood pressure tablets and your grandparents need compliance boxes to keep track of their various daily doses for osteoporosis, osteoarthritis, thyroid disease and sleep problems. The chances are that there is much more that you do not know about, even among your nearest and dearest; intimate and embarrassing things like irritable bowel syndrome (IBS), anxiety, cystitis, menorrhagia, psoriasis, bleeding piles, perhaps an eating disorder. Their GP might not be aware of these. Medical supplies can be got discretely by visiting the local chemists in rotation or via the Internet between visits to the health shop or acupuncturist, so they don't even have to go to the GP to restock.

Maybe you think most of these are not real chronic diseases. They do not incapacitate, cause much absence from work, necessitate much family comment or stop them having a good laugh. However, the lad with the epilepsy has had to give up his job in sales when he lost his driving licence; the IBS sufferer does not go on package holidays or undertake long journeys; the same applies to the cystitis lady, who no longer plays golf; a brother with psoriasis never goes to the gym or pool; the diabetic has problems getting cover for a mortgage; the anxious sister gave up teaching and has an office job far below her ability level. The parents and grandparents lead normal lives and regard themselves as healthy for their age and stage, close to or in retirement.

So what's remarkable about this family with regard to chronic disease? Clearly very little, from what has been thus far revealed. Medically they are functioning mostly 'below the radar' for illness. A few lifestyle adjustments enable each one to function and live, fulfilling their normal social roles. They live within their ability to compensate for the effects of the various conditions. They occupy the shallow end of society's pool of chronic disease. Yet it might not take much to move one or other of them into deeper water and any resulting turbulence to destabilise other members.

The diabetic suffers a sudden visual loss. The lad with epilepsy is stopped by the police, having been cajoled into driving home his inebriated friends, and he is charged with driving without a licence and insurance. The underemployed nervous sister is found to be a secret drinker. Father's stent blocks. Osteoporotic granny has a fall. The IBS sufferer has shown increased symptoms and has been reclassified as having Crohn's disease. The pressures of life increase sharply for everybody. Suddenly there is a burden of care, a rise in the communal level of anxiety, a sense of lost security bringing worry about the future. Role relationships change. We now have four patients, one criminal record, several carers and a drinker about to lose her job.

In terms of clinical diagnosis nothing very calamitous has happened. Zap a retina with laser, pin a fractured femur, arrange motivational counselling for the tippler, revisit the coronary angiography suite and equilibrium will be restored. A bad patch, admittedly, but all will be well. Of course, follow-ups will be necessary and medications will be adjusted to optimise secondary prevention, but these are routine enough. The GP will notice little. He or she probably will not know of and therefore not connect most of these events.

Why is the family devastated? Things have changed, utterly. Much of it they are aware of, but much is outside the sphere of their consciousness. There has been a huge financial transaction. If these 'routine' medical interventions had to be paid for fully by their recipients the bill would have been impressive, the equivalent of a year's national average salary. Fortunately, in most developed economies the provisions of the healthcare system offset this. For most of the world, and for over 40 million people in the United States, this is not the case. Even with health insurance there will be co-payments and benefit thresholds.

However, real and lasting change lies in the area of the social roles, self-image and family dynamics, and the risk status of several family members has increased substantially. The now unemployed sister will be watched and will be aware of the stigma of being under scrutiny; the lad with fits now has a criminal record and is having difficulties in getting a work visa to join his girlfriend who lives in United States; father is depressed following his second stent encounter and rising pressure to retire early; granny is unable to climb the stairs and the house has to be reconfigured to create a downstairs bedroom and toilet facilities. The financial impact of these is potentially significant.

But help is at hand. There are visits from the occupational therapist concerning home alterations with the possibility of funding by the social services. This leads to searching and intrusive inquiries by a social worker into family finances, care needs of the elders, and the capacity of the family to provide extra support for and attention to the grandparents. The restoration of equilibrium has required external input, an increase in problem-solving activity within the family, heightened awareness of vulnerability and the adoption of new roles, such as patient, carer, disabled person in need of social care and benefits, from a productive unit to a 'burden on society'.

These roles are elusive. There is no process of induction or training into them, such as there is, for example, into working life through apprenticeship, or into marriage through courtship and engagement, or into parenthood through pregnancy and postnatal care. One may dip into the patient role through minor encounters with illness throughout life, but this is not the same as being plunged into it through a crisis without any mentorship or preparation. The same thing applies when becoming a carer. Each person enters these roles without seeking them or having any handbook for the process. How to do it right? What skills, attitudes and knowledge are involved? Which family members can or will become the carers? What are the rights, duties and responsibilities inherent in the role? These are sociologically determined, have substantial psychological components and impinge profoundly on relationships, wealth, workplace and social functioning and the interface with the community. The medical model is but one facet of the encounter with disease, especially when it is chronic.

At the core of the illness episode is the matter of resources. When adversity strikes, often through clusters of events, there quickly arises the need to deploy resources, those of the individuals affected, their spouse and family, and of the society and community within which they subsist. This is the ecology of chronic disease management. The resources encompass the personal capacities of the patient to sustain stress, solve problems and seek help; the availability of support in the form of family or its proxies (friends, neighbours and colleagues); the financial status of the family unit; and the resources of society (medical and social welfare systems), both statutory and informal. As to the professionals involved, their training and experience endow them with social roles – the powers that go with expertise and authority, and the keys to the treasury of the common wealth. How these attributes are achieved, sustained and resourced constitute the complex pathways of professional qualification and practice, technical knowledge, experience, governance and contractual framework. None are comprehensive experts who can be free-standing. Assuming that they are professionally competent and adhere to codes of professionalism, however defined, there is much to be said about how they relate to the patient and one another and how they deploy the resources at their command to provide a seamless service for the benefit of the patient and family affected. In this context, for doctor please read 'therapist'. No doctor feels self-sufficient in the daily encounters with continuing illness. Multi-professional working and learning are integral to the work.

It is in the common ground, the interface between what both Hippocrates and Balint defined as the basic triad of care, the doctor, the patient and the illness, that these reflections on chronic disease will dwell. Schön[7] analysed the various ranks of professional in topographical terms. The high-altitude clarity of the mountain-top belongs to pure science and fundamental research, where the variables are eliminated to define problems that can be addressed through the empirical model. The upper slopes are where applied science refines and disseminates the fruits of the laboratory to tackle and solve defined practical clinical problems. The lower slopes and boggy lowland, where people carry on their lives, is where practitioners operate using theory and technology to manage complex 'messes', amid much uncertainty. These reflections are firmly placed on the valley floor, managing the messy and ill-defined realities that surround people's lives when they experience ongoing health problems within complex social units such as family, workplace and community.

And so far we have just been exploring the shallow end of the pool of illness and disease.

Dissertations on chronic diseases tend to focus on the slopes and peaks of individual 'mountains' – the fruits of research and development, and how these may be applied clinically. Every clinician is aware of the need for grounding in the bioscience of disease, and it would be false to underplay this. We are, on the whole, well versed in the applied science of our disciplines, and this will merit some mention in the chapters that follow. However, the intention is not to write another pathology book but to reflect on chronic disease commonalties, with some emphasis on sociology, epidemiology, health policy and the experiential dimension of illness.

Paradoxically, it seems that there is relatively little accessible literature that explores comprehensively the 'low ground between' (as in Schön's metaphor). This is the space where the expertise of the professionals and the experience of the patient and carer must join hands in a partnership of equity and mutual respect. To extend Schön's metaphor, we must now take up our backpack and compass, put on stout boots and explore the lowlands in order to map the territory. Ready-made maps are not easily available, as far as this therapist is aware, having blundered around in the boggy ground for many years. Your company on the journey will be most welcome.

SCENARIO: a consultation

Now, doctor, before I go … It's about my mother; she's not been able to come in herself. She's a lot worse and I can't cope with her.

Having recalled her mother's name and called up her file onscreen, my heart sinks as I scroll through the parallel lists of problems (major/continuing; minor/transient) and medications (routine repeats; recent/acutes), but I indicate that I am in receptive mode.

Well, doctor, you know, she's nearly eighty and we can't expect too much from her, but she doesn't get out of bed much anymore, except that she tends to wander during the night, and we're afraid of her falling; her breathing's terrible and she would fight with her shadow. She's all the time calling for her painkillers. When we try telling her she's just had them she won't believe us and when we go to give her insulin she thinks we're poisoning her. And we can't keep the bandages on her leg ulcers. She's giving your nurse a terrible time; she thinks the nurse is going to put her in a home. She's not far wrong there, but it's my husband who wants her put in a home. My husband and I are fighting all the time. He says she's the problem, but I don't know … He's not well himself, with his nerves and the drink … But you're going to have to do something about her. She's not the woman she used to be … always one to cope with things she was, up until my daddy died, that is.

My receptive mode is wearing thin. She had come in because she had received a computer-generated letter suggesting she have her blood pressure checked and her routine medications reviewed (with a footnote that we would like to discuss her recent requests for sleeping tablets). The inquiry about her sleep pattern had certainly opened the floodgates. However, as her eyes fill and tears appear, my diminishing receptive mode finds its balance with pragmatism. Direct questioning (Patient Health Questionnaire) establishes that she is moderately depressed but not suicidal; her sleeping tablets are reissued (for now), a review appointment for further assessment arranged and a home visit to her mother agreed. She dries the tears and appears somewhat relieved. As I hand over the scripts and begin to rise from my chair (consultation over) she remains firmly seated.

> Doctor, while I'm here can I have a certificate to get some time out of work, and my mother's prescriptions to save me coming all the way down again? It's hard to get through on the phone and we're nearly out of bandages and everything else too.

I subside into my chair, and begin to write. What happened to the 10-minute appointment? What can you do in 10 minutes? As she leaves I sincerely hope that the next case will be a sore throat or flu, something quick. I turn to the new trainee who has been observing this afternoon's surgery.

> We can't stop to discuss any of that just now. While I'm getting on with the next few patients why don't you have a coffee break and spend a few minutes listing all the issues raised during that consultation? We'll go over them during your tutorial tomorrow.

THE IMPACT OF CHRONIC DISEASE

> Chronic conditions: the health care challenge of the 21st century.[8]

Modern healthcare systems are victims of their own success. There is an ageing population that attests to past triumphs but is a conundrum for the future, since diseases are more prevalent as longevity and survival increase.[9] The implications of this are far-reaching. Let's begin with some facts related to chronic disease in selected regions in Europe and United States, with some observations from the WHO, but beginning with the UK.

The population of the UK is both growing and ageing. In 2012 it was 63.7 million and this is projected to increase to 67.2 million by 2020 and to 70 million by 2027.[10] Based on demographic trends, the number of people in the UK aged over 50 will grow from 20.3 million in 2005 to 26.2 million by 2025.[11] Life expectancy for men is 79 years and for women, 82 years.[12] By 2035, life expectancy at birth will be 83.4 years for males and 87 years for females.

The death rate from chronic disease in men is 440.6 per 100 000 and for women,

309.3 per 100 000. The rate of deaths occurring under the age of 60 is 13.1% for men and 8.2% for women. According to WHO, long-term conditions account for 88% of all deaths in the UK.[13]

Almost one-third of the adult population of England (17.5 million) is estimated to have a long-term condition, and 58% of those are aged over 60. Those with long-term conditions account for well over 50% of all appointments in general practice (elsewhere quoted as 80%),[14] 70% of all bed occupancy, and 70% of the primary and acute care budgets. This indicates that the one-third of the population with long-term conditions use over two-thirds of the health budget.[15] The costs associated with diabetes care alone are approaching 10% of the healthcare budget.

People who are entitled to benefits amount to 20 million, at a cost of £150 billion per annum and this is 50% more than the health budget; 7.5% of the working population receive incapacity benefits, and sickness absence from work costs the economy an estimated £100 billion.[16] This equates to the total cost of the NHS for England, which was £102 billion in the year 2010–11.

Long-term conditions correlate with poverty and deprivation. They are 60% more prevalent and 60% greater severity in social class 5 (least privileged group) compared with social class 1 (most privileged, as defined by the UK Registrar-General Classification)) and they reduce the probability of being in work by one-third.[17]

There are about 6.5 million carers in the UK, and this is expected to increase to nine million over the next 2 decades; the care they provide is estimated to be worth £119 billion annually.[18]

In the United States, according to the CDC, chronic diseases were the leading cause of death and disability in 2005. Chronic illness is the cause of 70% of deaths. One in every two adults, or 133 million, had at least one chronic illness, of whom one-quarter had one or more daily activity limitations, arthritis being the commonest cause of disability. Heart disease, stroke and cancers accounted for 50% of deaths.[19] Chronic conditions account for 50% of healthcare but 75% of healthcare costs and the chronically ill population is projected to rise to 171 million by 2030.[20]

In the European Union, World Bank figures show that public expenditure on healthcare should jump from 8% of GDP in the year 2000 to 14% by 2030, relating to increasing longevity and the rise in chronic disease. These account for 70% of health expenditure. Cost inflation is a substantial factor, relating to the sophisticated workforce required, rising expectations and technology costs. For example, between 1975 and 2006 the cost of bringing a new medicine to market rose tenfold (to $1.3 billion). The life expectancy of males born in 2030 is projected to be a decade longer than for those born in 1980. The proportion of Europeans aged 65 and over is set to increase from 16% in 2000 to 24% by the year 2030. One-third of Europe's population is estimated to have at least one chronic disease. However, healthy active life expectancy is 7–10 years short of life expectancy, so life will be longer but not necessarily healthier. These data on the EU are from a report by the Economist Intelligence Unit, which also summarised the factors that are 'drivers of the current crisis':[21]

- the ageing population
- unhealthy lifestyles
- an explosion of technology-based cures
- bureaucratic systems
- increased specialisation in medicine
- shrinking revenue base (tax, insurance premiums) due to shrinking proportion of working age people.

The Australian Institute of Health and Welfare analysis of the 2004–05 National Health Survey showed that just over seven million people (from a population of 23 million) had at least one chronic condition; of those aged over 65, 26.7% had two and 42% had three; more than half of all potentially preventable admissions were due to 'selected chronic conditions'.[22]

The World Health Organization's global report of 2002 warns that chronic disease is 'accelerating globally, undaunted by regions or social class' at 'an alarming rate' and will be the main cause of morbidity and mortality globally by 2020.[23] Noncommunicable disease and mental disorders accounted for 59% of total mortality and 40% of the global burden of disease in 2000. This will increase by 60% by the year 2020. Heart disease, stroke, depression and cancers will be the largest contributors. The cost burden falls upon all levels of society – on patients, their families, the health workforce, healthcare organisations and government. The global report asserts that

> chronic conditions are no longer viewed conventionally …, considered in isolation, or thought of as disparate disorders; the demands on patients, families and the health care systems are similar, and, in fact, comparable management strategies are effective across all chronic conditions making them seem more alike than different.[24]

This brief survey of data touches on and illustrates a variety of issues.

There is a marked increase in the prevalence of chronic conditions worldwide, which is causing alarm to nations and healthcare agencies everywhere, and to global watchdogs such as WHO, the World Bank and the OECD. In the wealthy economies of Europe, Australia and North America they dominate the scene. In poorer countries, still burdened with fundamental problems in healthcare, preoccupied with infectious disease and malnutrition, the rates of chronic conditions are expected to rise dramatically and disproportionately.

Illustrative figures presented here are not strictly comparable between sources. Rates cited are often reached by extrapolation from databases, and definitions of terms show variability. For a start, there is no universal agreement on what constitutes a chronic disease and no comprehensive list of long-term conditions. The very terms 'disease', 'illness' and 'condition' are often used synonymously although there are subtle distinctions between them; similarly for usage of 'long-term', 'chronic' and 'non-communicable' with regard to disease. Indeed, terms such as these are frequently used interchangeably. Any distinctions between them will be explored elsewhere in reflections on the sociology of illness.

It is sufficient for now to observe that they are increasing in prevalence and incidence as the population grows and ages, and the treatment of acute conditions improves. They increase markedly in the over-60s, where multiple pathology becomes common. Life expectancy and survival rates favour women over men. Chronic conditions have a major impact on economic productivity, national wealth and rates of dependency on state benefits. A commonly used measure of the contribution of age to the healthcare crisis is *the dependency ratio*: the proportion of over-65s and under-18s compared with that of the 18–65 age bands, those who are the workers and producers of wealth. One article, provocatively entitled 'Population Ageing: The Timebomb that Isn't?' suggested that the predicted crisis of a society top-heavy with disease-ridden elderly may be an unwarranted assumption; retired people are productive in their own ways, as volunteers, carers and childminders, and have made their contribution to the economy and to their own pension-pot. Life expectancy at 65 is growing steadily, and healthy life expectancy with it. Maximum call on services occurs in the final months of life, whenever that is. Thus, the authors suggest, the dependency ratio is misleading as a yardstick for future-scoping, at least in terms of health demand, and the prevalence of multi-morbidity is a more accurate test.[25]

It is difficult to assess the human cost of chronic illness. However, it clearly impinges on employability, earning capacity and the quality of life of the victim and the family unit. Family and friends undertake unquantified duties as carers, with consequences for their lives and lifestyles. If their contribution were factored into a total costing of social care the resulting budget could easily outstrip the costs of healthcare. The costs associated with social care arising from disease and disability have not been mentioned here, but they are widely regarded as one of the major unsolved problems in chronic care.

Respiratory disease, cardiovascular disease and diabetes, arthritis and mental illness are major contributors to the long-term disease burden. Others that feature as chronic diseases might seem more surprising at first sight. Conditions that were previously considered acute, critical or rapidly fatal, such as HIV/AIDS, cancers and stroke, can now be regarded as 'chronic diseases with episodes'. As survival rates increase, so does the cost of the supporting technology and manpower (health cost inflation).

A consistent theme that emerges from the data presented is **the generic view of long-term conditions and chronic disease**. WHO policy explicitly adopts this analysis. Progressive healthcare systems are adopting this view, including the UK Department of Health, the CDC, and think tanks such as the Economist Intelligence Unit and the World Bank.

It is significant that these bodies emphasise the view that **non-communicable diseases, many of them degenerative in nature, are potentially preventable**. They apply a comprehensive model of prevention (primary, secondary and tertiary). Chronic diseases generally are multifactorial and influenced by known risk factors. The CDC[26] indicates that there are four modifiable health-risk behaviours that are responsible for much of the illness, suffering and premature death associated with chronic disease: (1) lack of physical activity, (2) poor nutrition, (3) tobacco use and (4) excessive alcohol consumption. Addressing these may avoid or defer the onset of disease, relapse and recurrence rates may be reduced and complications may be minimised. This implies a preventive, trajectory-based model of the course of chronic disease, with points of significance that indicate interventions in order to modify outcomes.

Further support for the generic view of chronic disease is represented in various WHO global reports that were prompted by the 1979 Alma Ata Declaration (famous for the phrase 'Health for All by the year 2000'). In them the prevailing medical model of healthcare receives trenchant criticism, even blame, for the emerging crisis in healthcare. The characteristics of 'the medical model' are described as 'hospital-centrism, disease-centrism and hyper-specialisation'. WHO argues that this has failed to deliver affordable, accessible, equitable healthcare but has contributed to fragmented and fragmentary episodic care with strong commercial overtones.[27] This 'acute care model', it maintains, is ill-suited to the imminent demands that confront all countries and systems of health arising from the phenomenon of chronic disease. An alternative approach, which it calls **the paradigm shift**, is advocated, requiring person-centred, continuous care, best delivered by medical generalists in a community setting. It cites evidence of the effectiveness of the primary care-based approach, combined with harnessing community resources to support patient participation and self-care. It warned that, 'Without change, healthcare systems will grow increasingly inefficient and ineffective as the prevalence of chronic conditions grows.'[28]

Healthcare, especially for chronic disease, is both controversial and political. The Health and Social Care Act 2012 in England, which places a substantial proportion of the health budget in the hands of consortia of general practitioners, met with opposition from specialist medical groups and anticipation on the part of private commercial providers. 'Obamacare' represents the latest round in a deeply divisive

US health policy war. The WHO analysis is endorsed by Mark Pearson as head of the Health Division of the OECD:

> Healthcare systems in Europe look like they were designed for the 1950s. They are oriented around acute care. Medical education is oriented around hospitals. Payment systems are oriented around particular interventions. Biomedical research is still based on the assumption that people have single diseases at a time, but already the biggest challenge is multiple morbidities. These require a more longitudinal approach and payment systems that can cope with care provided in more than one setting. Success will mean finding some way to move on from the acute care model.[29]

SOME CHARACTERISTICS OF CHRONIC DISEASE

It will be clear by now that the agenda has three main headings: (1) the patient experiencing chronic illness, (2) the services that may be invoked and (3) the disease that is the common enemy. Furthermore, that this disease is being cast as the abstract archetype that represents the full range of chronic diseases. As such its characteristics should be amenable to scrutiny. Four aspects will be examined: (1) **disease trajectory**, (2) its implications for **prevention**, (3) chronic disease as a **psychosocial phenomenon** and (4) as a **system construct**.

The trajectory

The disease trajectory is a concept that has little currency in medical discourse. However, it is represented in the nursing literature over the past 2 decades, and it reflects the high profile accorded to chronic disease in nursing research, especially in the United States where chronic care is regarded as nursing territory. Prominent American authors, Larsen and Lubkin, go so far as to state that caring for someone with chronic illness is nursing, not medicine; that it is nursing's domain of practice.[30]

Modern nursing researchers in the United States, notably Corbin and Strauss,[31] developed a trajectory-based model for the nursing process, by which they mean the course of the illness for the patient plus the actions taken by those affected to manage the shape and course of the illness. There is little evidence that the nursing trajectory model is widely translated into medical thinking, apart from the literature of terminal care. A medical trajectory model of disease would visualise the activity and impact of the disease as a timeline, demonstrating sequential stages, or phases, as the condition runs its course. These phases have implications for the nature and timing of interventions, both preventive and therapeutic (*see* Appendix 2). The list of phases is descriptive rather than definitive.

Trajectory phases

- Pre-disease: risk factors and social antecedents of disease that define at-risk status.
- Pre-symptomatic: akin to the incubation period in infectious diseases; a disease process has begun but is latent; it may be detectable through screening (as with impaired glucose tolerance) and preventable through addressing risk factors (such as diet, exercise, hypertension or obesity).
- Early symptomatic (or onset) phase: the first detected manifestation of symptoms or dysfunction; this is often non-specific, or it may coincide with …
- Acute illness phase: sometimes a critical event that may terminate the timeline or which may be the first of a series of crises (as in stroke disease).
- Recovery phase: restoration of functioning; in chronic conditions recovery is often relative, with impairment occurring (as following a stroke).
- Plateau phase: a level segment of the curve; functional accommodation, even though subclinical progression may be continuing.
- Relapse: a repeat episode, frequently seen as therapeutic failure, but which is inherent to many disease trajectories (exacerbation; acute-on-chronic episode).
- Escalation, or transition phase: cycles of overt illness; increasing disability and decreasing interludes for recovery; progressive organ impairment.
- Crisis phase: perhaps with irreversible organ damage and cascades of events involving multiple organs and systems.
- Palliative phase: priorities shift from expectation of recovery towards damage limitation, symptom control and emotional support.
- Terminal phase: multi-organ failure, diminishing vital function, end-of-life issues.
- Posthumous phase: management of death and the consequences of life lost; attention to the needs of the bereaved (including carers) since they are fellow travellers on the illness path and have been affected by the disease.

What is the meaning of this?

The trajectory and its stages may be seen as merely a common-sense description. However, it does represent *the natural history of chronic disease*, and this may facilitate prediction and prognosis. In acute or self-limiting illness this may matter little, but Victorian literature was full of the intense night watch where the attending physician soberly pronounces, 'If she gets through the next few hours, all will be well' (it has to be lobar pneumonia). Medical interventions, however crucial or critical, are episodic. Doctors need to be aware of the big picture since point observations may not reveal progression. It is necessary to join the dots in order to be prognostic and directional, to act as a signpost for the patient and carers, and to institute proactive care. Case management requires the long view, based on knowledge of the natural history of disease, its trajectory, and how this might be shaped or altered through interventions. **Trajectory awareness facilitates prediction and prognosis**.

The essence of nursing may be, as Larsen said, caring for someone who is chronically ill, and the nurse is frequently well placed to observe the dynamics. For the 'continuity doctor', the GP, the essence of medicine lies with prevention, prognosis and intervention. The ancient word 'seer' covers all three – to foresee future problems, to read the situation and to respond promptly and appropriately. **Prevention lies at the core of chronic disease management** and on this is based much of the medical contribution.

The trajectory model will be explored further in Chapter 2, where the nature of chronic disease is examined in greater detail.

Prevention and the trajectory

> The goals of effective chronic disease management are preventive in orientation, to prevent exacerbations, complications, treatment side-effects and emotional distress …. The most preventable problems are iatrogenic.[32]

It is through prevention that we provide a health service rather than just a sickness service. Prevention may be dull in practice but it is life-giving and life-enhancing. This is the problem we have with epidemiology from student days. It seemed remote and unglamorous. Who celebrates a disease prevented? Who is even aware of it? Who rewards a non-event? We just have to trust the numbers, the epidemiologists and the evidence derived from studies amid the daily grind of surveillance, screening, secondary prevention, biometrics, systematic prescribing and rehabilitation; and as Paul of Tarsus advised, '*Be not weary of well doing.*' Keeping in mind the full natural history of the condition, aborting or modifying this or that event on the trajectory may involve the full palate of personal and technological resources. Even the most hopeless phases are full of preventive opportunity, both clinical and psychosocial. Palliative care is essentially anticipatory. We have to look far beyond primary prevention, and value the secondary and tertiary modes. In trajectory terms, primary merges through secondary and into tertiary, as rehabilitation, mitigating disability and symptom control gain prominence.

Chronic disease: a psychosocial condition

A great divide in the literature of long-term conditions is represented by terminology. This hints at the fundamental division between the so-called medical (disease-centred) and social (person and community-centred) models. Consider the following pairs of terms:

disease	illness
chronic	long-term

patient	service user
expert	experience
drugs	medicines
diagnosis	condition
handicap	disability
compliance	concordance.

These represent something of the cultural divide between medical and social domains, the former being seen as harsher and deterministic, and the latter as less threatening or oppressive. Semantics, maybe, but there are sets of values enshrined in these. Medical literature favours one, nursing and social work the other, even when covering the same territory. Medical professionals, as they are faced with increasing involvement in the management of people with long-term conditions, ought to be conversant with the social constructs and sociology, to seek to become increasingly patient centred, without compromising the essentials of their medical role.

Self-care is at the core of modern health policy. People know what they need and will tell us if we ask or if we will listen. Doing what we can to enhance this self-management is a key feature of the management of chronic disease. Our patients want to own their own illness, feel empowered through information and signposting to what services are available, to exercise autonomy and feel that they are more in control of the processes. This way lies concordance, as distinct from compliance, and leads to adherence to programmes of treatment. Chronic illness afflicts individuals, but in doing so affects profoundly their household and social circle. Most healthcare is self-care, according to the iceberg model of illness. Most of it goes on out of sight, with only the top 10% or so delivered by professionals. The disease resides with the family and is presented episodically to clinical view.

The family is an essential adjunct to self-care and these informal carers, along with any participating friends or neighbours, constitute the forgotten legion in health and social care. Their contribution is little-recognised, unremunerated and undervalued. Their needs reflect those of their dependant, but may be complicated by further issues of their own. All members of this 'caring unit' are liable to share in the social impairment and stigma that are features of illness and disability. These include loss of income, status, employment opportunity, freedom of movement, autonomy and self-expression. Carers span the age range from schoolchild to extreme elderly. Family resources are used up – leisure time, social life, emotional energy, relationship resilience and the ability to plan a future. These can be summed up as chronic stress, and lead to health risk and increasing dependency on external supports. The statutory supports are healthcare, social services, social security and employment support.

The instinct for self-care generates a need for participation and the creation of social support mechanisms. Civil society to a great extent rests on the voluntary sector, and the bulk of their personnel are volunteers (many of them fellow sufferers or veterans of illness). This is called 'the third sector'. Self-care generates self-help on a community development model – that is, finding local responses to locally identified needs. Long-term condition sufferers have found that, whatever their diagnosis, up to 80% of their need is generic.[33]

This third sector exhibits sophisticated levels of organisation through voluntary and non-governmental organisations. It is organic in its development and is based on valid expression of needs. Its reach extends to providing services, commissioning research and development, and advocating people's needs up to government and policy-making levels. In the UK National Health Service (NHS) chronic care services are widely contracted out by the NHS to the voluntary sector. Some self-help and voluntary bodies have an international profile. Examples include Alcoholics Anonymous, the International Diabetes Federation, Alzheimer's Disease International and the International Association for Hospice and Palliative Care. These merit respect from professional bodies and their work influences the knowledge and attitudes that enrich the formal health sector. Participation and inclusion are important pillars of health policy in the UK under the banner of personal and public involvement. The 'expert patient' is another emerging concept.

The needs expressed by people with long-term conditions and their carers may be summarised as:

- to live ordinary lives
- normalisation; minimise stigma
- to be treated with dignity and respect
- engagement on the part of professionals
- services that are user-friendly, accessible and streamlined
- ownership of their condition; empowerment
- information about their condition; signposting to services
- emotional support
- employment support
- youth support, for young patients and underage carers
- lifestyle support
- contribution: the ability to give something in return, as 'experts by experience'.[34]

What is the meaning of this?

Although doctors and other clinical workers are not social engineers they have powerful roles that are socially determined. The status of doctor, for example, confers command of resources, authority and, indeed, power. In taking this for granted doctors are strangely unaware of these attributes, but others perceive them, for good or ill. These privileges are not personal rights but are accorded to professionals because of their role-relationship with the sick and with society. It is they who validate us as professionals. This becomes apparent when we are faced with issues of accreditation and regulation. In daily life, however, professionals can abuse their position, through self-interest, or use it to enhance the lives of others. If we limit ourselves to a self-absorbed, medical focus we may be depriving patients and society of real benefits. When doctors fail and are criticised it is mostly through breakdown of performance of their social role rather than technical incompetence. Examples include failure to treat people with respect and dignity, mismanaged communication, or being inaccessible. Praise and gratitude follow the perception of providing support and demonstrating engagement with their patients. Doctors make important contributions to voluntary organisations and enhance their patients' capacities for self-help. There is a popular maxim, 'When you get it right you will always be remembered; when you get it wrong you will never be forgotten.'

Chronic disease: a system construct

Chronic disease management is central to healthcare policy at local, national and international levels. Here, without prejudice to patient centeredness, we turn towards a population denominator and embrace the public health and epidemiology perspective. This does not mean delving into esoteric knowledge or management-speak.

A technical or professional service is only as good as the vehicle that delivers it and no area of care is more systems dependent than that of chronic illness. Medical professionals are slow to engage with systems of delivery. We tend to be relatively unaware of their nature but if, for example, our computer systems in general practice broke down, we would be like fish out of water. In general practice there is much that is essentially public health medicine, where the good of society is the aim even, perhaps, at some expense to the individual. A prime example is in immunisation against infectious disease. Babies and mothers hate the baby clinic, but eradicating polio and controlling pertussis or measles avoids much morbidity, disability and mortality. The herd immunity trumps the personal pain (and even the element of risk). All our risk factor surveillance and cancer screening are directed at population health. The concept of risk is a statistical one. We do not know which individual patients will benefit. Reducing the disease burden saves lives and spares resources even though there will be consequences arising from the inevitable false negatives, false positives and side effects.

Resource is a dominant factor in the systems model of chronic disease – who pays, for what, how much and how? There is a grave threat to the capacity of health systems for a variety of reasons that we have seen, such as demographics, increased survival with impairment, and cost inflation. There are two basic kinds of health system – *consumer-driven*, usually disease centred and specialist delivered, or *generalist-based* with a socialised, community orientation. The former tends to be individualistic and privately funded; the latter tends to be centrally funded and based on risk-sharing. Most systems develop features of both or attempt to balance these polarities. There is a growing body of transnational evidence that systems based on a firm foundation of primary healthcare are the more cost-effective and deliver better population outcomes.[35] Countries where the generalist has been undervalued historically are finding it necessary to experiment with new systems of care that seek to bridge gaps in provision of services. Examples of this include programmes that are established in the United States such as the Veterans Health Administration and Kaiser Permanente models. On the other hand, those that have national health services that emphasise primary care are studying the US managed care models in order to drive down costs and enhance patient involvement as, for example, in the idea of commissioning in the UK. Macro systems show immense inertia to change, and professional interests and political pressures play a great part in this. There are few circumstances where nations can reinvent their healthcare system, as happened in the UK in the post-war years of national crisis.

Paradoxically, perhaps, it was in United States that the chronic care model was developed and it influenced fundamentally the WHO report *Innovative Care for Chronic Conditions*.[36] This emphasises an enhanced role for patients and their families in management of chronic conditions, supported by their healthcare teams and communities, based on six principles:[37]

1. evidence-based decision-making; effective, needs-based processes of care
2. population focus; long-term, proactive
3. prevention focus; informed, involved patients; lifestyle changes
4. quality focus
5. integration across settings and conditions
6. flexibility and adaptability; foresees and responds to changing demand.

This, it proposes, is the necessary paradigm shift, away from the individualistic, market-driven, fragmented, hospital-centred models of care. In order to implement this the WHO report identifies eight essential actions:

1. support the paradigm shift
2. manage the political environment
3. build integrated healthcare
4. align sectoral policies for health (across government departments)
5. use healthcare personnel more effectively
6. centre care on the patient and family
7. support patients in their communities
8. emphasise prevention.

These considerations operate within a national framework at three levels:

1. *micro* systems – patient, family, community organisations, local healthcare teams
2. *meso* systems – the healthcare organisations
3. *macro* systems – the political, policy-making, fiscal level.

WHO states that chronic conditions will be the leading cause of disability by 2020 and that, if not successfully managed, will become the most expensive problem for all healthcare systems.[38] All of this may be outside the 'need to know' area for the average clinician. However, forces like these are driving the agendas for change in healthcare delivery everywhere. What we experience as new, irksome local directives are the waves that come from storms far offshore, and therefore they are not without meaning.

While health policy giants in the United States and WHO are inventing structures to bridge gaps in systems of care, the centralised systems like the UK health service are struggling with interface problems, where areas of the organisation overlap, clash and reduplicate. One striking interface in the UK lies between GP and hospital; another lies between both and the social services. Integrated care is one solution that is proposed, whereby these sectors are mutually reinforcing and the care pathway of the patient with chronic illness is 'seamless'. This is problematic because of disparate chains of command, lines of management and streams of funding, not to mention the small matters of co-morbidity and complexity.

Complexity affects all the stakeholders and the patient bears a good deal of the consequences, particularly since their needs are liable to arise from multiple long-term conditions and adverse social circumstances. It is a truism that chronic conditions frequently coexist (multi-morbidity) and increase with ageing (cumulative disease burden combined with frailty) and social disadvantage (social determinants of health).

Much systems-related research and development is directed towards **vertical and horizontal integration** (dovetailing specialist and community care), through enhanced roles for GPs and their co-workers, **connected healthcare** (the use of electronic systems for patient monitoring) and **intermediate care** (as in 'hospital-at-home' and 'virtual ward'), based on chronic care specialist nurse teams for implementing care plans, and social workers for programmes of care in the community through case management. Such policies converge on the GP as the hub. They aim to achieve a synthesis that might be expressed as:

- multidisciplinary teams that function as learning organisations
- bonded together by managers, team meetings and enhanced IT
- working with patients and families across the range of their need
- cooperating with community partners and specialist services
- to care for the patient in the location of lowest intensity

- effecting smooth handover where interfaces exist ('revolving doors')
- creating clinical pathways that are characterised by:
  - minimum disruption for the patient
  - high quality of care
  - appropriate information and signposting regarding available services.

What is the meaning of this?

Our inherited systems of care tend to be linear and resemble line management in organisations. Chronic or complex illness, however, requires access to services that span general practice, hospital-based services that may be far away, and social services in the community, through repeated episodes of care, with monitoring of continuing treatments. This is not a linear function. Neither is it cyclical. It is more suggestive of a chaotic system that resembles a framework or network-based model. There are promising developments in connected health (telemedicine) and intermediate care that are being piloted, even if their evidence base is not yet fully established. All of this is a work in progress and a long way from delivering comprehensive solutions to the problems of chronic care but ideals, even elusive ones, have value. One way to reduce the mystique of complexity is to reduce the variables. For a start, we should **regard chronic disease as a composite construct and imaginatively design our systems of care accordingly, with the patient and family at their core**.

DISABILITY AS A CHRONIC CONDITION

A disability may not qualify as a disease, although the converse may be true. It may be regarded as an impairment of function at the level of the person, a chronic condition that is not normally regarded as a chronic disease although they share much common ground. Some definitions and further thoughts will appear in the section on disability, impairment and handicap in Chapter 2, but it deserves to be introduced at this stage for completeness. A person with severe osteoarthritis may be well, in the sense that they are not ill. However, they require clinical interventions, perhaps social ones too, and other supports in order for them to achieve the normal activities of life. The range of disability is wide, stemming from any number of impairments that may include:

- sensory organs (e.g. of hearing, seeing, sensory or pain pathways)
- mobility (e.g. limb amputation, arthritides, spasticity, tremor, coordination)
- organ function (e.g. brain injury, atresias)
- development (e.g. in intellectual disability, developmental delay)
- social functioning (e.g. autistic spectrum).

There is a wide range of aetiologies and risk factors, genetic, toxic, infective, traumatic, developmental and degenerative. As with other chronic conditions, much disability results from missed opportunities for prevention, therapeutic deficit and social disadvantage. There has to be great emphasis on the management of disability in childhood, since the consequences are life-shortening or lifelong. The priorities lie in early detection, timely diagnosis, assessment of needs, medical management (especially of co-morbidity and polypharmacy), multidisciplinary management, integrated care, crisis intervention, developmental monitoring, health promotion, assistive technology, social support, educational support and eventually employment support; and the needs of carers. These are so well managed by community paediatricians and those who care for the intellectually impaired that the GP can easily be unaware of the scope of the pathways of care, until children with complex needs reach the big transition into adulthood.

How closely this all resembles the provision required for managing the chronic diseases. Disability, impairment and handicap will not always receive special mention throughout the rest of these chapters, but they are very much part of the entire concern of chronic care. Disability is under-represented in the curricula of undergraduate and specialist training, even for general practice. Training in the generic approach to chronic conditions should redress this.

SCENARIO: tutorial time

Standing orders:
- regular weekly, uninterrupted, protected time
- informal (coffee and biscuits, comfortable chairs; laptop and PowerPoint)
- preparatory work by both trainer and trainee
- agreed topic or agenda; cross-referenced with the training curriculum.

I open by saying that, although there is an agreed topic for this tutorial, the previous evening's consultation merits the first half hour, not because it is unusual in its scope and content but because it is so representative of how general practice is going. I ask the trainee to analyse what was going on from her perspective.

It seemed to me that there were two consultations going on. The first was initiated by the practice to update her blood pressure record and review her medications, but that was complicated by her use of hypnotics. The consultation might have ended if you had just authorised continuing supply of her tablets, but exploring her sleep problem enabled her to go on to tell you about her mother, and that's when things really took off.

I admit that there was a moment when I regretted providing that opening for her, when I was completing my agenda. But I felt sure she would have turned back as soon as she touched the doorknob and given me phase two (her agenda) anyway; so it was better to manage the situation positively from the start. On to the list of issues raised.

> Well, my list may not be comprehensive, but she is hypertensive, has insomnia, she is depressed, has a list of repeat prescriptions and a few indirect ones, and she wanted a sick line. She lives with her husband and her mother who is very elderly, difficult, and has diabetes and leg ulcers that are probably related to the diabetes. Her mother may also be developing Alzheimer's, but she may be depressed following the death of her husband, her diabetes may be out of control or she may be overdosing on painkillers. The district nurse is attending her for dressings and, I presume, to monitor her diabetes. She will need a house call to review her diabetes and assess her mental state; she's probably on half a dozen different drugs that will need to be reviewed.

I have one reaction to this workman-like overview; that the new trainee should be the one to do the home visit to the mother while I undertake the review of the daughter. She should report back at the next tutorial, which will be devoted entirely to this case (we are getting into case-based learning more and more). She agrees. We proceed to look at preparation for the next tutorial by drawing up a list of the non-disease issues that had arisen from the consultation:

- who the patient is in this case
- how we manage complex consultations
- issues of professionalism: use of time; working under pressure; managing one's own feelings …
- patient centredness
- carers' needs
- certification of unfitness for work
- care in the community
- use of primary care team
- importance of home visits and domiciliary care
- family dynamics and marital problems
- addiction (alcohol, hypnotics, analgesics …)
- the computer and repeat prescribing (IT).

> That's a tall order; how can we fit all that into a tutorial? How am I going to prepare all that stuff? It looks like the whole curriculum – it could take us through to Christmas!

A clear communicator, our new trainee. She came highly recommended from her hospital posts. She is therefore probably well informed about diabetes and hypertension, but she may well be a bit vague on depression, addiction, Alzheimer's, insomnia and leg ulcers. The other, non-disease, factors did not figure on her list of issues at all. 'Soft GP stuff', she calls it; that's what has caused her to panic. Many of the topics are not in the clinical textbooks she has known.

I often wonder at the start of the training cycle how we are going to structure the process – how to open it up and unpack it in a way that grabs the attention of the newcomer to general practice. On the first day I had shown her the substantial file that contains the curriculum for general practice. Her eyes had glazed over. She was right. It is my job to know the curriculum and to render it accessible to the learner. She thinks I am now asking her to prepare nearly the whole GP curriculum for next week and, rightly, is appalled at the prospect.

So, I say to her, we have to start somewhere. What is the one thread that links all the factors we have identified in this case?

'General practice, is it?' – with a whimsical smile, after a considerable pause.

Not a bad gambit; she's got instinct, or is it sarcasm? We settle for chronic disease management. The woman, her husband and her mother all show aspects of chronic conditions, illnesses if you like, and their consequences.

She objects mildly that hypertension is a risk factor, not a disease, the husband's alcohol is a bad habit, and that his nerves and her insomnia are neurotic, learned behaviours that are probably personality related.

OK, good points, but let's leave for the moment definitions of what constitutes an illness and focus on the concept of chronic disease. It looks as if we are going to reinvent the wheel. Can I suggest options? You can read up on all these topics for next week, and see how far you get. Or you can carry out a search on chronic disease – you'll get a thousand hits (most of them about health policy), which is a problem in itself. What I suggest you do is to think general; consider the factors that might be common to managing all chronic diseases. Try to create a diagram or a mind map that enables you to think your way through all the different aspects of the practice and the services we provide that relate to people who have long-term conditions; how you might address the demands posed by any chronic disease. Let's not focus on what you know of each disease at this stage – they are too diverse. Think general, like doing a jigsaw puzzle to create a composite picture. I guarantee that this will take you into every aspect of primary care – what GPs do, how practices are run, including the finances and The Contract. Actually, inventing the wheel is not a bad image to keep in mind when you brainstorm this. Think hub, spokes, etc.

Now, back to today's tutorial topic. We still have an hour.

The following day I received a note from her:

Dear trainer,

I enclose my attempt to mind-map the things we were talking about yesterday. I'm not sure what you were looking for, but I hope this makes sense. See you tomorrow,

JB (associate in training)

(*see* Figure 1.2)

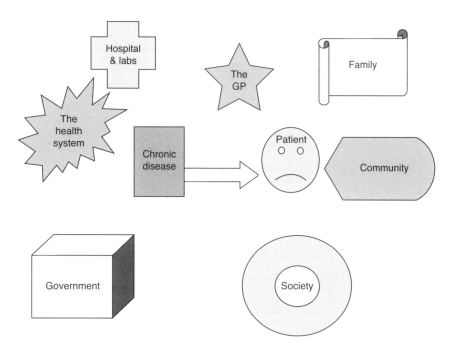

FIGURE 1.2 The new trainee's diagram

CONCLUSION AND REFLECTION

This chapter has been a preliminary map of the territory of chronic disease management. Chronic diseases should be seen as a collective, with common features in their natural history and trajectory, and the consequent needs of patients and their family carers. The generic model of chronic disease encompasses disability and other long term conditions. These indicate the need for prevention, patient centredness, planning of interventions and improved service delivery. They are represented in the chronic disease paradigm. Chronic care is a training priority that covers much of the curriculum of training for general practice. The paradigm change proposed by WHO reorients health systems towards service priorities.

POINTS FOR REFLECTION

- Can you carry out a computer search and compile a register for a particular chronic disease?
- For which key long-term conditions might it be useful to compile such a register? Are there particular, hidden conditions in your area or region (e.g. in Northern Ireland we have a relatively high prevalence of haemochromatosis and coeliac disease).
- Identify the 10 long-term conditions that are most common in your country. What is their incidence? Prevalence? How many of each might you expect to find in your practice population? Why not check?
- How is primary care defined in your country and system?
- Review the trajectory phases and identify them on the curve in Appendix 2.
- Create your own trajectory graph for a patient you know well. What is the prognosis (the trajectory projection) in the short and longer term for your patient?
- Review the list of wants for patients and carers. In what ways do you contribute to any of these items?
- Collate the sentences in this chapter that are in bold type. What message do they convey?

REFERENCES

1. World Health Organization. *30th World Health Assembly: the Alma Ata International Conference on Primary Health Care.* Geneva: WHO/UNICEF; 1978.
2. World Health Organization. *Innovative Care for Chronic Conditions: building blocks for action; global report.* Geneva: WHO; 2002.
3. Starfield B, Shi L, Macinko J. Contribution of primary care to health systems and health. *Milbank Q.* 2005; **83**(3): 457–502.
4. World Health Organization, 2002, op. cit.
5. Verbrugge L, Jette A. The disablement process. *Soc Sci Med.* 1994; **38**(1): 1–14.
6. Starfield B. William Pickles Lecture. Primary and specialty care interfaces: the imperative of disease continuity. *Br J Gen Pract.* 2003; **53**(494): 723–9.
7. Schön D. *The Reflective Practitioner.* London: Temple Smith; 1983.
8. World Health Organization, 2002, op. cit.
9. The Economist Intelligence Unit. *The Future of Healthcare in Europe (Foreword).* Geneva: The Economist Intelligence Unit; 2011. p. 1. Available at: www.janssen-emea.com/future-of-healthcare-in-europe (accessed 20 April 2014).
10. Office for National Statistics. *Summary: UK population projected to reach 70 million by mid-2027.* London: Office for National Statistics, 26 October 2011.
11. Adshead F. Foreword. In: Alder J, Mayhew L, Moody S, *et al. The Chronic Disease Burden: an analysis.* London: Cass Business School; 2005. p. 1.

12. World Health Organization. *Countries: United Kingdom*. Available at: www.who.int/countries/gbr/en/ (accessed 26 November 2013).

13. Ibid.

14. Belfield G, Colin-Thomé D. *Improving Chronic Disease Management*. Available at: www.natpact.info/uploads/ChronicDiseaseDHNote.pdf (accessed 8 April 2014).

15. Department of Health. *Ten Things You Need to Know about Long Term Conditions*. 2012. Available at: webarchive.nationalarchives.gov.uk/+/www.dh.gov.uk/en/Healthcare/Longtermconditions/DH_084294 (accessed 08 April 2014).

16. Bland P. Helping patients back to work. *Practitioner*. 2010; **254**(1729): 7.

17. Department of Health, 2012. op. cit.

18. Carers UK. *Facts about Carers 2012*. London: Carers UK; 2012. Available at: www.carersuk.org/media/k2/attachments/Facts_about_carers_Dec_2012.pdf (accessed 26 November 2013).

19. Centers for Disease Control and Prevention. *Chronic Disease Prevention and Health Promotion*. Available at: www.cdc.gov/nccdphp/overview.htm (accessed 26 October 2013).

20. Hardy GE Jr. The burden of chronic disease: the future is prevention. Introduction to Dr. James Marks' presentation, 'The Burden of Chronic Disease and the Future of Public Health'. *Prev Chronic Dis*. 2004; **1**(2): A04.

21. The Economist Intelligence Unit, op. cit.

22. Australian Institute of Health and Welfare. *Chronic Diseases*. Available at: www.aihw.gov.au/chronic-diseases/ (accessed 15 November 2013).

23. World Health Organization, 2002, op. cit. p. 10.

24. World Health Organization, 2002, op. cit. p. 11.

25. Spijker J, MacInnes J. Population ageing, the timebomb that isn't? *BMJ*. 2013; **347**: f6598.

26. Centers for Disease Control and Prevention, op. cit.

27. World Health Organization. *World Health Report 2008: primary health care, now more than ever*. Geneva: WHO; 2008.

28. World Health Organization, 2002, op. cit.

29. The Economist Intelligence Unit, op. cit.

30. Larsen P, Lubkin I. *Chronic Illness: impact and intervention*. 7th ed. Sudbury, MA: Jones & Bartlett; 2009.

31. Corbin JM, Strauss A. A nursing model for chronic disease management based on the trajectory framework. *Res Theory Nurs Pract*. 2001; **5**(3): 155–74.

32. Glasgow R, Orleans T, Wagner E, *et al*. Does the chronic care model serve also as a template for improving prevention? *Millbank Q*. 2001; **79**(4): 579–612.

33. McEvoy PJ. Patients with long-term conditions, their carers, and advocates. *Br J Gen Pract*. 2013; **63**(608): 148–9.

34. Ibid.

35. Starfield B, Shi L, Makinko J. The contribution of primary care to health systems and health. *Milbank Q*. 2005: **83**(3): 457–502.

36. Wagner EH, Austin BT, von Korff M. Care for patients with chronic illness. *Milbank Q*. 1996: **74**(4): 511–44.

37. World Health Organization, 2002, op. cit.

38. World Health Organization, 2002, op.cit. p. 1.

CHAPTER 2

The story of chronic disease (the disease complex)

Contents

CHAPTER OVERVIEW

An outline of chronic disease has been emerging through Chapter 1. Time, now, to examine the chronic disease story in more detail. I call this a story because chronic disease lends itself more to imagery than scientific discourse, and this chapter will follow that approach. It is personified as a predatory genus that occupies the same eco-space as *Homo sapiens*. The characteristics of this genus, as with any virulent organism, manifest an epidemiological profile – that is, it has a natural history, course, impact, and social and environmental determinants that constitute its habitat. From this can be deduced possible avenues for countermeasures, aimed at controlling it, since it seems impossible to eradicate it. This leads into a summary of epidemiology, which will be complemented by a review of sociology in the following chapter. Both of these merit attention as fundamental health sciences, although perhaps dimly remembered from student days, if at all.

The villain of the story is the collective threat posed by long-term conditions, the imminent and immanent challenges that confront our complex healthcare systems. We need a 'Hero', like a St George, to pit himself against this Dragon. In the legend he felled the Dragon with a single dramatic intervention. The image of St George slaying the Dragon is a familiar one from fable, heraldry, coinage, cartoons and children's books. The legend is ancient, with origins in Armenia or Cappadocia (he was only adopted by England in late mediaeval times as her suitably martial but benevolent champion). The story, however, was set in the deserts of Libya. It offers an early example of a multinational collaborative report on a venture in public health and safety.

SCENARIO: story time

Once upon a time, a plague-bearing Dragon dwelt in a lake close to the city of Lasia and, as Wikipedia states, 'envenomed the whole countryside'. It reaped a tally of two sheep every day to appease its virulent appetites and meeting this costly toll threatened the viability of the local economy. In an early instance of escalating virulence through jumping the species barrier, the Dragon took a fancy to children. Initially one child a day fell victim, with fatal outcome, in what may have been a postcode lottery. Inevitably, the time came when the next chosen victim was Sabra, the daughter of the king. St George, a soldier (perhaps Roman) happened on the scene and without hesitation intervened to prevent the Dragon's attack, saving Sabra at the moment of crisis. This example of the inverse care law illustrates how the privileged are first in line to take advantage of any available preventive interventions. St George's spear shatters against the Dragon's defences, his sword bounces off its scaly torso but he stabs it in its one vulnerable area, the axilla, immobilising it. St George calls on the princess to let him borrow her girdle (there being no hint of deviant behaviour) and, using it as a halter, she is able to lead the Dragon like a lapdog into the city, where the arrival of this plague vector causes panic. St George tells the city council that if, through a change of heart, the whole population mend their ways and live wholesomely, the Dragon will die. They do, and it does.

The ending of our modern story of struggle is not yet within view. We do not yet know the kind of miracle we hope for. But, like St George, we size up the adversary, scrutinise it for possible weak points and deploy the weapons of mobility and relative simplicity, with much at stake. And now our enemy is in sight. Like a Dragon moving forward as a looming threat, it is becoming definable. As we have seen, it has been described with apocalyptic metaphors – the tsunami, the asteroid strike, the iceberg, the epidemic, the healthcare challenge of the twenty-first century …

CHRONIC DISEASE, THE ENEMY WITHIN

Probably the most formidable and growing threat among the ranks of chronic diseases is diabetes. In a press interview in 2012 Baroness Young (chief executive of Diabetes UK) described type 2 diabetes as:

> The perfect storm, a potent combination of increasing numbers with diabetes and NHS pressures that threatens to bankrupt the NHS.

She went on to say that at least 90% of all diabetic cases are type 2, fuelled by obesity, too much alcohol, a lack of exercise and generally unhealthy living. As in Edward Gibbon's *The History of the Decline and Fall of the Roman Empire*, it seems we are succumbing to decadence and unpreparedness to defend ourselves.

But the chronic disease threat is not a disaster story where one obscure scientist with arcane but vital knowledge would get the ear of the all-powerful president, who would mobilise a brave and clever task force to avert the disaster at the last moment. Unlike the Dragon of Lasia, this adversary will not be overcome with one judicious thrust. Neither is it a story of alien invasion. There is little we do not know about the forces that threaten. It is more like the enemy within that we have to come to terms with eventually through managed coexistence. Chronic disease lurks in our genes, incubates in our own modes of behaviour, is endemic in our environment and accompanies each stage of the human life cycle. Yet it has all the elements of drama – threat, fear, conflict, hope, suffering, a challenge to the human spirit, contending with a personalised and dire entity that nevertheless has universal implications. However, what we are doing, and have been doing, about it is reckoned to be insufficient and inappropriate,[1] and in fact, this is feeding its frenzy. This enemy, which can be characterised as a mythical, predatory genus of beast – like the Dragon – is *Big, Bad and Ugly*, and rapidly getting more so. We cannot ignore this force, and to do nothing is not an option.

Big and getting bigger: our part in its increase

Population growth means more mouths to feed, and lives to tend and protect; we enjoy enhanced longevity as we are better fed, housed and our welfare secured; we survive acute threats. *Good medical and social care prolong life and defer death*. The population pyramid is becoming top-heavy. Much of the life extension is not added years of health but is subject to accumulated morbidity and degenerative disease. Increasingly, *we live with rather than die from chronic disease*. Healthcare activity and expenditure cluster in three areas, the very young, those with severe disabilities and the final few months of life. All are areas of expanding need. Diagnostic and clinical interventions reveal more and earlier pathology, and convert acute pathology into long-term conditions, thus increasing prevalence. The cost of medical technology is growing (health inflation) faster than national economies.

Bad and getting worse: our contribution

Chronic conditions are frequently multiple, coexisting and cumulative. Survivors of disease onslaught require intrusive 'life-support systems' of continuing care for residual disabilities and defence against recurrence. As societies age, the burden of care increases but the economically productive base of 'healthy' population which generates tax revenues and provides caring manpower narrows. Are the young and fit willing to carry this burden? The NHS is the largest enterprise, and biggest employer, in the UK and around 60% of its costs are in manpower, which, too, is subject to cost inflation. To keep pace with its workforce requirements the UK has raided the health services of much poorer countries, recruiting large numbers of their trained staff, especially nurses. Even prevention as a coping strategy gets costlier since it relates to whole population medicine, which is labour intensive.

Ugly and getting uglier: partly because of our good intentions

The longer people live and survive with impairment the more they encounter multi-morbidity and age-related conditions, degenerative diseases, organ failure (notably of brain, kidney and heart) and frailness. We mean well but we prolong the agony. Many of our countermeasures cause collateral damage through onerous treatment pathways, polypharmacy, toxic treatments, heroic surgery and other iatrogenic hazards – the slow death by a thousand cuts of enthusiastic rescue and maintenance measures. In the home care setting there is often the problem of 'the old and infirm caring for the old and infirm'. Chronic illness breeds poverty, and the costs of social care can deprive the elderly of their homes and their life savings.

Chronic disease is out of control

Chronic disease is out of control. It always was, it could well continue to be so, but we are losing ground. It grows faster than our resources and we can no longer afford to provide or purchase the full potential fruits of our technology, even at its present state of development. Even if we could, our delivery systems are not efficient or correctly targeted. They are prisoners of historical development, with a focus on the acute and infectious diseases, concentrated in 'silos' of specialisms and hospitals, mostly urban based, fragmented and slow to respond to patterns of need.[2] In most countries only the very privileged can reap the full benefit, and then usually at the expense of the less well-off, directly or indirectly. At the same time the expectations on the part of everyone are rising to unrealistic levels (no one should ever die!) and the affluence gap between the wealthy and the poor is growing. The economic chill post 2007 that affected the United States and most of Europe has magnified the problems the less well-off have in accessing affordable care. Where national health services attenuate this expense factor through risk-sharing strategies the public funding pot is shrinking. To counter the rapid growth of chronic disease, therefore, requires health and social care professionals and systems everywhere to work smarter, not just harder, to understand and embrace what needs to be done and why, and be able to communicate this to others – notably, their patients and team workers; to participate in innovation and change. At the same time those at the front line have to retain optimism in the face of rising workload and worsening statistics. It is not our fault. The levers of real change reside at the *meso* and *macro* levels – that is, at system and government level. It is there that real leadership and inspiration are required.

PROFILING CHRONIC DISEASE: CHRONIC VERSUS ACUTE DISEASE

We all know what we mean by infectious disease, which is mostly acute. Other acute medicine is largely the focused management of crises that occur within the trajectory of chronic disease. The term 'acute condition' has been defined by the US National Center for Health Statistics as one that lasts less than 3 months, involves medical attention or causes restricted activity.[3] Kane *et al.*[4] define as chronic an illness or condition that has persistent or recurrent health consequences lasting for a substantial period of time (variously identified as at least 3 months, 6 months or longer), is not self-limiting, waxes and wanes in terms of severity, and typically cannot be cured. In the absence of any better definition of chronic disease it may be useful to compare characteristics of both acute and chronic disease, to create a profile of both to illustrate the contrasting dynamics of each. These are summarised in Figure 2.1.

There is a middle ground that overlaps both and is of considerable importance. Patients, whether with acute or long-term conditions, experience a high prevalence of *non-disease conditions*. Examples include anxiety and depression, fatigue, pain, constipation, itch, dyspnoea, sleep problems, dyspepsia and weight disorders. Although many of these are transient they are very likely to be recurrent and therefore to rank as truly chronic conditions. They particularly oppress the elderly who are, in addition, plagued by 'the Five Big I's' (also known as the 'Geriatric Giants'): Incontinence, Immobility, Instability (falling), Intellectual impairment and Isolation. These contribute to a chronic condition of old age called frailty.

	Acute disease	Chronic disease
Examples	Appendicitis Pneumonia	Arthritis Diabetes Heart disease
Causes	Single (e.g. organism) Preventable	Multiple Risk factors Limited prevention
Diagnosis	Clear, clinical Single Test results definitive	Early diagnosis difficult Delays in diagnosis Time as a diagnostic tool Multi- or co-morbid
Duration	Brief or circumscribed	Lifelong
Effect of treatment	Curative aim High primary prevention role Definitive medical or surgical intervention	Aims not curative Prevention secondary or tertiary Episodic interventions (medical or surgical) Modified progression Palliation

FIGURE 2.1 Comparing acute and chronic disease

Chronic disease is a new conceptual space. It is not regarded as a specialism in its own right and has not featured specially in the formal curricula of learning. It lacks a succinct definition. Simple temporal definitions such as 'Any condition that is present for 3–6 months or more' are too reductionist to be satisfactory, and that is why it is described as a *conceptual space*. This notion respects the relative absence of boundaries, of exclusive territory or ownership (except by the individual patient). A host of professionals operate within this space. Clinical generalists are accustomed to the absence of boundaries, however challenging this may be. Foremost among these is the GP, although *generalism* may also be claimed by the geriatrician, the paediatrician or, in the United States, the general internist (or 'hospitalist'). Managing chronic disease is not new to the GP but the growing focus on this has brought within his or her orbit a host of new responsibilities, perspectives and methodologies. This erstwhile 'Lone Ranger' of primary care is refashioned as the agent of prevention, the early warning system, case finder, multidisciplinary coordinator, conductor of an orchestra of specialists, guide/mentor/interpreter for the patient and the front line of health services, who has public health concerns in addition to those of personalised primary care. GPs really have to struggle to maintain their perspective and vision for the complete campaign against chronic disease, especially when overcome by an avalanche of constant, detailed, repetitive and 'menial' tasks. This vision for the final product is vital if they are to sustain the heavy responsibilities of safe, person-centred practice in the face of the volume and diversity of disease, and an increasingly complex health system.

The conceptual space of chronic disease needs to be rendered comprehensible and explored. I propose to populate this place with the mythical genus Dragon, to represent the collective disease that shares this ecology with humans, including those professionals who (like field biologists) seek to study, analyse and, where possible, bring it under control. We will presently examine a few different notions or *models of disease* that have a bearing on the nature of this Dragon.

> Whoever fights monsters should see to it that in the process one does not become a monster.
>
> Friedrich Nietzsche

THE NATURAL HISTORY OF CHRONIC DISEASE: THE LIFE CYCLE OF THE DRAGON

Much of the natural history of chronic disease will be apparent from what has gone before. As we have seen, this refers to the life cycle of the condition as its course unfolds, unfettered by the interference of external agency. It may be described in epidemiological terms, beginning with a general description, and continuing with its impact, risk factors, at-risk population and course. What we are addressing is well summarised in the WHO 2002 report that, as we have seen in Chapter 1, refers to, 'Chronic conditions; the health care challenge of the 21st century', and defines chronic disease as:

> an enormously broad category of what could appear on the surface as disparate health concerns. The category consists of:
> - persistent communicable diseases, e.g. HIV/AIDS
> - non-communicable diseases, e.g. cardiovascular disease, cancers, diabetes
> - certain mental disorders, e.g. depression, schizophrenia
> - ongoing impairments of structure, e.g. amputations, blindness, joint disorders.
>
> All fit within the chronic disease category and share fundamental themes:
> - persistent
> - require some level of healthcare management over years or decades
> - increasing prevalence worldwide
> - seriously challenge the efficiency and effectiveness of current health care systems and test our abilities to organise systems to meet imminent demands

- engender serious economic and social consequences in all regions and threaten health care resources in every country
- can be curtailed if leaders in Government and health care embrace change and innovation.[5]

PAUSE FOR REMINISCENCE

Dr Bill McCormick, a revered teacher of psychiatry in Belfast, was fond of telling us, his students, of 'the Seven Cs' of clinically significant and serious conditions that merited our particular study and attention, which he characterised as: Common, Chronic, Communicable, 'Crippling', Catastrophic (lethal), Costly and Childhood onset. Most of these seem apt as descriptors of the impact of our Dragon on the human life cycle. Incidentally, his brother, Professor James McCormick of Trinity College, Dublin, achieved renown as a teacher of community medicine, a GP and author of an early book on general practice theory (*The Doctor: Father Figure or Plumber?*), and along with Petr Skrabanek as an exponent of critical interpretation of epidemiological data and the limitations of screening programmes, through their classic book *Follies and Fallacies in Medicine* (*see* 'Screening and Wilson's Criteria' later in this chapter).

As do all diseases, the Dragon exhibits the usual epidemiological characteristics, such as a natural history, risk factors and an at-risk population, prevalence, impact on society and specific, individual effects. Chronic disease is universal, affecting all populations and societies. Genetic predisposition plays a substantial role in the genesis of most chronic conditions. A small number of risk factors are common to very many chronic conditions. The predominant one is age. Risk from the Dragon increases into old age and the prevalence of multi-morbidity rises in all age groups, but there is marked clustering of diseases in the under-20 age group. Young people are likely to have very good health or else to suffer multiple related conditions that reduce their life expectancy. The multi-morbidity risk curve is U-shaped rather than linear, rising at either end of the human lifespan.[6] Chronic disease is not randomly distributed. It is not simply a matter of ageing but affects 'the seven ages of man'.

The long-term conditions that afflict *early life* are mostly congenital, genetic, the consequences of trauma (including birth trauma), social deprivation, and associated with developmental delay and disabilities. This stage of life has benefited from the major success stories of prevention through improved maternity care, neonatal screening and immunisation against the serious acute infections that are such potent causes of long-term disability.

Moving into *early childhood*, the main additional problems in affluent nations are asthma and epilepsy. Both are modifiable through continuing surveillance and medications, although at some considerable cost to the childhood of the child and the peace of mind of parents. The increase in childhood obesity is causing much concern as a long-term health issue. A notable non-disease chronic condition that plagues childhood is chronic constipation. Significantly, the experience of emotional trauma in childhood is positively correlated with the subsequent rates of smoking, alcohol misuse, drug addiction, sexual promiscuity, depression and attempted suicide; it also correlates with high rates of morbid obesity, emphysema, diabetes and heart disease, and death 20 years earlier than those who have not experienced a significant adverse event in childhood.[7] A meta-analysis in 2012 reported that children with disabilities experienced high rates of sexual and physical violence, emotional abuse and neglect.[8]

Given survival beyond the early years of life, the chronic disease risk factors that beset the *teen population* are predominantly lifestyle related. They are heavily influenced by risk-taking behaviours, vehicle accidents, sports injuries and other trauma, experimentation with substances of abuse, exercise avoidance, and nutritional and appetite disorders. The effects of these are frequently lifelong. This stage, following adolescence, is also associated with the early onset of chronic mental illness, which blights many promising careers. The age band 16–18 experience a little-remarked disjunction in health and social care in chronic conditions. Young people in social care are cast adrift upon the world. Those with unstable epilepsy, diabetes or asthma lose their paediatrician as a kind of parent figure and have to join the general melee of chronic needs sufferers in the queues to access services. No longer cosseted in the children's wards with their peer age group, they find themselves in wards that are effectively geriatric. This transition point of care is disruptive, frequently turbulent and needs to be managed by parents, hospitals and GPs.

Thereafter, factors that beset the early years carry into *adult life*. They include social deprivation, smoking disease, hyperlipidaemia, hypertension, alcohol abuse and obesity. In *senior years* involutional trends such as loss of mobility, isolation, depression, cognitive decline, malnutrition, osteoporosis and falls are distinctive features.

Awareness of risk status bestows the capacity to intervene preventively through surveillance, screening, early diagnosis and anticipatory action. The prevalence, morbidity and mortality due to the Dragon would be greatly reduced by effective health education directed at lifestyle choice and focusing on a range of risk factors, such as body mass optimisation, positive nutrition, exercise, dealing with addictions, enhanced socialisation and trauma prevention. This shortlist of modifiable factors, combined with the aforementioned list of preventive actions, is at the core of any generic management model for combating the genus Dragon.

MODELS OF DISEASE

It is quite fashionable to speak of disease in terms of models. A model of disease is an abstraction, a generalisation that illustrates an aspect of disease in a metaphorical way that helps us bridge the gap between the particular and the general, and to speculate concerning the nature of disease. Different models can be simultaneously valid; they are not mutually exclusive, nor are any comprehensive. Chronic disease, itself, is a model of disease. Models of disease can be useful and indeed influential in analysing and understanding, which in turn may lead to policy and programmes structured around valid general concepts. Chronic disease will be addressed through four models that will be described: the natural history model, the medical model, the chronic illness model and the trajectory model.

The natural history model

The natural history model operates at the historical and clinical level, that of descriptive observation. It is important since a lot of valuable information and scientific advance is represented by the recording of the course of disease, unmodified by interventions. This descriptive model is most clearly exemplified in the major progressive neurological conditions – notably, multiple sclerosis and Huntington's, Alzheimer's and Parkinson's diseases – for which no specific preventive or curative measures are yet available. Nevertheless, there is much to learn from the taxonomy and nomenclature of conditions and the observational capacity, therefore, to make diagnosis and prognosis. In this it has much in common with the trajectory model and paves the way for the medical model.

Characteristics

- Observational, descriptive, taxonomy-based; facilitates diagnosis and prognosis; foundational to epidemiology and the beginnings of preventive medicine; identifies points of possible intervention and opportunities for fundamental research.

Consequences

Our textbooks of pathology and epidemiology are based on a foundation of the natural history of disease. If we do not value the perspective lent by the natural history model of disease we lose familiarity with the fingerprints of disease. Forming a differential diagnosis is based on case history-taking plus the physician's instinct for probability based on prevalence. This is related to clinical acumen, the pattern recognition that breeds vigilance for unfamiliar diseases. Many common diseases are becoming unfamiliar in some countries, such as tuberculosis, measles and pertussis, and this may lead to missed diagnoses, misdiagnosis or diagnostic delay. Modern medicine is tempted to rely excessively on clinical technology rather than clinical method.

Detection and treatment at any stage can alter the natural history of a disease, but the effects of treatment can only be determined if the natural history of the disease in the absence of treatment is known.[9]

The medical model

The medical model is the most familiar to practitioners of 'Western medicine'. It has been described as Cartesian; that is, based on cause and effect rationalism, that every ailment has a (single) basis that is organic and amenable to diagnosis in terms of aetiology, pathology and symptomatology; it should be remediable by rational means based on chemical, tissue or functional pathology, with the expectation of cure or relief.

Characteristics

- Rational-deductive; cause and effect; linear; disease-centred and physician-reliant; it is the dominant model through which doctors operate, patients perceive and the media portray medical care; its simplicity makes it attractive, easily commercialised and marketed.

Consequences

- A rational management plan
- The patient is a passive host or victim; needs to follow 'doctors' orders'
- Expertise and technology-based responses ('the magic bullet')
- Technology-driven, expensive and resource-intensive
- Need bigger, better and more complex institutions and machines to combat disease
- Specialisation and differentiation
- Commoditisation of healthcare
- Well suited to acute illness, trauma, and critical and emergency care
- Ill-suited for chronic, recurrent, multi-morbid or psychosocial conditions

The chronic illness model

The chronic illness model takes account of the patient's experience of persistent, multiple and recurring disease over an extended timeline. It highlights the needs of the patient in the context of his or her social and family setting, in ways that are responsive to health events, against a background of one or more disease entities and where clear-cut disease resolution is not anticipated. It emphasises prevention, health maintenance and problem-solving. It recognises the realities of co- and multi-morbidity, complex interventions, progressive decline and expects relapses and crises as intrinsic features of the patient's pathway of experience.

Characteristics

- Humanistic, reflective, continuing, patient-centred, problem-oriented; it emphasises the full range of preventive, ambulatory and interventional action, including
  lifestyle modification and social/welfare support; it is community-based, with
  planned care, patient and family involvement, and public participation.
- It envisages complex clinical and care pathways, management responses that are
  multi-layered, including medical and social interventions, integrated and connected health (*see* Chapter 5).
- Where appropriate it enlists the strengths of the medical model.

Consequences

- Long-term perspective; aim to modify the symptoms and disease progression
- Patient and professional partnership
- Realistic patient expectations based on involvement and information
- Valuing the goal of functional capacity as highly as clinical ones
- Institutions and technology that serve the patient's continuing support network
  in the community
- Integration of the patient's medical and social needs
- Generalist-led and multidisciplinary

There are two extremely influential constructs whose titles appear similar and suggest a close connection: Wagner's Chronic Care Model and the Chronic Disease
Model.

Wagner's Chronic Care Model[10] is a specific framework for health policy in
respect of long-term conditions. It was created through Wagner's analysis of best
practice in US chronic care, formulating what are the most beneficial aspects of the
programmes of the time (1990s, the United States). Its key contribution to health
policy is described in Chapter 6.

The US Centers for Disease Control and Prevention in Atlanta, Georgia, have
formulated a related set of principles that they call **the Chronic Disease Model**.[11]
Its headlines are:

- the crucial importance of prevention
- much of prevention in chronic disease lies with behaviours, social circumstances
  and institutional policies
- intervention must be based on evidence of effectiveness
- the importance of population measures in addressing risk factors for chronic
  disease.

The perspective here is one of epidemiology, aimed at health maintenance and health
promotion.

The trajectory model

The trajectory model is a new paradigm disease concept based on the natural history of disease. It reflects the patient's journey through a serious long-term condition. It proposes that:

- long-term conditions can be seen to evolve through a series of definable stages, from pre-disease through terminal, and beyond (*see* Appendix 2)
- these stages suggest points and types of intervention, and prognosis
- charting the patient's timeline progress (trajectory) can enhance anticipatory care and provide useful orientation and guidance for patients and their carers as the disease evolves
- there are benefits for family and carers, and for psychosocial dimensions.

It resembles the *Trajectory Framework* that was conceived by Corbin and Strauss[12] in the United States to guide the nursing process in chronic care and which will be discussed further. The trajectory is represented by a timeline that illustrates the course of the unfolding natural history of the target condition, demonstrating the various degrees of clinical activity of the disease as it goes through successive phases. Concurrent diseases, each with its individual trajectory, may give rise to complex patterns. Interpretation is required in order to deduce appropriate interventions, provide guidance and prognosis. This model does not appear to figure much in medical literature. I have found it useful as a framework for teaching and learning through case discussion.

Characteristics

- Observational, evolutionary, continuous, biographical and patient centred; facilitates anticipatory care; emphasises the value of observation and charting as a basis for interpretation and prognosis.

Consequences

- Acknowledges the natural history of the of long-term conditions
- 'Joins the dots', reveals patterns and interprets them as trends
- Facilitates holistic care and realistic expectations
- Personalised, centred on the patient's biography and narrative
- Emphasises continuing care, continuity of care and teamwork
- Combats fragmentary and fragmented care
- Contributes to case management and integrated care
- Useful teaching framework

The trajectory of disease will be discussed in more detail later in this chapter.

CO-MORBIDITY AND MULTI-MORBIDITY

The simultaneous presence of multiple conditions is one of the striking features of the genus Dragon. However fashionable it is to ascribe the chronic disease crisis to the ageing population, age does not appear to be the chief culprit. Spijker and MacInnes[13] cite evidence that the economic costs of old age dependency appear to have been exaggerated and that age, although important, is less influential than *multi-morbidity*. Demand for services will rise but driven mainly through the progress of medical knowledge and technology, and the increasing complexity of co-morbid, age-related conditions. The term *age-related* here does not equate to geriatric but refers to any given point on the trajectory of age. It is, then, co-morbidity that will be the main stressor on the health services. Although the prevalence of disability and other chronic conditions increases with age successful ageing is widespread and the elderly are generally healthy; indeed, the prevalence of disability among the elderly is declining in some developed economies.[14] The costs of care accrue chiefly in the last few months of life, at whatever age death occurs, and the probability curve of multi-morbidity is U-shaped, rising at either end of the age spectrum.[15] Over 50% of older people have three or more concurrent conditions. The prevalence of multi-morbidity is 10% among those under 20, 80% among those aged 80 or over, and 30% overall.[16] Not all chronic conditions are equally likely to predispose to co-morbidity. A study of people who suffered from the five commonest chronic conditions in the United States (mood disorders, diabetes, heart disease, asthma and hypertension) showed that co-morbidity was most common among those with diabetes or heart disease, at 56% and 61%, respectively; especially and predominantly affecting patients who were females or the deprived, with 15%–20% living below the poverty level.[17] The high prevalence of multi-morbidity among children has been remarked upon as unexpected, but it is in this cohort that complex needs related to disability, multiple handicap and genetic syndromes arise and impinge on the peak developmental period of life. Co-morbidity is particularly striking among people with intellectual disability; these include sensory disabilities, seizures, spasticity/dystonia, dental problems, risk of sexual and physical abuse, social impairments and the effects of stigma.

Are co-morbidity and multi-morbidity the same thing? They are frequently used interchangeably, especially in the early literature definitions, which favoured the generic use of co-morbidity. Definitions by Starfield[18] make a valid distinction between them:

> Co-morbidity is the simultaneous presence of multiple health conditions when there is an index condition and other unrelated conditions. Multi-morbidity is the simultaneous presence of multiple conditions when no one condition is identified as an index condition.

The consequences of co-morbidity are not surprising. Starfield cites: increased risk of premature death; poorer prognosis for co-morbid conditions (notably cardiovascular); poorer quality of life; more health service usage (especially hospital admission) and increased physical impairment or disability. She states that co-morbidity is the rule rather than the exception in primary care; and, except in the case of rare conditions, that is where they attend for care.

THE ECOLOGY OF THE DRAGON

Any consideration of a natural history must include the ecological perspective. Like all organisms, the Dragon thrives within a wider context of habitat factors, biodiversity, homeostasis (or resistance to change) and adaptation. The field biologist looks beyond any narrow, exclusive focus on the organism and takes account of these wider factors. To know our enemy, in an ecological sense, is to know the factors that sustain it, its place in the foodchain, what it feeds on, its predators and defences, its vulnerabilities to toxic factors. Even virulent organisms may make a positive contribution to the ecosystem. After all, is it not the soil bacteria that cause infections that also provide us with us antibacterials? Study of its habitat is essential to developing any countermeasures, remembering that all ecological interferences are subject to unintended consequences.

With regard to the Dragon, the inherent diversity of the genus dictates that any interference should adopt a holistic approach, to be prepared for unintended and unexpected consequence or chain reactions that create new challenges, and plan for a prolonged process rather than a quick fix. This is iterative rather than definitive. Resources must be deployed, safety-netting must take account of possible confounding factors and possible 'melt-down scenarios', and collateral damage minimised.

Ecology is about complex networks of interaction rather than linear pathways. Crucially, the Dragon and *Homo sapiens* occupy the same ecosystem, within which all components interact continually. If we apply the wrong countermeasures we could be harming our own interests.

Twelve ecological thoughts
1. Respect the inter-connectedness of the ecosystem
2. Keep in mind the natural history of all its components
3. Value biodiversity
4. Intervene reflectively, not impulsively
5. Expect unintended consequences from interference
6. Be vigilant for intercurrent eco-threats
7. Respect the bottom of the foodchain, however slimy

8. Remember that even predators and slugs have their place
9. Organisms need fundamental nutrients (such as water, air and energy sources)
10. Deal with waste effectively and creatively
11. The human survival capsule needs communications and energy resources
12. Clean up your act and mend your ways

Formidable as it is, the Dragon depends on habitat needs in order to express itself. Even some intrinsic human vulnerabilities that we cannot as yet change, such as some genetic diseases, may find their expression only in the presence of environmental factors. These are represented by the big behavioural risk factors, listed by WHO,[19] that act as the 'nutrients' in the 'substrate' on which the Dragon thrives – tobacco use, prolonged and unhealthy nutrition, physical inactivity, unsafe sexual practices and unmanaged psychosocial stress. Even among these there are linkages of causation and association. They are broadly preventable and subject to being 'engineered' or modified.

For example: while there is a genetic predisposition to diabetes, the consequences can be attenuated through control of weight, reduction in blood pressure, nutritional care, exercise and smoking cessation. We have technologies to address all of these. This package is cost-neutral (potentially even money-saving) and achievable by the person, with suitable guidance. This is the key ecological message: 'Pay attention to the foodchain that feeds the Dragon.'

The Dragon thrives on human misbehaviour and ecological malfunction. Correcting these starves the Dragon. Environmental health is fundamental, and countering air pollution has changed dramatically the experience of people with respiratory diseases. Clean water supply and effective sewage disposal are indispensible for urban living, and over half the world's population are now urban dwellers. Clean, cheap and reliable energy makes possible our thermal survival, distribution of essential goods and our information-hungry society. In a blackout people die in cold houses and our IT systems grind to a halt.

We should cherish the fundamentals of our own environmental complex. Water, sanitation, air, transport and communications are the logistic base of our campaign against the Dragon. These exemplify the base level of Abraham Maslow's hierarchy of needs.[20] Further up the pyramid of needs is the generation of wealth and its rational distribution. Housing plays an essential role also, not just for our thermoregulation but also as the survival capsule of the family. Even the so-called 'sink estate' is a quantum leap from the favela. At this level dwell most of the social antecedents of disease. There is much scope for preventive action. At the upper level of organisation come health and social care professionals. These expensively trained, high-maintenance and interdependent experts are extremely vulnerable to systems failure, which is a characteristic of complex systems. The more differentiated and sophisticated they are, the more resource-intensive their requirements in order to function, and the more fragility is built into the system.

At an individual level there is a clear tendency for people towards self-destruction. Is it radical to propose that most people die from their own hand (or, perhaps their own knife and fork); that unhealthy lifestyle is the norm; that addiction of some kind is the rule rather than the exception; that we do the Dragon's work for it? The lesson from health experts, from WHO level down, is clear and perennial, dating from the wisdom literature of our traditions, religions and cultures – **clean up your act and mend your ways**.

Going green

The concept of *intermediate (or appropriate) technology* is an essentially environmental one. It derives from the Third World aid and developmental literature, under the auspices of two Geneva-based international authorities, WHO and the Christian Medical Commission. It is based on the experience of a century of development and healthcare work in the poorer nations, that when money and trained manpower are scarce you have to get the 'best bang for your buck'. It is based on a few simple truths, outlined here.

- Simplicity is robust, affordable and replaceable; embrace the lowest level of technology that will do the job.
- A small benefit for the many is more productive than a large one for a few.
- Devolve tasks as far down the skill ladder as effectively possible; lower-skilled operatives can be trained more economically and dispersed more widely.
- Use locally available resources where possible; this is doubly beneficial – to the local economy and for ready availability.
- Make do and mend; do not waste resources; recycle where possible; minimise 'use and throw away' behaviour.
- Facilitating self-help is better than making donations.

These principles validate the crucial role of primary healthcare in serving population health. They have wide applicability to medical practice where all the historical trends appear to embrace complexity, based on vulnerable high-tech systems, and where much resource is squandered in overkill treatments and multilayered bureaucracy.

ENTERING THE DRAGON'S DEN

Examining the trajectory of chronic disease

The characteristic phases of the trajectory of chronic disease, as shown in Appendix 2, suggest a framework and a challenge. The framework represents the behaviour of the

Dragon, its mode of action, natural history and virulence. The challenge is to deduce areas where it is vulnerable to countermeasures and explore what interventions might be applied – the action points. Clearly, the further one looks along the disease trajectory curve the more irreversible the effects of disease become. Tissue damage occurs and accumulates, homeostatic mechanisms become stressed, relapses multiply, organ failure sets in and multi-system involvement results. In parallel with this the victim is ageing, accumulating wear and tear in all tissues, defence competency and cellular repair decline, along with progressive cell loss; risk from complications increases, as does the probability of developing additional, unrelated diseases.

This, as we have seen, does not mean that the timeline simply describes the ageing process rather than the characteristic effects of the disease at work. The Dragon attacks all stages of the human life cycle and there is overwhelming evidence that good medical care can turn back the clock. The ageing process is but one of the factors that cause susceptibility. There is nothing to be gained by regarding chronic disease as inevitable and intractable. Prevention is every bit as crucial here as it is in the case of acute and infectious disease, and arguably more so. In the course of the next few pages some characteristics of the various stages of the chronic disease trajectory will be described and some action points appended to illustrate implications for practice that may be drawn from the model. Appendix 2 illustrates the trajectory model of chronic disease: a timeline of progression in disease activity in relation to a baseline, phases of change and (dotted line) corresponding loss of functional capacity.

Pre-disease

There is a prequel to chronic disease that deserves to be included in the overall trajectory view. The more or less environmentally based issues that incubate the Dragon genus may be seen as the pre-disease territory. These have been alluded to elsewhere, and their prevention (that is, attempting to starve the Dragon) lies in the domains of politics, policy, and the policing of health and safety regulation in society as a whole. This 'primordial prevention' means not only taking steps to ensure that the Dragon does not strike, but better still, does not come into being in the first place. This core of pre-emptive measures includes, as we have seen, provision of clean air, sanitation, water, food, housing and promotion of healthy living habits – that is, addressing the social antecedents of disease. These are most influential early in the human life cycle. Poor nutritional and addictive behaviours, and toxic influences in early life, are powerful risk factors that carry lifelong significance.

Common infectious diseases of childhood often cause lasting tissue damage or have residual effects that predict long-term conditions of the cardiorespiratory systems, sense organ disability and impairment of full developmental potential. Childhood immunisation and acute illness management form a large proportion of the daily toil of general practice but they are essential to the lifelong campaign against long-term conditions. Even where control of acute childhood infectious diseases is good, vigilance is of crucial importance. Would I now reliably recognise the early signs of polio, pertussis, measles, tuberculosis or meningitis? It is so long since I last saw any of these that I cannot afford to be complacent. There is too much at stake.

Practice action points: primordial and primary prevention. Immunisation of the young and developmental surveillance in childhood; maintain enthusiasm for jabbing babies, and even for treating children's wheezes, coughs and fevers (among these lurk occasional immature Dragons); continuing and opportunistic health promotion for all patients; smoking and alcohol awareness; nutritional health, obesity prevention. The extensive consequences of childhood mental trauma require preventive medical or social intervention to promote developmental and emotional health.

Pre-symptomatic phase

The Dragon may be hatching out long before illness becomes overt. Changes at cellular level, where detectible, provide the next point of timely intervention. This is where primary prevention merges into secondary prevention. Examples of such action include cervical screening for dysplasia, selective colonoscopy to detect premalignant polyposis, or checking moles for melanoma, where prompt intervention is effective in aborting malignant change. Detection of hypertension is effective in preventing vascular and renal diseases. As a theoretical point it may be argued that the life cycle of the respective diseases has already begun and these are no longer purely primary prevention. However, the pathogenesis of chronic diseases is a process, not an identifiable event. We recognise a gradient of cervical dysplasia that puts in place a ladder of escalating intervention procedures. Who ever said prevention is simple and boring? One 'by the way' example that is of clinical significance arises from diagnosing hypertension. Patients seem to find it helpful to be told that this is not really a disease; that they are well people who happen to have a risk factor that is not of their making; what therefore appears to be heavy-handed *medicalisation* that makes demands on them is preventive medicine and health promotion; to perhaps regard their medication more as a 'food supplement' than a drug; that their periodic hypertension review facilitates opportunistic screening for related (co-morbid) disorders of renal function and glucose metabolism or metabolic syndrome.

Practice action points: screening for early cancer, hypertension, hyperlipidaemia, diabetes; opportunistic screening and health promotion; surveillance of those with genetic risk; explaining risk to patients.

Onset phase: early symptomatic and initial event

Reliable blood and tissue markers are not available in many chronic diseases (*see* 'Screening and Wilson's Criteria' later in this chapter). Frequently therefore, the first clear point of intervention is when the disease becomes an illness. The 'initial event', when acute, is the very stuff of medical melodrama – the chest tightness, the show of blood, acute breathlessness, loss of power – that rapidly escalates into a full-blown, life-changing 'Dragon attack'. Hospitals and disease specialists are wonderful at coping with these, and lives are saved. Less attention-grabbing, but no less significant are the follow-on processes, away from camera: fire-proofing bundles of medicines to be taken, classes for cardiac or pulmonary or neurological rehabilitation, followed by permanent surveillance. This has taken the place of a seemingly now redundant phase, that of convalescence (which was in former times the best that could be offered, a period of rest and enhanced nourishment, following a serious illness). Reviewing and addressing risk factors form the basis of programmes of shared care (by hospital specialist and GP) that would also include fostering lifestyle changes, monitoring biomarkers and targets, providing personalised information that addresses immediate concerns – for example, self-care, the course of the illness and alerting the patient to possible 'red-flag' symptoms.

The registered patient (healthy, with sporadic contact) is transformed into the chronic disease patient (regular contact, 'service user' with daily life impact) even though his ('his' for the sake of this example) acute illness has been overcome. **The purpose of definitive intervention early in the disease trajectory is to enable the person to survive so that acute illness gives way to the long-term condition.** Having survived the crisis and achieved recovery the patient may experience a substantial period of restored stability, and perhaps remission.

This is a time of normalising, which does not mean that all is well. Life has changed utterly for the survivor of the Dragon attack. Well and fully functioning he may be, but his family will tell you otherwise. In this phase secondary preventive measures become embedded. The cycle of change precipitated by the initial event rolls right through the patient's home and family life, occupation, social life and, less visibly, in his interior life. **Normalising is not restoration of normality, but the creation of new norms.** This is sociology territory. Experiences such as reactive depression, anxiety or depressive illness are common and are frequently accompanied by sleep disorder or other of the non-disease conditions outlined earlier.

Medication side effects are experienced and addressed, reminders of his new health status. Stigma is felt, along with guilt and insecurity. This is akin to the grief cycle. The person has not died, but death has loomed. Cosy assumptions about healthy longevity are challenged. Family members may begin to count their blessings but the index patient begins to count his probabilities, take stock of his resources and wonder 'what if …?' Everyone around revises their assessment of him, including the actuaries who determine his insurances. His spouse experiences a parallel crisis (thoughts of widowhood or financial insecurity). This adjustment period is turbulent and the manner in which people respond to 'the changeling' have far-reaching consequences that will colour any remaining phases of the journey along the disease trajectory. Denial ('cured and fire-proofed'), complacency (non-compliance), overprotectiveness ('sit down there and rest yourself'), hyper-vigilance and health anxiety (hypochondriasis), all are examples of behavioural responses that may be rectified, if detected early. These are the psychosocial tasks involved in recovery from acute illness, especially the acute onset of a chronic disease.

> *Practice action points*: awareness on the part of the clinicians that the disease has not gone away; patient enrolled in a disease register; follow-up support and surveillance; reinforce positive, normalising adjustment to change; detect and correct negative influences and attitudes; inform, involve, support; signpost to helping agencies in the voluntary or community sector.

Relapsing and remitting phase

In chronic disease the occurrence of relapse or recurrence should not be interpreted as personal failure. It is the nature of the Dragon. In multiple sclerosis this phase can dominate the disease trajectory.

Prochaska and DiClemente[21] established the model of change out of addiction through their work on smoking cessation. This has been generalised to include much behaviour, and identifies relapse as an inherent feature of the cycle of change. They found that subjects completed the cycle of change up to half a dozen times before achieving stability in indefinite remission, or once again succumbing to their condition (smoking disease) and returned to being 'pre-contemplators'. Addressing risk factors depends heavily on successful behaviour change. Relapse and non-compliance are common. The same perspective should be accorded to clinical setbacks in the course of chronic disease. Blame may be apportioned and guilt radiated in all directions (frequently at the doctor), but these are negative energies and cause further kinds of damage of their own. The Dragon has not gone away; it may have been tamed or caged, for now, but it is still restless and may break out. Relapse is one of the new norms, a feature of the Dragon's natural history. Therapists must achieve a degree of tolerance of this and model this perspective to the patient with positivity. This is not the same thing as complacency or fatalism, but familiarisation, so that the signs of recurrence will be recognised and acted upon promptly.

Recurrences may symbolise disease progression, with incomplete resolution and cumulative loss of functional ability. Knowing this, active and prompt intervention is important to limit damage and re-emphasise the secondary prevention measures. A 'catastrophic response' is one to avoid. Both patient and GP are liable to the sense of failure, with loss of morale and impaired motivation. 'We will get through this; get up and move on again' is a positive response that enlists the efforts of all players, emphasises the positive energy, mobilises further supportive measures and restores confidence. It is stock-taking time, an opportunity to audit the treatment to date and to problem-solve. Confounding factors may come to light. A common one is non-compliance with the treatment regimen; another is iatrogenesis. A further one, alluded to earlier, is the maladaptive response to the index event: the patient may start drinking heavily or smoke more, denial that leads to complacency, family attitudes of mothering or smothering the patient, and other kinds of collusions. Of course there may have been a *therapeutic deficit* – that is, insufficient or inappropriate early medical measures. Initial clinical management decisions may have to be reviewed and previously discarded options revisited. Assessment of any new clinical impairment should be carried out and action taken. The relapse is a 'wake-up call' for all concerned. Secondary and tertiary preventive measures must be emphasised, such as regaining fitness through a guided programme of self-help, or physiotherapy to restore lost function. Knowing that further episodes are likely to occur, measures to reduce risk to the patient should begin early. Are there implications for the patient's social functioning, employment or other co-morbid health issues that need to be addressed?

Practice action points: anticipate and respond with positivity to relapse or recurrence of disease; inform, involve and support; review management decisions, medication, and lifestyle issues. Reinforce preventive measures – tertiary prevention begins; combat dependency and low morale; promote healthy living in all domains; invoke voluntary sector and social support; promote self-management (*see* disease self-management programmes, Chapter 4).

The plateau phase

Many chronic diseases exhibit plateau phases. Disease activity appears to have diminished or been modified by therapy and homeostatic mechanisms, both physiological and psychosocial. A period of stability is achieved. Medical and team involvement with this phase is concerned with 'keeping the plates spinning'. Patients **should be managed in the least intensive setting** that is compatible with safety, effectiveness and quality of care. Routines and protocols apply, and must be applied.

- Regular attendance at reviews, ideally through their GP's *practice-based clinic* where the service is convenient to the patient and the process is evidence-based, protocol-driven, and regularly audited for quality and performance indicators. Frequently these are nurse-led with multidisciplinary input where appropriate.
- Periodic medication review is a contractual requirement of the GP in the UK, an essential maintenance activity that involves updating and 'weeding' the list of continuing medications. Otherwise the list grows longer, especially where there is multi-morbidity. Separate guidelines that govern coexisting long-term conditions can lead to overlapping or incompatible clinical protocols. Clearly the medication load must be minimised and manageable routines of administration agreed. The inclusion of a pharmacist advisor is an increasingly valued resource employed within the primary healthcare team for medicines management.
- Regular biometric monitoring gives rise to much routine, supportive work – for example, tracking blood pressure, weight and, spirometry, and blood sampling for essential continuous variables.
- These activities are additional to, or shared with, secondary care specialists; this reduces the need for expensive hospital specialist review and monitoring activity, and helps streamline the patient's clinical pathway.

Managing the activities that arise creates a high level of continuing workload for the primary care team. Much of the routine is shared among team members but interpreting and acting on the flood of laboratory reports requires high-level skills in clinical decision-making. Every diabetic or vascular disease clinic is beset by a torrent of numerical data. Decision support technology and paradigms are employed to reduce risk, not to save time; they don't. This is all very busy and routine, but there is value in the routine; it keeps the plates spinning safely, 'keeps the Dragon in his box', and defers the end of the plateau.

It is also onerous for the patient to keep pace with the demands that issue from disparate recall systems. Each co-morbid condition and risk factor is hedged around with evidence-based protocols that are driven by guidelines, and dictate interval-led actions that seem to defy attempts to streamline, amalgamate or rationalise them into neat bundles. They tend to be computer-generated and the bits of the system that trigger action do not yet talk to one another. As Dr Isabel Hodkinson (Royal College of General Practitioners clinical lead for Care Planning) said:

Patient feedback is clear: they do not want multiple annual reviews for their various different comorbidities but unitary management … to broaden out from a single disease model.[22]

CASE REPORT 1

A woman aged 55 who has diabetes, depression, smokes and has early chronic obstructive pulmonary disease attends two hospital specialist appointments, the nurse practitioner's smoking-cessation clinic and the GP's treatment room to have the phlebotomist draw blood prior to her diabetic clinic visit, all in the same month as she is prompted to attend for a medication review and a routine cervical smear and receives a recall notice from the mammography screening programme.

Health maintenance can become a part-time job for this patient who is at an age when she is still in employment and has family commitments. And we wonder why non-compliance and appointment default rates are high! Ways must be found to reduce the burden of health maintenance care for the stable patient with long-term conditions. It is important to revise guideline-derived protocols to enable them to mesh, especially for people who have jobs, the elderly, those with restricted mobility and people who have complex health needs. That may account for the majority of people with long-term conditions. There are increasing calls for the practice of **minimally disruptive medicine**.

Of course, even in the plateau phase there are likely to be intrusive and distressing symptoms that are persistent. *Holding work* is the term applied to the considerable effort involved in providing *ongoing support* to people through protracted times of distress, to maintain motivation and morale. Health maintenance is also necessary, since reducing broader risk factors may contribute to regression of the actual disease. Other things can happen and intercurrent illnesses, such as influenza, pose additional risk and should be vigorously combated.

CASE REPORT 2

A middle-aged widow has stable ischaemic heart disease; she is the lone carer for a dependent adult son with muscular dystrophy who has complex needs. One Sunday morning she develops acute, crushing chest pain and contacts the out-of-hours GP. On visiting the home he diagnoses an acute coronary event, but she declines hospital admission, because of her son's care needs. The cardiac ambulance is called anyway and the cardiology team confirm the diagnosis of a coronary. The hospital switchboard operator is contacted with a request for the contact number of the duty social worker, whose prompt response to an outline account of the situation enables the lady to agree to be admitted to coronary care immediately. The social worker attends, arranges for the son's urgent admission to respite care in a nursing home. Since they live in an area subject to a high level of crime, the police are alerted that the house has been vacated. They attend, secure the premises and promise to check on it during the next few days. The lady survives a major myocardial infarction and following stent insertion returns home to continue caring for her son, both supported with an enhanced package of community care as arranged by the social worker. Some years later both are alive and in a stable, although more advanced, state with their respective long-term conditions.

Patient involvement is another major contributor on the plateau. This does not just mean patient participation in the managerial sense, although there is much that can be said on this too (*see* Chapter 4). It refers to enabling patients to take ownership of their condition, to become well informed about its course, and to take responsibility for maintaining and promoting their own health. The doctor–patient consultation becomes a meeting of experts, the one by qualification and social role, and the other as an 'expert by experience'. To pool the knowledge they both bring is to create a three-dimensional database that informs and sustains the long-term management process. The doctor, the patient and the illness are all present to be interrogated through needs-assessment, problem-solving and generating ideas (ideas like attending and participating in the local branch of a disease-interest organisation or a local self-help group; or consulting the practice website, the internet or a library for condition-specific information). Patient autonomy and self-help are the foundation of healthcare. On this is built the pyramid of further levels of service and sources of help (*see* Chapter 4).

Practice action points: a time of apparent stability for health maintenance through teamwork and monitoring according to reasonable protocols; streamline these where possible, especially through editing and rationalising continuing therapies; facilitate patient involvement and self-management; minimise the intensity of management and disruption for the patient; intermediate and e-connected health technologies may contribute; holding work, with vigorous management of intercurrent health challenges (e.g. influenza) and other preventive measures.

Advanced disease phase

The plateau phase may not be as tranquil as it sounds. Homeostasis is an active process. Defences are working hard under the surface to counter disease inroads. However successful this might be, body systems are stressed. Declining function may be occurring because of neuronal damage, vascular degeneration, loss of functioning nephrons or collapse of alveoli. A point of instability meets a triggering factor such as an acute infection and a crisis occurs. When homeostatic and cellular repair mechanisms cease to compensate 'dis-integration' occurs and this tends to be rapid. Cascade effects occur and negative feedback loops give way to positive feedback chain reactions. (Ask any engineer or economist about the dynamics of systems failure). Crisis intervention has to be prompt, focused and radical if a new equilibrium is to be achieved. This should be anticipated through treatment planning and practised emergency care procedures. In the UK there is a contractual requirement on GPs for annual cardiopulmonary resuscitation (CPR) training certification. **Acute care skills training is an essential element of chronic disease methodology.** The patient may have to be admitted to hospital or intensive domiciliary team support applied. In managed care systems in the United States, unforeseen admission is even regarded as a failure of anticipatory care and sanctions may be applied. In parallel with clinical care, psychosocial interventions are necessary because critical illness occurs in an ecology that includes social and family resources.

At some stage the degree of irreversible damage is such that the therapeutic aims have to be revised. When the full range of secondary preventive measures and rescue treatments have been exhausted the options narrow. The palliative phase has been reached. In some cases of advanced disease with organ failure, tertiary specialists may offer hope of regaining stability – for example, through renal dialysis or transplantation.

> *Practice action points*: multidisciplinary and intersectoral teamwork; anticipatory care; integrated care (including social support); maintain acute and crisis care skills (CPR, infusion skills), use of secondary care services and intermediate care; specialist medical and surgical options explored, directed at tertiary prevention and restoration of functional capacity.

Palliative phase

This is not the same as the terminal phase, although the two may overlap. Palliative care is directed at symptom control and supporting whatever degree of function remains (both physiological and psychosocial), rather than on curative or restorative aims. A consensus on this among the stakeholders should be negotiated. This does not mean loss of objectives on the part of the clinicians. The preventive perspective is as relevant as ever. Having fought the Dragon with primary and secondary prevention, tertiary prevention becomes the mainstay of management. This aims at conserving mobility and social capacities, the anticipatory care of pain and other troublesome symptoms, respiratory support, and skin care for pressure points. All of these represent productive effort to preserve and maintain a quality of life that is the best possible given that the circumstances are unlikely to abate. Valid medical hazard concerns – for example, fear of opioid, psychotropic or corticosteroid dependency – may be relaxed in favour of shorter-term pragmatism. Nevertheless, this period can be a prolonged one with its own kind of plateau of minimal intervention and maximum support. The initiative may pass to those members of the primary health-care team whose skills lie in the provision of domiciliary-based support and nursing care – the district nurse (advanced primary care nurse in the United States) backed up as necessary by the physiotherapist, occupational therapist and care assistants in conjunction with the social services. The GP retains the role as clinical overseer, problem-solver and crisis resource. At this stage, especially for cancer sufferers, the hospice team may be alerted concerning anticipated needs or initial assessment. The patient may need assistance in facing the end of life, making provision and dealing with unfinished business while he or she is capable of so doing. The Dragon is winning the chess game, but checkmate has not yet been declared.

Practice action points: integrated care, multidisciplinary team-based, full domiciliary care where the patient is not ambulant, close oversight with crisis intervention plans; use of the range of social care provision; support to patient and family; information needs addressed.

Terminal phase

There is extensive overlap between palliative and terminal care approaches. In the UK, the hospice movement pioneered both. Its impressive track record in developing supportive procedures has only been matched by its success in transforming attitudes and values in relation to the management of advanced disease – notably, cancer. Its comprehensive philosophy regarding end-of-life care emphasises the value of life to its end, the dignity of the person, and concern for the well-being of immediate relatives and carers in physical, psychological and spiritual domains. It seeks to provide patient-centred services in whatever setting the patient elects to be, whether at home, in a hospice unit, or both – on a 'revolving door' basis. Hospice care provides support, symptom management, respite and problem-solving. The insights derived by hospice care have influenced greatly the provision of end-of-life care within mainstream hospital services. These now employ palliative care physicians, specialist nurses, symptom-control teams and bereavement counsellors with a cross-departmental brief, who facilitate and train general staff in matters related to end-of-life care.

Practice action points: implement the Gold Standards Framework on palliative care management;[23] promote clear communication with patient and family carers to explore the patient's ideas, information needs, concerns, consent issues and views on place of death; anticipatory care and symptom control, practical skills such as appropriate opioid administration and infusion pump use; high-level domiciliary care nursing skills; teamwork within general practice, with hospice involvement; psychosocial and spiritual support to include the needs of relatives and carers.

LAYING THE FOUNDATION STONE OF THE CHRONIC DISEASE PARADIGM

Through the trajectory pathway we have seen many of the threads that connect the general narrative – the commonalities that characterise the Dragon genus. End-of-life care is a microcosm of the full field of chronic disease management. The challenge for the future of chronic care is **to bring the attitudes, skills and high ideals that characterise end-of-life care to bear on the full trajectory course of long-term conditions**, in accordance with the needs of the patient.

So there it is: the natural history of the Dragon of chronic disease, interpreted as an environmental and trajectory-based model. It defines the disease complex, one element of the chronic disease paradigm. The *practice action points* that arose from our exploration of the trajectory model of chronic disease suggest an action list that bears some resemblance to established job descriptions for general practice (such as that of the Leeuwenhorst Group's statement from 1974).[24]

- The GP and primary healthcare team are key workers in chronic care
- Employing their preventive, diagnostic, therapeutic and palliative capacity
- Through supportive, continuing and interventional action
- Sustainably over protracted periods of time
- Aware of the significance of the trajectory phases
- In a comprehensive and inclusive, patient-centred way
- Addressing psychosocial issues, including the needs of carers
- Invoking or coordinating all necessary levels of health and social care
- To promote the best interests of the individual
- Supplementing the patient's self-care and participation
- Intervening proactively and responsively
- To combat the threats arising from chronic disease.

To this keystone will be added, in the subsequent chapters, description of the complexes of issues that surround the patient, the social supports, the clinical tools, the policy framework and implications for training. Together these constitute the chronic disease paradigm (*see* Appendix 1).

SUMMARY: THE STORY TO DATE

Chronic disease is a major and growing phenomenon. Universal demographic changes, population growth, improved life expectancy and illness survival all create an expanding at-risk population, and diverse subgroups many of whom live with impairment and cumulative illness. Long-term conditions represent the preponderance of healthcare activity and expenditure. Policymakers and politicians are particularly wary of these trends. The news media and medical literature both refer frequently to chronic disease in lurid terms – tsunami, epidemic, and so forth. The contributory diseases that comprise the genus Dragon have little in common pathologically but they are now regarded as a collective threat, like a complex family of organisms that function within an ecological space. They have much in common in terms of shared risk factors, possible countermeasures and management approaches, and the issues experienced by their victims. There are a number of terms in use that are more or less synonymous – chronic disease, chronic illness, non-communicable diseases and long-term conditions.

A chronic illness model is gaining currency. This is reflected in a growing public health perspective, a paradigm shift from, on the one hand, reliance on curative and acute care towards, on the other hand, prevention, health maintenance, palliation and integration of clinical with social care services; from disease-centred towards patient-centred programmes of care. They are best and most comprehensively addressed at primary care level, through public health medicine and general practice.

These perspectives are not currently reflected in the training of health professionals, notably medical ones. They should be, because a unitary model draws attention to generic, transferrable knowledge and method. Lack of awareness of the chronic disease models and frameworks fragments the work of an already hard-pressed workforce, disadvantages primary healthcare and reduces our attentiveness to major areas such as disability.

The Dragon can be portrayed within our existing, disease-based framework of understanding, which enables us to describe an epidemiology, a natural history, therapeutic and management responses (and, indeed, medical sociology in the next chapter). Much terminology has been employed during the telling of the Dragon story that derives from basic concepts in epidemiology.

This merits some further exploration. Clinical epidemiology will now be presented at some length because of its significance in the management of chronic disease with special reference to prevention, surveillance, screening and measurement. Essential as this is to the story of chronic disease, some readers may opt to move directly to Chapter 3, where we will encounter in more detail the journey of the patient through chronic illness.

A BIT OF EPIDEMIOLOGY

> The function of protecting and developing health must rank even above that of restoring it when it is impaired.
>
> Hippocrates

How much epidemiology do you need to know? Probably a lot less than you may by now have forgotten, and just enough to rehabilitate it in your esteem as a fundamental medical science. Much chronic disease management is predicated on population medicine. Clinicians employ epidemiology constantly, when they read a paper critically, implement a guideline or advise a patient about choice and risk. It provides the link between biological sciences and the clinical setting, from pathology to praxis. It is generally under-represented in curricula at student and graduate level. It challenges the time-honoured medical model of the individual hosting a particular disease. It ensures that there is wider community awareness on the part of clinicians. It advocates that fairness and distributive justice must attenuate the extremes of market-based models of care and it seeks to enhance the health of the whole population. This is not a new perspective. Cicero, in a treatise on Roman Law, states:

> *Salus populi suprema lex esto*
> ('The well-being of the People is paramount').

Progressive healthcare policy is based on *the population perspective*. This encounters and reveals political and ethical dilemmas such as the rationing of resources (and therefore of care), the balance between preventive and curative endeavour, and tension between public and personal rights. It challenges the validity of professional boundaries, the meaning of quality of care, addresses the limits of consumption and upholds the values of equity, accessibility, efficacy, affordability and human dignity.

Some years ago the Royal College of General Practitioners introduced a new kind of paper to their Membership Examination. It was called 'the Critical Reading Paper', and it was designed to, among other aims, test the candidates' grasp of evidence-based practice, the understanding that goes beyond what we do, to question why we do it and upon what authority. This caused a deal of consternation among the candidates and, it must be said, among their teachers too. Many training programmes responded with a study module entitled 'Hot Topics'. This relied on promptings from the editorials and news sections of journals, popular magazines and other media, and issues raised by patients, to create a learning agenda. The task was to identify issues of note and explore current evidence, either for consensus or discussion of dilemmas. Like a medical journalist piecing together a story.

The evidential consensus that underlies the practice of medicine evolves erratically through twists and reversals. What constitutes best practice today may be seen as reprehensible in retrospect, and therein lies the story. Whose work is seminal? Who replicated a crucial finding or validated it in different populations so that it may be generalised and applied? This 'storytelling approach' was well suited to exploring the range of issues that underlie the evidence base of practice. It humanised a lot of technical stuff, employed lateral and sequential thinking, historical perspective, identified unanswered questions, explored the political and economic framework, and even made statistical method seem relevant.

EXAMPLE

A controversial paper published in the 1990s claimed that there was a causal link between a vaccine for children (against measles, mumps and rubella) and chronic disease (colitis and autism). The ensuing controversies have resurfaced intermittently over the years (indeed, an outbreak of measles in Wales in 2013 among teenagers and young adults was directly attributable to the damage to parental confidence that resulted from this incident). The critical evaluation of scientific data, consequences of intense media coverage on the attitudes of parents, the impact of reduced uptake on 'herd immunity', research ethics, consent and counselling with regard to risk, the difficulty of proving a negative, these all provided enough material to keep the trainee group busy for ages. This was problem-based learning, and the narrative became increasingly diverse and complex.

There was a 'eureka moment' when the group realised that this was clinical epidemiology. No other word encompassed what we were doing. Epidemiology was rediscovered and redeemed from the nether world of undergraduate indifference, recast as the science of health. There was a job to be done in reviving the dormant concepts and converting them into evidence-based primary care. We revisited the statement from the Leeuwenhorst group from 1974, the earliest internationally agreed definition of general practice, to find that much of the work of the GP is epidemiologically based. So much of primary care centres on the management of chronic conditions, prevention and the early diagnosis of evolving illness and its therapeutics that epidemiological literacy is important.

> Epidemiology is the distribution of disease plus the determinants of disease.
>
> Sir Michael Marmot

Epidemiology, the natural experiment

Epidemiology has been described as '*the field of observation of disease under natural conditions in whole populations, (and as) medical ecology that deals with the natural relations between man and his environment*'.[25] Our image of epidemiology is split between dry 'number-crunching' and 'fire fighting' in far-off places. Not something GPs do (unless you are a John Snow, John Fry, or a Will Pickles, to mention just a few jobbing physicians who rank as epidemiologists having made vital contributions from community-based practice).

CASE STUDY: JOHN SNOW

The story of John Snow and his pump is an epidemiological classic that provides a useful case study in epidemiological method. Snow observed cholera outbreaks in mid-nineteenth-century London, noting incidence, prevalence, distribution and associations through case-finding and mapping new cases. Current theories of miasma, contagion and social factors did not fit his plot. There were outlying, sporadic cases in more affluent neighbourhoods. These turned out to be due to a liking on the part of yuppies for the fizzy appearance of water that was, in fact, polluted with fermenting organic matter. One side of a street of poor houses was unaffected since it drew its water from a different supplier from the other, affected, side. A large cluster centred on the Broad Street Pump.

He did not, as many suppose, vandalise the pump handle. He collated, analysed and presented his data and conclusions to the competent authority, the Board of Guardians, who then decommissioned the pump. The outbreak subsided before long. Pressure from local interests and public opinion quickly forced them to reinstate it, with recurrence of cholera.

Snow did not see the end of the story. Years passed before further published evidence confirmed his view of cholera as a waterborne disease. Still later, new technology (in bacteriology) discovered the causative organism and identified it as *Vibrio cholerae*.

In a nutshell: observation, case-finding, measurement, distribution plotting, collating and analysing observational data, noting correlations, making and testing hypotheses, presenting and publishing conclusions, political action, policy implementation, the effects of public opinion, the value of a control study (upon reversal of the policy), evaluation and confirmation of findings through further research, the impact of new thinking (the microbe, Koch's postulates) and new science (pathology, microbiology). The natural experiment methods of epidemiology created the bridge between a public health threat of unknown aetiology and full pathological understanding. Epidemiology can provide the diagnosis and prognosis and define a plan of action, including preventive measures, all based on a natural history model and long before full scientific discovery of causation.

Until public health medicine and the widespread use of vaccines and antibiotics radically altered perceptions of threat to health, epidemiology was regarded as the study of the natural history of infectious disease. The pharmacological revolution following the 1960s led to a broader understanding that included evaluation of treatments applied to diseases, and their prevention and prognosis. Koplan *et al.*[26] saw this progress as placing epidemiology and public health in the front rank of medical science,

> recognising, measuring and countering health challenges through population based interventions in infectious as well as chronic disease by improving environmental health, occupational health, mental health, reduce injuries and improve systems for delivering these *(sic)*; additionally to prepare for unanticipated problems and emergencies such as national disasters and bioterrorism.

This is clinical epidemiology, the prevention of non-communicable disease through the study of risk and risk factors, their modification, the evaluation of medical interventions that reduce risk in selected study populations and the promotion of evidence-based practice. The great prospective studies, some now continuing over 50 years, give us salient examples of this at work: the Framingham Study, Veterans Administration Study, the Whitehall Studies, Nurses' Study, Million Women Study and others carried out in the population laboratory. They inform our everyday clinical practice of secondary prevention, and our wealth of guidelines and protocols for the management of chronic disease.

For our purposes, the GP's 'need to know' limits apply. Accordingly the remainder of this section will focus on a shortlist of headings: prevention, surveillance, screening and a brief look at measurement. Since measurement is largely a matter of definitions and formulae, these will make up a short glossary of epidemiological terms later in this chapter. In the pages that follow I draw heavily on a WHO publication, *Basic Epidemiology*, with gratitude for its clear, succinct and accessible style.[27]

Prevention and chronic disease

Prevention is where the battle against nature really is waged, the prolonged counter-attack against the territory of serious long-term illness. Modern, neo-romantic trends lead many people to regard nature as a benign goddess-figure, whose providence merely has to be invoked and nurtured to create health. Nothing could be further from the truth. Biological systems are, indeed, self-righting mechanisms that seek stability (homeostasis). However, they are full of goblins that seek to subvert this stability. This, I suppose, is the basis for evolutionary theory, dependent as it is on natural mistakes. So, we are, at some level warriors against the natural order (or rather, disorder). For all our sophisticated prevention, there are few enough areas where a disease is truly prevented and only one example of eradication (smallpox), although we were nearly there with polio until effective prevention was subverted by political upheavals.

The classic triad of primary, secondary and tertiary prevention has become common parlance, though lots of us might struggle to define them. It is only in recent years that a fourth one, primordial prevention, has been added, a bedrock concept that tends to be out of sight, for that is where bedrock tends to be.

Primordial prevention aims to 'avoid the emergence and establishment of the social, economic and cultural patterns of living that are known to contribute to an elevated risk of disease'.[28] As the scourges of infectious disease become more amenable to control, specific remedy and even eradication, the non-communicable diseases achieve prominence and priority as threats. This is sometimes called disease substitution. Some are degenerative. Many, such as traumatic injury, accidents, cancers and cardiorespiratory disease, are closely related to environmental risks arising from traffic, machinery use, carcinogens, radiation, environmental pollution and lifestyles. These are concerns that must be addressed at the level of national politics and the time-response curve of effective corrective action on such risk factors is prolonged. Reform and change demand resources, and to change public policy takes time. Appropriate measures tend to be introduced late in the cycle of social change, so benefits are derived a generation or more later. Political will to apply costly levers of change is accordingly weakened. Thus, the work of Doll on smoking disease bore fruit in changing the smoking culture in the UK within 2 decades. By contrast, in developing countries, where scarce resources correlate with weak regulatory frameworks, smoking rates are still climbing steadily, two generations later.

> All countries need to avoid the spread of unhealthy lifestyles and consumption patterns before they become ingrained in society and culture.[29]

Primordial preventive measures may address traffic accidents (e.g. enforceable seatbelt use), industrial hazards, nutritional practice, smoking, hypertension management and healthy exercise. It is directed at the pre-disease trajectory point and is applied to whole populations through public health, trans-sectoral policy-making and enforcement of regulation.

Primary prevention is the control of causes and risk factors in individuals and communities to limit the incidence of diseases. It is directed at populations, specific groups and individuals who are at risk; its focus is the pre-disease phase of the trajectory. It rests on two strategies.

1. *The population strategy*: aimed at whole populations to reduce personal as well as average risk. For example, systematic immunisation where, additionally, 'herd immunity' is enhanced through reduction in risk of exposure.
2. *The individual strategy*: the focus on people with high risk or special exposure. However effective for the individual, this makes little contribution to the burden of disease in society; an example is the elective treatment of those with familial hypercholesterolaemia.

Secondary prevention refers to the early identification and treatment of patients who have developed the disease, to reduce either the risk of it recurring or of the disease becoming established. It is applied to at-risk populations and individuals and is directed at the early disease points on the trajectory – pre-symptomatic, early symptomatic and primary episode. Two main methodologies apply: programmes of *screening* and those of *surveillance*. The former has limitations to its suitability. It is appropriate where there is an identifiable test that marks the latent or early phase of disease that is curable or modifiable. The latter is very widely applied in vascular disease following the initial event of symptomatic ischaemia, cardiac or cerebral.

Tertiary prevention aims to reduce disease progression, complications and any consequent disability from established disease. This represents a high proportion of the clinical work of GPs and of many specialists, and includes rehabilitation. It applies in established disease, at various trajectory phases that follow onset of overt disease. It is the chief mode of preventive action in advanced disease and established disability, and is the essence of palliative and terminal care.

> Tertiary prevention is often difficult to separate from treatment since the treatment of chronic disease has, as one of its central aims, the prevention of recurrence.[30]

Surveillance

This is a more or less continuous preventive measure directed at specific at-risk groups. Often it employs multiple observations simultaneously. An example is child health surveillance, which addresses numerous developmental milestones in pre-school children, aimed at early diagnosis of deviance from healthy norms, and early intervention. General practice abounds in routine programmes of secondary and tertiary prevention – for example, the monitoring and continuing management of hypertension, vascular disease, diabetes and chronic respiratory disease. It relies on periodic measurement and recording of biomarkers. Deviation from standard limits prompts review and corrective action. It provides the opportunity to impart information, signpost to supplementary services, screen opportunistically for co-morbid disease, provide valuable support and impart additional primary prevention (e.g. influenza vaccine). It creates the possibility of modifying the disease trajectory through early detection and prompt intervention, for example the early use of steroid inhalation in childhood asthma. Surveillance is supported through two requirements: (1) *the IT system capability for* holding patient details, disease registers, call-and-recall functions and biometric data and (2) *a 'management machine'* that ensures the quality of services provided. Frequently surveillance takes place through a regular, GP- or nurse-led, specific session, the 'general practice mini-clinic' (*see* Chapter 4). The characteristics of surveillance in general practice include:

- *continuing* – at appropriate intervals
- *comprehensive* – that is, involving all persons within the catchment who have the condition or conform to selection criteria
- *multi-professional* – involving skill levels and skills mix
- *patient involvement* – in the interests of adherence
- *protocol-driven*, so that observations and data sets are collected and collated uniformly by all involved
- *reliable systems* – for processing lab reports, scrutinising results, noting trends in laboratory data and acting on prompts that arise
- *alertness to trends* – and to deviances
- *quality managed* – by an identified lead.

Some ethical considerations apply. Since surveillance is clinician led, and not by the patient's initiative, there is a great onus on the clinician to make the processes user-friendly, be painstakingly thorough and to communicate with skill. One cannot be vigilant for everything all the time and the tools are imperfect. Risk is inherent in biometric testing and screening. They deal in risk. At the interface between population medicine and patient centredness it is important to respect the autonomy of the individual, backed up with informed consent.

The logistic and information management tasks involved are formidable. Multi-professional working requires that the different system 'silos' communicate with one another. This means meetings and information sharing. Protocols should be safe, agreed, evidence-based yet realistic. There are crucial features to processing numerical data that have to be considered. Lab returns measure mainly continuous variables (e.g. the concentration of electrolytes). The limits of normal are statistically set in terms of standard deviation. Cut-off points defining normality are not, then, definitive. Borderline reports are frequent and require problem-solving decisions. Any significant un-actioned data can have heavy consequences for both the patient and the team. Surveillance saves lives and reduces illness. It is worth doing well, but it is a lot of work!

Screening and Wilson's Criteria

Like surveillance, screening is a public health exercise directed at selected at-risk populations. It aims to identify an early disease or pre-disease state and refer those identified for definitive investigation and treatment. It is predicated on three factors: (1) the target *disease*, (2) the *screening test* and (3) *what can be done* about it. These have been codified in a WHO publication in 1968, and are now known as *Wilson's Criteria*.[31]

1. The *disease* is serious, has a natural history that is well understood, with a protracted identifiable preclinical phase and affects a population that can be defined.
2. There exists a *reliable diagnostic test* that can be administered economically and easily on a large scale, is ethical, safe, acceptable, minimally invasive, sensitive and specific; preferably the test should not require high levels of skill.
3. There is a *curative procedure*, backed up by systems for investigation, treatment and follow-up for those who test positive.

As with all public health interventions in healthy people, safety and quality assurance are crucial. This is because the initiative arises from public policy through the health system, and the individual subjects are healthy but liable to experience negative consequences from the process. It is clear from Wilson's criteria that any formal screening programme must conform to exacting specifications. And very few match up to these.

Screening can be bad for your health, according to the work of Skrabanek and McCormick.[32] Their work in Trinity College Dublin in the 1980s drew early attention to the adverse effects of the false result, complications that arise from administering screening tests and, furthermore, from the subsequent procedures that are mandated on the basis of unsatisfactory samples and borderline test results. While screening applies to many clinical situations, the more emotive ones surround cancer detection. Very early diagnosis prolongs the time period during which the person is aware of the disease and this increases measured prevalence (as well as stress). This is called length/time bias. An *interval onset cancer* is one that arises within the standard period between screening points. This interval is one decreed in consideration of the risk of disease occurrence and the logistics of screening. Broad intervals reduce cost but increase the risks from undetected disease and delay in diagnosis. Narrow intervals increase the detection of early disease but are onerous for the patient, are resource intensive and carry risk (e.g. increased radiation exposure and over-investigation). Thus different national programmes vary in their protocols. Setting the screening interval is a compromise between economic practicalities and safety, informed by the natural history of the disease.

Very early diagnosis often relies on the interpretation of subtle changes, perhaps subjective classification of criteria of cell type or assay-based measurements that can fluctuate. These introduce uncertainties of the false negative/positive kind. It is taxing enough to inform patients that their test is positive and needs action. It is more difficult to convey that the 'positive test' was a false alarm; still more so to find retrospectively that a 'negative test' had provided false reassurance in the presence of disease. Imperfect knowledge about the natural history of the target disease may mean that a true positive test may set in train formidable interventions geared towards a worst-case outcome, whereas the condition may, in reality, be a relatively benign variant. Examples of this include prostate and breast cancer, which, in many instances, turn out to be indolent, as epidemiological studies show. A variety of motivations towards definitive clinical intervention can give rise to overtreatment, the consequences of which mean that the treatment can become the disease.

Glossary of epidemiological terms

With reference to the four cells that make up the grid in Figure 2.2, the letter (a) represents a true positive result; the disease is present and the test shows positive. The letter (d) represents a true negative; the result correctly indicates the absence of disease. But we know that biological test results are not clear-cut.

	Positive	Negative
Disease present	a	b
Disease absent	c	d

FIGURE 2.2 Grid for defining the characteristics of tests for disease

False positive is a positive result in the absence of actual disease (c)
False negative is a negative result in the presence of actual disease (b)
Sensitivity is the probability of a positive test in people with the disease (a/a+c)
Specificity is the probability of negative result in people who are disease-free (d/b+d)
The *predictive value* of a test depends on its sensitivity, specificity and prevalence in
the test population; low prevalence degrades the value of even highly valid tests
Positive predictive value is the probability of the person having the disease when the
test is positive (a/a+b)

Negative predictive value is the probability of the person not having the disease when the test is negative (d/c+d).

Accuracy: the proportion of all tested samples where the test provided the correct result (a+b/a+b+c+d)

An analogous grid can be constructed for evaluating clinical interventions to come up with values such as *number needed to treat*.

Complex interactive systems

> In complexity, the dominant metaphor is the living system – organic, dynamic, unpredictable and constantly adapting to its environment. This is more suited to a large, complex organisation like the NHS.[33]

Statistics as a subject is beyond the reach of this author and not strictly relevant to this work. *Complexity*, though, is highly relevant. It deals with large populations of interacting and interdependent elements that may not behave randomly. It is not the same thing as *complicated*, which refers to mechanistic systems that can be designed and controlled to achieve a defined output, like the steam engine. The health service, on the other hand, is a complex system that has to adapt itself constantly to changing political, social and financial environments, interact with professionals and patients, and is prone to non-linear change.

Understanding *complex adaptive systems* requires knowledge of the components and how they relate to one another, and the initial conditions; they are *non-linear*, capable of *self-organisation* and resulting behaviour (emergence) is *unpredictable*. The act of observation in a complex adaptive system implies participation in it. There are *positive feedback* loops, where any of a number of possible equilibriums may emerge, and *negative feedback* where there is a single *equilibrium point* – restoration of the original state. *Connectivity* refers to the *inter-connectedness* and *interdependence* of the components, resulting in complex behaviour. The behaviour of epidemics is one example. The SARS outbreak in 2002–03 did not sweep China, but it popped up in Toronto and 37 other countries because of the connectivity of air travel before appearing to vanish. The new social media is a complex system; there is much that is chaotic but (some would say) not without meaning. Mathematical and computer modelling illuminate complex systems in an emergent fashion that is not predictive. Continuous surveillance combined with modelling can identify the probabilities attached to outcomes, for example, in forecasting the behaviour of weather systems.

In healthcare organisations multidisciplinary working is subject to complexity. Populations of ill people, often with multiple ailments which may or may not be interdependent, are actively managed by disparate teams all applying their respective complicated inputs, within a NHS that is subject to external influences and an ecosystem that injects random events. Welcome to NHS chronic care. Not chaotic, just complex.

CONCLUSION AND REFLECTION

Quality and safety assurance in preventive medicine entails risk to the individual and creates demands on patients that are mysterious and confusing for them. They need clear communication, information and guidance to enlist their informed participation and adherence. The relevance for chronic disease management of this venture into epidemiology includes:

- the statistical nature of normality, deviance in biometrics and complexity
- the implications of case-finding, early diagnosis and disease prevention
- safety implications of the systems employed in programmes of prevention
- the adverse experiences for patients in the course of their clinical pathway
- workload implications, especially in primary care.

Awareness of risk status bestows the capacity to intervene preventively through surveillance, screening, early diagnosis and anticipatory action. The prevalence, morbidity and mortality due to the Dragon would be greatly reduced by effective health education directed at lifestyle choice and focusing on body mass optimisation, positive nutrition and exercise, dealing with addictions, enhanced socialisation and trauma prevention. This shortlist of modifiable factors, combined with the above list of preventive actions, is at the core of any generic management model for combating the genus Dragon.

POINTS FOR REFLECTION

- List the commonest chronic diseases you encounter in order of (a) frequency, (b) challenge for you and (c) challenge for the patient.
- Review the practice action points provided in this chapter; collate them and edit down to a minimum set of tasks or skills; you may wish to add some of your own.
- Which aspects of palliative/terminal care would enhance most the care of non-cancer patients who are in the mid-trajectory phases of a serious chronic disease?

REFERENCES

1. World Health Organization. *World Health Report 2008: primary health care, now more than ever*. Geneva: WHO; 2008.
2. Ibid.
3. US National Center for Health Statistics. Available at: www.nationalhealthcouncil.org/NHC_Files/pdf_Files/AboutChronicDisease.pdf (accessed 10 April 2014).
4. Kane RL, Priester R, Totten AM. *Meeting the Challenge of Chronic Illness*. Baltimore, MD: The Johns Hopkins University Press; 2005.
5. World Health Organization. *Innovative Care for Chronic Conditions: building blocks for action: global report*. Geneva: WHO; 2002.
6. Van den Akker M, Buntinx F, Metsemakers JFM, *et al*. Multimorbidity in general practice: prevalence, incidence, and determinants of co-occurring chronic and recurrent diseases. *J Clin Epidemiol*. 1998; **51**(5): 367–75.
7. Loxterkamp D. Humanism in the time of metrics. *BMJ*. 2013: **347**: f5539.
8. Research News. *BMJ*. 2012; **345**: e4799.
9. Bonita R, Beaglehole R, Kjellstrom T. *Basic Epidemiology*. 2nd ed. Geneva: World Health Organization; 2006.
10. Wagner EH, Austin BT, von Korff M. Organising care for patients with chronic illness. *Millbank Q*. 1996; **74**(940): 511–44.
11. Centers for Disease Control and Prevention. *Promising Practices in Chronic Disease Prevention and Control*. Atlanta, GA: US Department of Health and Human Services; 2003. Available at: http://stacks.cdc.gov/view/cdc/11310/ (accessed 21 April 2014).
12. Corbin J, Strauss A. *Unending Work and Care: managing chronic illness at home*. San Francisco, CA: Jossey-Bass; 1988.
13. Spijker J, MacInnes J. Population ageing: the timebomb that isn't? *BMJ*. 2013; **347**: f6598.
14. Rice DP, Fineman N. Economic implications of increased longevity in the United States. *Annu Rev Public Health*. 2004; **25**: 457–73.
15. Van den Akker, Buntinx, Metsemakers, op. cit.
16. Ibid.
17. Druss B, Marcus S, Olfson L, *et al*. Comparing the national economic burden of five chronic conditions. *Health Aff (Millwood)*. 2001; **20**(6): 233–41.
18. Starfield B. Threads and yarns: weaving the rich tapestry of comorbidity. *Ann Fam Med*. 2006; **4**(2): 101–3.
19. World Health Organization, 2002, op. cit.
20. Maslow AH. A theory of human motivation. *Psychol Rev*. 1943; **50**(4): 370–96.
21. Prochaska JO, DiClemente CC. *The Transtheoretical Approach: crossing the boundaries of therapy*. Melbourne, FL: Krieger; 1984.
22. Hodkinson I. Care planning. *RCGP News*. 2012; (March): 6.
23. www.goldstandardsframework.org.uk/ (accessed 21 April 2014).
24. Allen J, Gay B Crebolder H, *et al*. *The European Definition of General Practice/Family Medicine*. WONCA, Europe; 2005. p. 29.
25. Plunkett and Gordon. 1960. Cited in: Macmahon B, Trichopoulos D. *Epidemiology, Principles and Methods*. 2nd ed. Boston, MA: Little Brown & Company; 1996. p. 5.
26. Koplan J, Dusenbury C, Jousilahti P, *et al*. The role of national public health institutes in health infrastructure development. *BMJ*. 2007; **335**(7625): 384–5.
27. Bonita, Beaglehole, Kjellström, op. cit.

28. Ibid. p. 103.
29. Ibid.
30. Ibid.
31. Wilson JMG, Jungner G. *Principles and Practice of Screening for Disease*. Geneva: WHO; 1968.
32. Skrabanek P, McCormick J. *Follies and Fallacies in Medicine*. Dublin: Tarragon Press; 1992.
33. Sweeney K, Mannion R. Complexity and clinical governance: using insights to develop the strategy. *Br J Gen Pract*. 2002; **52**(Suppl.): S4–9.

CHAPTER 3

The journey through chronic disease (the patient complex)

Contents

CHAPTER OVERVIEW

The patient's story comes third in the chapter sequence. This is regrettable in terms of the priorities I seek to present since patients should always come first, but they have not been absent from the story to date. There is such an intimate relationship between patients and their diseases that, in this narrative, both are contenders for the spotlight. This becomes apparent through the discussion on sociology, which points out that, while ***disease manifests itself objectively through effects on people, it is what patients experience that defines illness.*** Here we examine some personal consequences of disease, trace the patient's pathway through chronic disease using a simplified form of the trajectory model before going on to look at implications of illness for people through the medium of sociology. The use of the term *patient complex* as subtitle to this chapter also prompts a word of explanation. In acute disease, the patient occupies a singular and transient state, subjected to focused therapies aimed at cure and exit. By contrast, in chronic disease the patient is not the sole occupant of the stage. The prolonged pathway draws in a solar system of participants that revolves around him or her. These include the family, social circle, workplace and intimate carers. The patient complex is not a state of mind but the reality of all those who experience the disease complex. There are dangers in telling people's stories for them; in objectifying them as sociology subjects, or philosophising at them on the meaning of their suffering. I think the former is the lesser evil and it is better to err in that direction. If meaning is to be found through or in their suffering, this is a path for the individual, to discover what meaning they can for themselves and share this with fellow sufferers. For the sake of the continuing story the identity of the patient is prioritised. The details of sociology, and the social determinants of health and disease, are deferred to the latter part of the chapter, which concludes with a scenario that summarises the testimony of patients and carers.

> Illness is the night-side of life, a more onerous citizenship. Everyone who is born holds dual citizenship, in the kingdom of the well and in the kingdom of the sick. Although we all prefer to use only the good passport, sooner or later each of us is obligated, at least for a spell, to identify ourselves as citizens of that other place.[1]
>
> Susan Sontag

WHAT IS IT LIKE TO LIVE WITH CHRONIC DISEASE?

Professionals in healthcare tend to assume that they know a lot about chronic disease, and so they do. In reality though, our knowledge is confined to our point of contact with diseases, the features of this or that condition, how to recognise the fingerprints of diseases and how to respond within our respective professional disciplines with available resources. Expertise, however, is not the same as experience. As a GP my encounters with a typical chronic condition sufferer amount to little more than an hour or so annually, spread over any number of encounters, direct and indirect. My *experience* of chronic disease is composed of extrapolations from many such circumscribed encounters.

This stands in contrast with the lot of individual sufferers who experience their disease and its myriad effects 24 hours a day, year in, year out. It 'lives with' the patient full-time, in their being, their home and their family. It resides at their address with various degrees of visibility, impact and impairment. The household and family have to accommodate to it as best they can. It is like an unwelcome guest who declines to depart their home, even accompanying them on outings and holidays. And very often it does not come singly.

But first, a report of a training exercise.

SCENARIO: a case study

The new trainee has been asked to make a home visit, conduct an interview and write a reflective account of her observations of a family struggling with a chronic illness. This is the extended narrative that emerged following our lengthy discussion in tutorial.

It is a typical three-bedroom, semi-detached, suburban, owner-occupied house – small garden front and rear. It appears well kept. The family comprises a couple in their forties with two school-age children, one still at primary level. The father has been diagnosed with multiple sclerosis and several years ago he had to give up his job as a civil servant, having been pensioned off on health grounds. In the Department of Agriculture his duties included fieldwork, driving to forestry and fishery projects, and this had become increasingly unrealistic. His wife, a classroom assistant in a primary school, is in good health. Their joint income, including his incapacity benefits and pension, is about the national average. They receive housing benefit and personal independence payments. They experience a good deal of financial anxiety because her job lacks long-term security.

On entering the house there was a distinct tang of disinfectant, which, one suspects, disguises a uriniferous odour. The stairway is partly obstructed by a bulky chairlift. The small downstairs toilet has an elevated toilet seat appliance surrounded by a tubular metal frame with handgrips. The upstairs bathroom is the same, only more so. There are handrails everywhere; the bath has been removed in favour of an ugly shower cubicle that contains a high plastic seat as a permanent feature. These, the second-most-visited rooms in the house, bear the clear stigma of disability.

In the main bedroom the first impression is the decor, bright, clean and cheerful. There are twin beds, however, that symbolise the degree to which disability is triumphing over intimacy. A bedside locker is functional and capacious enough to serve as a repository for the many accoutrements and appliances required by someone on lots of medication who spends a more than average amount of time in bed. Then on to the living room, where the furnishings are comfortable and quietly elegant with the exception of the incongruously large reclining high chair in a clashing colour. The other dominant feature of the room is the unit containing the disproportionately bulky television, its massive plasma screen telling of the amount of time and attention it receives and its centrality as a resource for the household.

Customary greetings elicit that the couple are both quite well today. One suspects that this is not the full truth but accepts this at face value, knowing the capacity of people with long-term conditions to normalise their disability and adjust the calibration of their expectations from life. He is experiencing a plateau, a period of stability (but not yet remission) in the trajectory of his disease. Apart from his usual weakness, tiredness and intermittent muscle spasms he claims to be 'ok'. He is going out more now as a deliberate response to a period of depression that followed a bad relapse last year when he was housebound for months after flu. He had become socially isolated, spending large amounts of time in bed or in front of the television and had put on a lot of weight. Now he takes his anti-depressants and goes to the day centre, where he is bored with the bingo and country music but enjoys the classes in art and 'gardening with disability'. He finds physiotherapy and the exercise facility there challenging, but necessary in view of his weight. In the evening, while his wife supervises the children's homework, he is able to walk to the local pub, provided the man next door is going too. He does this to reduce his former tendency to watch television, drink carry-outs at home and smoke ('it's hard to give them up when you have few pleasures in life and not a lot to fill your time').

When things are bad he finds it hard to concentrate enough to read. Over the years he has learned to use the computer. On bad days he plays the same computer game over and over. In better times he can surf the Web and keep in contact by e-mail, Facebook and Skype with his far-flung family and circle of friends, many of whom are fellow sufferers encountered through a self-help support network. One thing he misses is the banter he used to have with his workmates. He enjoys pottering about in the garden and watching sport on television.

His wife was born and brought up locally but she mixes little with the local community. Although well, she finds it ironic that she is married to a husband who is progressively disabled. As she explains, her mother had rheumatoid arthritis from an early age and her father had 'found solace elsewhere', leaving his wife and children to fend for themselves. She, herself, is the only one of her siblings to remain living locally, her two sisters having departed 'to get a life' elsewhere as soon as they could break free. She had felt obligated, perhaps trapped, to provide as much care as she could for her disabled and dependent mother. She was dismayed by her husband's diagnosis of multiple sclerosis that crept up on them in the early years of their marriage.

'I wish I could do more for my mother but it's hard to juggle everything – her, my husband, my job, the house, and at the same time give the kids a normal childhood.

I just hope my health holds out. I can see myself having to give up my job some time if it all gets too much. Just now I'm trying to cut down my hours at the school, but with less money it will be hard. I just hope we can hold on to the car – it's a lifeline.'

What she finds strange is that she is the healthy one. She kept expecting to be the one with disability, to become a victim of arthritis like her mother. She still finds it hard to shake off the fear, and every backache or joint pain ignites the terror that she feels lurks in her genes.

'My young sisters made bad marriages to get away', she says. 'I married a strong healthy man and now I have to cope with everything on my own.'

But, she reflects, growing up with disability has prepared her for this. She became accustomed in childhood to walking at a snail's pace with her mum, to not being allowed to run off out of reach by herself, to being mother's helper, missing school to get her mother to hospital appointments, to being responsible at all times. Everybody said she was so good and she had to keep on being good even when she felt embarrassed at her mother not being active, smart and elegant at the school gate or parents' meetings. Growing up as a 'child carer' she had little time for friends or fun. When her sisters visit now occasionally from afar, they are of little help. They recount their own unsatisfactory lives, find fault with the care their mother is receiving and depart leaving behind a trail of discontent and guilt.

'Sometimes I think I'm going to explode. My mother has always had panic attacks and I had to cope with her moods. My husband keeps getting depressed and I have to stay cheerful for him and the children.'

And now, once again, she has to take time out of school for her husband's clinic appointments, walk at a snail's pace, be responsible and good all the time, and has no time for herself, few friends and little fun.

'Sick people are not easy to live with; they keep reminding me that I am the lucky one; I have my health and what do I have to complain about? I think I'll get sick too; then we'll all be in the same boat! But I can't afford to be thinking like that. I just wish we could go away on a holiday, somewhere sunny, give us all a change of scenery; but whenever I think about that something always happens and the dream is gone. I can't plan ahead for anything.'

'This is what my life's all about – looking after sick people. I just hope for better things for the children. What keeps me going? Maybe it's the company at work, my faith, my kids.'

'I just wish there was more laughter.
I wish I didn't feel tired all the time;
I wish I could fix it for my husband and mother;
I wish I didn't feel guilty all the time;
I wish I didn't feel so helpless;
I wish I knew what the future holds for us, but I don't really want to think ahead.'

Her husband's eyes are moist, and he becomes agitated.

'Why didn't you tell me all this before? It's as if you have to wait for a stranger to come into the house before you can open up. I thought I was the one with the illness, the useless one not able to earn the bread for the table, play football with the kids, sick and tired of being sick, sore and tired. I feel like a burden on society and not even able to pull my weight at home. Don't feel guilty on my account; I have enough guilty feeling for both of us. This thing is not going to go away, so maybe I should just take myself out of it. You'd be better off then. I'm the one with the dribbling, the spasms and all the pills. I'm expendable so don't waste your pity and guilt on me. Look at our kids; what do they say when the other kids at school ask them what their daddy does?'

As he subsides, slumping in his massive chair, his wife looks at him in silence, impassive.

It made the new trainee wonder about the wisdom of this visit, penetrating the locked-in circle of a stressed family, inviting them to talk. The weight of the silence, the ring of truth, the feeling that there is no right thing to say, all brought to her mind a phrase from a classic television series, 'Beam me up …!' As the one in the room not overwhelmed with disease she felt she had no right to comment or offer advice. She had, without really trying to do so, opened up something that she felt inadequate to deal with, but as the professional she felt the urge to do something, to say something, to make it better!

At points in this narrative, our new trainee admitted, a sense of restlessness set in.

'Touchy/feely stuff' is all very well but that's for social workers, shrinks and clergy; we have a job to do back at the surgery and that is complicated enough without getting bogged down in the details of how people live. Isn't it time we moved on to firmer ground and got to grips with a few diseases?

This is the very real distinction between the words *disease* and *illness*, the objective of scientific and the experiential dimensions. But these are two sides of the same coin. There is a balance to be achieved between the disease-oriented approach and person centredness. Diseases are fascinating, just as flora and fauna are intriguing to the field biologist. However, every biologist will agree that the ecological analysis is crucial to the understanding of organisms and is every bit as important as their morphology. We as clinicians have a more rounded grasp of the disease if we take account of its ecology as an essential component of the natural history – how diseases behave, interact or coexist, and affect their host and environment. This should lead to a more holistic capacity to observe, analyse and intervene creatively. It also helpfully dispels our illusions that manipulating one disease at a time is a rational and sufficient approach. It confronts our delusions as clinicians that we are in control of the situation.

With respect to chronic disease in particular, the patient-centred perspective, how his or her daily life is affected and how this affects others, is the essential backdrop to our more focused everyday concerns, those of clinical assessment, diagnosis, prescribing and rescue when crises strike.

THE PATIENT'S JOURNEY THROUGH CHRONIC DISEASE

> The chief business of chronically ill persons is not just to stay alive or keep their symptoms under control, but to live as normally as possible despite the symptoms of the disease.
>
> **Anselm Strauss[2]**

The path of chronic disease, the journey with continuing or recurrent illness, is a normal human experience. Just under half of all adults, two-thirds of all aged over 65 and three-quarters of those aged over 75 live with a long-term condition, and 45% of them have more than one condition.[3] As a correlate of the ageing process it may be seen as developmental. It is a rare person who presents late in life with a thin folder.

Chronicity is not the same thing as severity. Any condition that extends beyond 3–6 months can be said to be a chronic condition. Many persistent disorders are not life-threatening and may be compatible with a relatively normal way of life. Very few chronic diseases are truly curable, even today, although most can be modified from the expression of their natural history, and their trajectory and impact significantly altered. Most chronic diseases are lifelong from their point of onset and in that sense incurable. People with chronic illness often feel stigmatised, unclean ('How do I know I do not smell?') and need to be reassured that they are not contagious. Chronic diseases are often referred to as non-communicable disease (although there are some infections that describe a prolonged timeline). The experiences of people with long-term conditions are as diverse as their respective conditions, personalities and circumstances, even though there is a core of commonality. David Locker,[4] writing about the consequences of chronic illness, observed:

> In other respects the problems faced by people with chronic illness may be common to all, irrespective of the nature of their disorder.

These problems include unemployment or reduced career prospects, social isolation, estrangement from family and friends, loss of important roles, changed physical appearance, and problems with self-esteem and identity. Locker concluded:

> When chronic illness becomes severe, daily life may be entirely consumed in coping with its symptoms, the medical regimens intended to control it and its social consequences.

Previous generations suffering long-term conditions were destined to enact the natural history, the timeline and trajectory of their disease. Our medical and nursing forebears presided over illnesses in which they had no real control. Support, guidance and palliation were their stock-in-trade, and these remain fundamental to what people need, and powerful in what professionals can offer. It is important to remember this when our science and our tools fail us at any stage on the patient's journey. There is always something that can be done to alleviate or address suffering. That is what palliative and terminal care are all about, and hope should never be quenched on the basis of a technological assessment. Clinical practice is full of unexpected outcomes and confounded prognoses. As we have seen, **the management of chronic disease may be regarded as bringing to the complete disease trajectory the skills and insights we already practise with confidence in dealing with those who are terminally ill**.

Although the diagnoses of people with long-term conditions are diverse, there are recurring themes, additional to those social ones listed by Locker, which reflect the common ground of chronic disease. One of these themes is the *trajectory* that points to stages along the way, as set out in Chapter 2. The trajectory model of disease will now be reinterpreted to represent the disease progression, through the eyes of the patient as he or she might experience it, condensed into three stages, with particular emphasis on the importance of the diagnosis.

Early stage:	onset and diagnosis
Middle stage:	moving towards self-sufficiency
	living with continuing illness

	points of progression
	points of transition
Advanced stage:	palliative care
	facing end of life

For the one on the journey, each of these brings its own challenges and issues, and clinicians need to be alert to these. After all, we will have seen these many times over and our experience should have something to offer; for the wayfarer it is all new territory every time.

THE EARLY DAYS: THE IMPORTANCE OF DIAGNOSIS

The onset of disease is the period of time that leads up to diagnosis, including the patient's response to this. It can be very brief, as with critical presentation or trauma – for example, the initial grand mal seizure, classical coronary or spinal injury; from onset to diagnosis in a matter of moments, when every minute counts. With good acute care survival is followed by evaluation, rehabilitation and secondary prevention. The triumph of modern acute medicine has been to turn a fatal acute condition into a chronic one, thus buying time to institute management and preventive interventions. In developed health systems very few children must now die in an asthma attack or status epilepticus. A fatal outcome to a coronary is perceived as shocking and potentially preventable. As one patient remarked *'Having a chronic disease isn't so bad, if you think about the alternative.'*

Of course, the disease may have begun long before it impinges on the consciousness of the patient. For example, it has been shown that undiagnosed diabetes type 2 is not a benign condition. Clinically significant morbidity, such as retinopathy, is present at diagnosis in many cases. The natural history of diabetes indicates that it takes around 5 years for retinopathy to develop. It is estimated that the true onset of diabetes occurs 7 years before clinical diagnosis, or perhaps longer.[5] Organ damage may be taking place during this latent phase.

More commonly, long-term conditions show a gradual onset, as with progressive angina pain, the spit and dyspnoea of chronic obstructive pulmonary disease, the polyarthralgia of rheumatoid disease. Insidious onset is one characteristic of the major neurological diseases multiple sclerosis, Parkinson's, Alzheimer's and motor neurone disease. Clearly, the mode of onset greatly influences the diagnostic process and this has consequences for all concerned. The patient needs to know what is going on, and so does the clinician, each for his or her respective reasons. This point is fraught with hazards for both: the over-investigation of non-specific presentations in the hope of achieving an early diagnosis of a treatable condition (great kudos), the retrospective failure to make an improbable diagnosis (unreasonable expectations), taking a long time to come up with the right answer (diagnostic delay), and empirical treatments to try to cover all the possibilities (overtreatment).

The onset of episodic or non-specific events such as paraesthesiae, fatigue or dizziness bears a significance that is different from the sudden, definitive one. The connection between episodes may not be apparent. To clinicians, diagnostic error and delay are understandable. Time itself is often used as a diagnostic tool. Pattern recognition takes time. Diagnosis is a process rather than an event, and is a statement of probability rather than certainty. This is less apparent to the patient. Communication has to be good in order to manage anxiety and uncertainty, and to forestall disillusionment and loss of confidence on the part of the patient and family carers. Receiving a diagnosis impinges on the patient's identity (I am now a diabetic, an epileptic, a schizophrenic, a cancer sufferer …), and confers a social label. He or she has to be able to justify any complaints, disabilities and incapacity with the name of a disease. '*My doctor doesn't know yet*' isn't good enough. In making a diagnosis a doctor validates the social role of sickness, and identifies any external agent that is responsible.

> When a diagnosis is finally obtained, it often comes as a relief; it legitimates the person's complaints and experiences and brings to an end conflicts with others over the reality of the symptoms.[6]

But it does not always come with the expected outcome.

CASE REPORT: MRS JB

Mrs JB lived well and actively until the age of 75. Following a 'check-up' a full blood count showed lymphocytosis. This was investigated and she was diagnosed with chronic lymphatic leukaemia. She came home from hospital, announced to her family that she had leukaemia and took to bed. She declined to leave her home for any appointments and she was eventually lost to hospital follow-up. Her family tended to her needs assiduously. She resisted opportunistic efforts by her GP to mobilise her back to a more normal lifestyle and her family concurred with her that she was an ill woman. A status quo of collusion was established and the sick role entrenched. The family adopted the carer role despite the GP's advice. Mrs JB lived quietly at home and died nearly 10 years later from bronchopneumonia following flu.

For some elderly people the sick role provides an excuse for being dependent.[7] There are limits to the realm of rational, evidence-based practice.

From the diagnostic point of view it is better to present with a crisis when early hospital admission is the high road to the full panoply of technical investigation that may be brought to bear. Investigative capacity is concentrated in the inpatient setting and many patients are admitted only to expedite urgent investigation. Reasons for diagnostic delay are summarised in Figure 3.1.

The patient	The doctor	The illness
Symptoms subtle or absent	Lack of urgency	Signs subtle or absent
Denial	Lack of recognition	Stigmatised disease
Ignorance	System failure	Insidious onset
Fear	Collusion of anonymity	Episodic
Stigma	Dilution of responsibility	Interval onset
Self-treatment	Overload	Modifiable?
Complacency		Diagnostic tests available?
Hyper-vigilance		

FIGURE 3.1 Factors that may cause delay in diagnosis and therapeutic response

EXAMPLE 1

It is now recognised that rheumatoid arthritis needs to be diagnosed and treatment instituted within about 4–6 months from onset if permanent synovial damage is to be averted. The average time from onset to treatment is 6 months and much of the delay is due to patients being slow to present. The introduction of a more sensitive and specific test for rheumatoid arthritis and the introduction of disease-modifying drugs have highlighted this particular watershed in the natural history of the disease. This is an example of an intervention marker that gained significance following a technological advance. Until then the significance of this action point was not critical.

Alertness, risk-assessment and prompt, decisive action are required if the aims of early diagnosis are to be achieved. Good records are fundamental to 'joining the dots' of pattern recognition, especially within large practices and diverse clinical teams (dilution of responsibility), where there is likely to be a corresponding loss of continuity of personal care (collusion of anonymity). Over-investigation, on the other hand, of non-specific complaints has very damaging effects and this is a systemic fault in health systems that are specialist delivered.

Gerada[8] has drawn attention to the opposite extreme – that of 'the unworried unwell' who present with advanced disease after long periods of denial or self-medication. A major health promotion task confronts society in order to achieve an informed and motivated populace without engendering the spread of fear. As Chesterton[9] said,

> The trouble with always trying to preserve the health of the body is that it is so difficult to do without destroying the health of the mind.

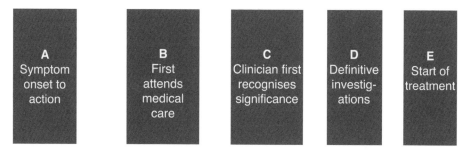

FIGURE 3.2 Trajectory-based model of diagnostic delay: the clinical pathway stages where delay may occur

The phenomenon of diagnostic delay as a timeline trajectory is illustrated in Figure 3.2. From the first experience of symptoms by the patient at point A to first attendance at medical care (B) is the *delay in presentation*, mostly due to patient factors and access issues. From that to start of definitive treatment is the *diagnostic interval*. This comprises the time it takes for the doctor to grasp the significance of the patient's state (B to C); add to that any interval for initiation and outcome of investigations (C and D), plus any waiting time to start of treatment (E). Many conditions, such as cancers or diabetes, have a pre-symptomatic stage of disease activity prior to point A. Clearly there is much scope for loss of time due to human factors, circumstances, access and other systemic delay. It has been calculated that between 7500 and 10 000 lives may be lost in the UK from late diagnosis.[10] The final part of the diagnostic phase of the patient's path frequently takes place at hospital. He or she enters this arena as a person and emerges as a patient – having a defined diagnosis. The process is rocky, however humane the professionals may be. Symbolically, there is the familiar frisson of dread at the periodic arrival through the post of the bland letter in a brown envelope with the portentous clinic appointment message:

Hospital number XXX,
Your time for clinic A is XX on DD/MM/YYYY
The entry code for the patients' car park is XXXX
Please attend on time, with a full bladder and fasting.
Please bring a family member or carer ....

The portents of doom and gloom, already addressing the person's private and intimate functions, bestowing a file number and PIN code; the process of depersonalising has begun.

To most people the initial contact with hospital is daunting, bleak, impersonal and alien. Doctors who themselves encounter this in the patient role are spared a portion of the impact because, to them, going to hospital is a bit like revisiting their old home (however, they have other issues of their own, such as foreknowledge of what lies in store). Procedures and processes take over and it is all like a surreal experience – a blur of unclarity. This is why it is recommended that patients bring with them a relative, someone who will have some detachment, some clarity and will be able to seek answers to questions that arise, and have some memory of what took place.

The breaking of bad news is not easy, simple or universally well carried out by professionals. There is a general consensus about guidelines for conveying bad news to people. It is necessary to create a proper space and time, explore the information needs, sensitively introduce the facts and invite questions. There are also consequences for the professional, usually a senior doctor or a specialist nurse; when done well the benefit this brings to people reflects the cost of it to the professional:

● it demands empathy, actively to explore the depths of the person's layers of emotion and tune in to them
● it causes the professional to participate in the necessary distress of the recipient
● it demands time to permit the patient to raise questions
● it implies the willingness to respond to any issues that may arise
● it suggests that some follow-on arrangement is envisaged.

All this requires great skill, both in communication and at the level of emotional quotient. Not uncommonly the scene is repeated at the GP's surgery. The distressed person and spouse make an urgent appointment to seek clarification on all the issues they could not put to 'the Big Doctor' (no slight is intended; indeed, perhaps, the reverse). One problem here is that the necessary information may not yet have reached the GP, to whom the experience of being the last to know what has transpired is a familiar one. This disadvantage can be turned to paradoxical use in that it enables one to focus on the 'messenger' rather than on the 'message', on the emotional state of the couple as an exercise in empathy and support, unclouded by medical technicalities. Matters of fact and detail may then be tabled for a further meeting.

The response to receiving bad news was analysed by Kübler-Ross[11] who described the classic five-stage model of anticipatory grief (denial, anger, bargaining, depression and acceptance). It is a cause of grief to learn that you are under threat, that you face suffering, and perhaps death. Grief is the behavioural and emotional outworking of fundamental loss. What has been lost?

- a sense of security
- sense of self as normal
- sense of integrity and wholeness of being; stigma attaches to the state of being ill
- ability to predict the future, plan and dream
- privacy and self-sufficiency
- modesty and 'dignity' – having to relate to bodily functions and organs that usually remain occult
- self-respect; there is a sense of failure and guilt; letting down those who depend on you
- autonomy, being free to plan a holiday, be mobile, swim, have sex …
- financial security – will I be able to get back to work, get a mortgage for a house, get travel insurance to visit family overseas?

Only death is a greater grief than the loss of the everyday concomitants of healthy life. '*Nothing matters, so long as you have your health*', is a frequent saying. Health has been defined as an absence of disease. Ill-health diagnosis entails the loss of wholeness. In the words of Charmaz,[12] 'The loss of self is a powerful form of suffering experienced by the chronically ill'. On the other hand, as we have seen, the confirmation of the diagnosis, when it is finally obtained, paradoxically can be a relief since it legitimises the person's complaints and experiences; it also ends conflict with others over reality of the symptoms.[13]

Johnny McEvoy, a well known Irish singer, shared his personal experience during an, interview on RTÉ Radio 1 in 2004:

> 'The day I was given my diagnosis was a turning point in my life. I felt relieved.
> I thought I was just bad. Then I was told I had manic-depression and that it was
> treatable; I should give up alcohol and take the tablets and have check-ups. I gave
> up the drink, took my medicine and life has been a lot easier since.'

For him, the grief was over when the diagnosis brought structure and form to prior chaos. Then, uncertainty resolved, systems of care begin to be formalised and a cathartic response paves the way for coming to terms with new realities. Initial therapeutic responses are applied and tested for effect. It is a busy period. Programmes of care alleviate initial suffering and this may succeed in distracting the person from fears of a longer-term nature. The sense of busyness and things that have to be done create an atmosphere of pragmatism after the initial shock factor. Personhood gives way to 'patient-hood' or 'subject-hood'. The patient feels relieved of responsibilities and decision-making when, for example, the 'sausage machine' of acute cancer care swings into action, or the rheumatology clinic begins to apply all its resources towards symptom control and disease modifying measures.

Diagnosis, as has already been seen, is not a simple matter of naming a disease. Its root meaning implies insight (Greek, *dia-gnosis*, meaning understanding in depth) and it should be not only shocking but also revelatory. In this it resembles the term 'crisis' (again Greek, for a turning point). Crisis theorists have defined this, not in terms of threat or catastrophe, but as '*an opportunity for change*'. It is widely recognised through the work of Prochaska and DiClemente[14] that change does not take place simply through the wish for change. Rather, the determination to change is precipitated by circumstances and events that make changed behaviour possible. A crisis may be beneficial.

The entry point into the world of chronic disease is a crisis in every sense. It dictates changes, such as:
- no more smoking
- you have to go on a diet
- take the following tablets …
- you should not drive a car for the next X months
- you will need to have regular check-ups and tests.

Other kinds of change also occur:
- 'It has brought us closer together'
- 'He's a nicer person since his illness'
- 'It made me realise that I have friends'
- 'I began to see that my business difficulties were just that; there are other important things in life'
- 'I have decided to retire and make the most of life while I have it'.

Shock is instant; positive realisations take longer to formulate. This is where the counselling skills that every GP should seek to perfect come into play, especially those of listening, interpreting or 'just being there'.

What sort of contract emerges from the stormy weather that accompanies diagnosis? This phrase brings to mind Tuckman's[15] description of the stages of small group work:
- forming ('ice-breaking', getting to know, establishing relationships)
- storming (disagreement, anger, casting around for direction)
- norming (exploring common ground, aligning thinking, setting goals)
- performing (getting on with it).

The relevance of this lies in establishing a new set of relationships; the person's 'new self' and the people whom he or she is going to have to work with and get to know within the new role as patient, including family carers, care workers, doctors, nurses and extended teams. Even the disease and 'the health system' assume quasi-identities that make them players in the group process as it unfolds. After a stormy start the team-forming begins and performing ensues, tackling aims and goals, and problem-solving.

And then there's the middle phase.

THE MIDDLE PASSAGE: ILLNESS PROGRESSION AND TRANSITIONS

> The fact that personal and social resources must be allocated to solving mundane practical matters is part of the handicap that flows from chronic disease.[16]

In the middle phase the bouquets of flowers no longer arrive at your door; the boss expects you back at the office, on time, and you have to answer your letters and e-mails and pay your bills. Ordinary life demands reassert themselves. The challenges are to normalise, maximise self-care and establish a modus vivendi with the continuing illness.

Moving towards self-sufficiency

It is a big step, and a significant one, following the early phase of the illness journey to take responsibility for one's own illness and the practicalities it generates. Self-sufficiency relates to overcoming denial, moving out of dependency, reclaiming autonomy and coming to terms with the reality of altered health status – stigma, disfigurement and stress.

CASE REPORT: LIAM

Liam comes out of hospital with a stoma following a diagnosis of cancer. At first he does not want even to acknowledge that it is there, let alone look at it or change the bag. The stoma nurse plans to help him move gradually from 'let's pretend she is just changing a dressing' towards fully autonomous self-management of the stoma and all the implications, including that of going to the pharmacy to get the appropriate supplies, a symbolic point of public acknowledgement.

This shift to self-care is more complex than it may appear and it can founder at various levels. The *emotional journey* is significant, from denial and dismay, to acceptance and adjustment to altered body image. The *information journey* ranges from not wanting to know, to perhaps being able to instruct and support others who become similarly afflicted. The *skills journey* involves communication, applying and reordering materials, dealing with malfunction and knowing what to do when things go wrong ('have the stoma nurse's mobile number'). The *self-efficacy journey* creates an attitude of 'I can do … and I want to …', and with enhanced confidence. These are components of the process of *normalisation*.

Living with continuing illness

It is in the stage of living with continuing illness that the personal needs of the chronic sick begin to crystallise. In addition to the fundamentals of healthcare and the activities of daily living (the basic level of Maslow's hierarchy of needs[17]), a definable menu of requirements emerges that is common to most chronic condition sufferers irrespective of their disease diagnosis and any requirements that are disease specific:

- peer support
- ownership and involvement in the care programme
- emotional support
- socialising
- information needs
- employment support
- welfare rights advice
- self-management programmes
- reach out and give back.[18]

Clearly professionals do not dominate, or even figure highly, on this agenda. Still less is it about textbook medicine. It expresses the need for partnership between the diagnosed person, the community resources, and the healthcare and social care sectors of the public services – that is, integrated care.

The agenda of self-care becomes of major interest in the narrative at this stage. The voice of the patient is impressively clear.

- They do not wish to be sleeping partners in the venture of their own healthcare.
- They wish to have their human dignity respected and safeguarded in all contacts with service providers and within the community.
- They wish to be in the cockpit of the care plan and processes – involved, responsible and active ('no decision about me without me').
- They wish to receive, and give to others, support in the areas of life that define normality – that is, the self-image and social role: self-worth, significant relationships, work and economic issues.[19]

Hjortdahl[20] sums up what people want from doctors as *security*, the components of which he lists as coherence, trust, confidence and accessibility. The expressed wants of patients and their carers are summarised in Figure 3.3, and feature in the 'Scenario: a reflective learning diary' later in this chapter. It is in pursuing these goals that people's capacity to organise themselves into collectives comes into being. Self-care takes on a mutual care dimension. Weakness and strengths are pooled, the single voices merge into a collective message, consciousness is raised, patients become a political force and solutions are found, and shared around. Some self-help groups also reflect

> a subversive readiness to question the knowledge of doctors and to assert that experiential knowledge has value ... to challenge and interrogate the medical perspective.[21]

In Chapter 1 we have already encountered that vibrant sector of civil society that includes self-help and non-governmental organisations (*the third sector*) and manifests these just, deeply felt and clear demands. There are very many disease-specific help and self-help organisations; there seems to be one (or more) for every imaginable long-term condition. In addition to providing socialising opportunities for peer support, they distribute and gather information, and formulate and represent the needs of their adherents. They also become service providers in their own right, often through voluntary action. A growing awareness of the common ground they share, and the negative consequences of competing for resources, has prompted many organisations to band together as federations of representative organisations. They have considerable success in shaping public policy and are consulted by local and central government, as exemplified by the title of a major official report:

> 'Towards a Million Change Agents': a review of the social movements literature; implications for large scale change in the NHS.[22]

Many people are lulled into a false sense of security following their successful efforts in addressing the onset of their illness and their adjustment to unwellness and disability. They have, to an extent, normalised their condition during the stage of living with continuing illness. They and their families have made adjustments in their lifestyle, explored the nature of the illness, socialised with fellow sufferers through peer support and self-help groups and thus have become familiar with the illness role and all that this entails. Initial treatment measures have moved from acute interventions and settled to a maintenance pattern.

Patients speak for themselves:

> 'When I received my diagnosis of juvenile arthritis I was unimpressed; I just had sore joints. But my mother was in tears. Now I know why.'

> 'I'm not medically trained but by *** I know about joints, pains and medication.'

'If you're going to the same clinic year after year you know what works; you have a lot to contribute.'

'I've lost my benefits and I never had a job; what can I do?'

'The best prescription my GP ever gave me was to recommend a Challenging Arthritis course.'

'GPs don't seem to know what services are out there.'

'Specialists are special but all patients are generalists.'

'We are not just patients; we are experts by experience.'

'My GP insisted on seeing me about the back pain … I sat waiting there for hours but all I wanted was a prescription for pain-killers.'

'I know a lot of people who died young; I'm just glad to be a person with a long-term condition.'

'I still have a lot of things I want to do …'

Illness progression

Then things begin to fall apart.

Relapse is one of the characteristic features of chronic disease. Temporary recurrence or fluctuation of symptoms can be assimilated into the new state of normality without causing undue dismay. But false alarms are frequent. The patient has been sensitised to risks and possibilities (although few have a grasp of probability) and any health-related deviation is like the 'crack of doom' and is liable to be endowed with great significance. The new crisis might turn out to be a run-of-the mill incident of non-specific pain or a viral infection. Of course, even flu can be the trigger for an exacerbation of their index disease. It prompts instant responses. Paradoxically, a common one is denial, resulting in inactivity – the reluctance to encounter again the paraphernalia of medicalisation. Frequently it prompts self-referral to the GP, *'just in case …'*. It has to be declared. Hopefully it will turn out to be nothing more than a trivial episode.

Encounters with medical professionals in these circumstances can be disconcerting. Even if the GP agrees that this appears to be a simple episode, he or she is likely to want to investigate it more thoroughly than average, *'with a few wee tests, just in case*'. Then there is the wait for results before life can resume its accustomed rhythm. It is important, they are told, not to let this false alarm lead to complacency; that it is important to look after their health, after all. Living with a chronic condition can be an emotional roller-coaster ride with risk, even in the plateau phase of a compensated, well-managed condition.

> The physical and functional limitations created by chronic illness will always be central to its experience but, with the passage of time social and emotional consequences may come to be more important especially for the family.[23]

Every plateau has edges. Increase in disease activity, recurrence of episodes of illness, with increasing severity and with shorter intervals that allow for only incomplete recovery, these all herald the progression of the disease. Further and more radical adjustments in lifestyle are put in place, along with additional supportive measures and awareness that the struggle has moved into a new phase with adverse effects on morale, mood and self-image.

Transition

Points of transition are the milestones on the path of illness. Loss of capacity may be marked by loss of driving licence, early retirement from work, supply of a wheelchair, moving the bed downstairs, admission to care or specialised accommodation. All represent a retreat from the trappings of residual normality, autonomy and relative well-being. There is an accompanying diminution of status, of sense of self-worth and of confidence for the future. Many people find themselves re-evaluating their life's course and priorities, *reflecting on unfinished business* and making provision for disposal of the clutter of their life. Nevertheless, many seriously ill people are capable of a great deal of autonomy, mobility and self-sufficiency, and are able to achieve a remarkable quality of life.

The GP has much to contribute in terms of guidance and support through this part of the journey. For the patient and family the course is unique, the waymarkers may be virtual and only definable in retrospect. The attempt to map the process is the province of the experienced clinician. This is where understanding and familiarity with the dynamics of the disease, its trajectory and natural history, become invaluable and enable him or her to act as 'navigator' for the patient and family unit, and to be aware of the indications for enhanced team intervention and preventive action.

ADVANCED DISEASE: THE PALLIATIVE PHASE AND END OF LIFE
The palliative phase
One of the major transition points is to the palliative phase. This may be gradual

rather than definitive. It is common for people themselves to recognise that '*there is no betterment for me now*'. In endorsing this, physicians may indicate, or be interpreted as indicating, that '*there is nothing more we can do for you*'. Such a message should never be promulgated in family medicine. Much of the most valued and rewarding work GPs do is in palliative care. Indeed, the history of medicine is immersed in palliation. Hospitals have now introduced widely the specialism of palliative medicine with symptom control specialist nurses and pain management clinics. Close attention to symptom relief and maximising autonomy are reassuring and highly valued by patients and their families. For those with advanced disease and immobility the provision of domiciliary-based care is an essential service. Active prevention (that is, anticipatory care) is a key strategy in the palliative phase.

End of life

The transition from ambulatory to domiciliary care is one of the markers of progression through the palliative phase and towards terminal care. Home visiting by doctors has been on the decline for decades and is indeed rare in some countries. Multidisciplinary home-based care is, nevertheless, essential for those many with advanced illness who have expressed a preference to die at home. There is a huge body of literature on end-of-life care that reflects the complex sensibilities and dynamics that surround the final phase of the disease pathway. This phase involves family and carers even more intimately than do the earlier phases. Symptom control, spiritual and emotional support, the practicalities of daily living, and provision of information and guidance for carers are all essential features of multi-professional teamwork when the person is dying. Recurring references to spiritual support in terminal care literature raises the question as to why it appears to be the great unmentionable elsewhere in the literature of chronic disease management. The Liverpool Care Pathway identified and described the characteristic features of impending death, and strategies to manage this.[24] As a result of reported instances of misapplication it came under a great deal of public criticism, much of it undeserved. A public inquiry in 2013 put in place further guidelines.[25] The Princess Alice Trust certificate in palliative and terminal care[26] accredits a training programme for health and social care professionals that is increasingly taken up in the UK and is rapidly acquiring an international profile.

The five-stage model of grief conceived by Kübler-Ross refers to the anticipatory grief work stages of facing death, even though they are more commonly considered to be the stages of grief following bereavement, where the model is equally applicable. The GP, more than any other clinician, is involved in bereavement support for family carers, since this is the follow-up work of caring for the person through chronic disease.

THE CLINICIAN'S JOURNEY WITH THE PATIENT

It is important not to romanticise the pathway of the patient and family through chronic disease or project it as ennobling suffering. There is risk in objectifying it as '*the patient complex*' and describing it in the somewhat dry terms of sociology and waymarkers. To do justice to this journey, these should be filled out with testimonies from the 'experts by experience'. Most people, including doctors, can claim direct personal experience of chronic disease, if not in themselves then within their family or friends. Protracted pain, mobility limitations, breathlessness, lymphoedema, hallucinations, gut cramps, messiness and demoralisation – suffering takes an infinity of forms, and so also do the ways in which people manage their illness. Attending clinicians participate in all of this through empathy, but it is the patient and family who bear the brunt of it. It behoves all clinicians to remember this when ill people weep, snap, complain and 'pester' them. But doctors do little service to patients if they allow themselves to become overwhelmed by the illness and suffering they witness. It is not necessary to have experienced the diseases we manage in order to be authentic healers, but it helps. Accompanying a close relative, or treading the path oneself, through cancer treatment, for example, is a highly instructive experience. Among the aims of training should be to induct young professionals into the empathic model, to learn by proxy what suffering feels like as an approximation to first-hand experience. There are several ways of doing this:

- make a point of occasional, in-depth, longitudinal, real-time observation and involvement through a particular case study for reflective learning
- take time to ask yourself, *How does this person feel and what is his or her everyday life like?*
- attend a Balint group as a way of getting 'inside the skin' of a challenging 'case' by exploring the rhetoric, the story, both lay and professional.

Compassion means 'suffering alongside' and this kind of suffering is a lot easier than being the victim. Problem-solving is a valid and necessary clinical stance but it can be a distancing mechanism that protects us from true understanding. And, not uncommonly, true understanding redefines the problems that need to be solved. But there have to be safeguards for the mental health of the doctor and to prevent compassion fatigue. Self-care for clinicians will reappear in Chapter 8.

The *BMJ* publishes an occasional series under the title 'Patient Journeys', each one an autobiographical account of experience of a disease, with commentary by the physician involved. These are recommended reading.

Time as the measure of chronic illness

It would be odd to write of chronic care without mention of time itself (Chronos) as a key player, albeit an under-examined one, in the drama of chronic illness.

Chronological time is not the same thing as biographical time for any of us, but especially not for those who suffer serious, protracted illness. It all depends on what is happening. A weekend goes by in a flash, but the visit to the dental chair can elongate time. As a whimsical graffito asserted, 'Time is Nature's way of ensuring that everything doesn't happen at once.' It is the commodity that doctors are least inclined, or equipped, to lavish on their patients. Hospitals are geared towards providing acute, technical, short-term care, where time is costly. GPs are constrained by the constant volume of brief encounters but this is where continuity is prized because of the cumulative effect. There is a myth that nurses are there to give time to patients but this is true only in special circumstances. 'Giving time' to patients is a curious concept, since time is not normally what they are short of as they negotiate the trajectory of their illness. To each party time has a different meaning. For the patient it is the quality and purposefulness of the face-to-face time given by their clinicians that matters. They do not often say thank you for your brain, or your drugs; most often it is 'thank you for your time'.

Time is the essence of the trajectory model of disease. The aim of therapy and management in chronic diseases is to seek to alter the trajectory of an illness, the course of its natural history expressed over time. This word trajectory conjures the image of a passive projectile that follows a pre-determined path. In a few diseases this may be an adequate enough metaphor, but in chronic conditions it should be more like a guided missile or, rather, a smart cruise missile that is capable of self-adjusting the course of its flight to accommodate change. For the doctor and nurse, the significance of trajectory is *prognosis plus management*, to modulate both outcome and course. These have been called *trajectory projection* and *trajectory scheme*. In this brief synopsis of trajectory theory I wish to acknowledge the wisdom of Corbin and Strauss,[27] their original thinking on the trajectory framework in the nursing process and their seminal book *Unending Work and Care*, which is recommended reading. For the patient, the trajectory is biographical, the cumulative experience that takes place *in their time*. Corbin and Strauss discern patterns in 'patient time', elegantly expressed as:

- the lost past ('the person I once was but left behind')
- the overbearing present (the painful situation where time seems to stand still)
- the urgent present ('time is running out')
- the eternal present (devoid of hope for positive change)
- the foreclosed future (the lost years of expectation)
- 'living on borrowed time'.

This is *biography*, that internal conversation on the part of the patient that projects past and present changes into the future and formulates conceptions around these. The timeline projections for them become radically distorted in the light of what they experience happening to their body (including their mind and ability to perform) and their identity (the cumulative experiences of body failure and impaired performance) and this creates new *biographical projections. 'Who I was in the past and hoped to be in the future are rendered discontinuous with who I am in the present.'*

To some extent biographical disruption is mirrored by others in the intimate circle of caring. All are faced with *'illness work'*, the attempts to repair the broken chain of, what Corbin and Strauss term, *biographical body conceptions*, or *BBC*. This is reminiscent of Freud's concept of 'grief work', that unavoidable total process over time that attempts to reconstruct, to achieve a new reality of meaning and living following change and loss. Clinicians can assist this process, but they cannot bring it about. The biographical work involved, they suggest, has stages (much like the grief stages of Kübler-Ross), which may be represented as follows.

- **Contextualisation**: incorporating the illness trajectory into the story – 'it is part of me, but there is more to me than the disease'.
- **Coming to terms**: seeking to understand and accept the consequences of failing performance; systems of personal belief may play an important part.
- **Reconstructing identity**: reintegrating an altered concept of wholeness around limitations of performance – 'grieve and move on', or embracing new values.
- **Recasting biography**: giving it new direction, attempting to take some control over the illness and its course, 'owning' the illness, participating in the therapeutic process, perhaps taking control.
- **Making a comeback**: moving on with a reconstructed but modified identity.

Naturally, as with grief, reconstruction of the BBC chain is not a smooth, sequential process; it can get stuck and then require external assistance to move on – perhaps with counselling, or measures to combat depression and other obstacles. As Corbin and Strauss advise, people with severe chronic illness cannot be regarded as merely in need of medical treatment. Often when people are ready to burst with anxiety, frustration and the like, one only has to listen. And this, perhaps, is among the time-gifts that a busy professional can bestow upon a person who is on the journey. The poet Rainer Maria Rilke[28] wrote to his depressed friend in these terms:

> In you, dear Mr Kappus, so much is happening now; you must be patient like someone who is sick, and confident like someone who is recovering, for perhaps you are both …. In every sickness there are many days where the doctor can do nothing but watch. And that is what you, insofar as you are your own doctor, must do now, more than anything else.

What do patients want?

A bit of fieldwork, asking people about their experience of life with chronic illness, along with a foray into a conference of patients' organisations, led to a compilation of items that they said would be like a 'big birthday present wish list', and this is shown in Figure 3.3.

- To be treated with dignity and respect, as 'people not patients'
- To live as normally as possible, and to be treated accordingly
- Empowerment, especially towards self-care
- Ownership, of their own condition
- Information about their condition(s), the right input at the right time and sign-posting to services available
- Services that are accessible and user-friendly
- Engagement on the part of professionals
- Streamlining of services and episodes of care; seamless pathways of care
- Poverty support; welfare rights advice
- Employment support
- Lifestyle support
- Emotional support
- Youth support, for young chronic sick and underage carers
- Contribution: the sense that they have something to give in return to society, to fellow-sufferers; some aspire to be Expert Patients

---

FIGURE 3.3 The Big Birthday Present List (*source*: McEvoy,[29] reproduced with permission of the *British Journal of General Practice*)

THE SOCIOLOGY OF HEALTH AND DISEASE

Sociology, the study of human social behaviour, has much to tell us about health and illness, and especially chronic illness. Despite our clinical expertise and experience, there is much about the experience and meaning of illness that is over the horizon of our awareness in the midst of the daily clinical grind. Sociology tends to be undervalued in medical training and thinking. It is not everyone's cup of tea and it may not make you a greater diagnostician but it could benefit your role as practitioner or therapist. It has much relevance to the pathway and experiences of people who suffer long-term conditions. Since medical sociology concerns itself with the patient, family and society, it has special relevance for GPs but should be of interest also to other clinical professionals and students. The sociology of chronic disease addresses three main areas:

1. *relationship complexity* that so frequently complicates ill-health
2. the *sick role*, which may be categorised as:
   - the person and illness behaviour
   - the meaning of health, disease and illness
   - disability, impairment and handicap
   - the doctor or healer role
   - social roles.
3. The *social determinants of health*

Relationship complexity

> There is clear evidence that chronic illness can place intolerable strain on families ... marital breakdown is not uncommon in these instances.[30]

Among the co-morbidities of chronic disease, one that must rank highly is its effects on family dynamics. In sociological terms a family is a social unit based on kinship, sharing economic resources, reciprocity, mutual security, emotional interdependence and providing a secure environment for the socialisation and nurture of children.

The role of the family in the care of the sick is fundamental. If there is no family support, a substitute has to be invented – for example, a care home or sheltered accommodation. For the sick and disabled the family is the survival suit within which they live, providing the essential Maslow requirements of food, shelter, protection and so forth. Significantly, the sociological definition of the family does not specify structure. The conventional pattern of father, mother and 2.1 children in many societies is on the point of being outnumbered by new patterns dictated by social change. Declining numbers of multigenerational households along with an increase in single parent units and complex families, built around successive partnerships and informal relationships, are notable factors. Whatever its structure, family plays a pivotal role in health and social care. Such factors as mood, marital relationship, family and social support are better predictors of quality of life after a stroke than degree of physical disability.[31] People with chronic illness and disabilities frequently feel that they are a burden, or may be perceived as such. Poor quality of relationship and social life are prime causes of stress in carers.[32] Families react in complex ways, ranging from avoidance to overprotectiveness, 'mothering to smothering', and often with a mixture of these. Within the intimate circle there is much that is experienced as loss as a consequence of chronic illness:

- **economic loss** – loss of employment, reduced income and increased expenditure due to illness requirements
- **loss of security**, sense of future, resilience and increased emotional demand

- **loss of sexual capacity** between spouses with, perhaps, loss of emotional intimacy resulting from pain, effects of medication, depression, debility and disability; these may lead to relationship breakdown and separation
- **isolation** may accompany prolonged illness; the family energies are consumed by the *illness work*; with diminishing outward reach the family becomes *encapsulated*
- **loss of opportunity** through reduced mobility, carers' loss of freedom to work or develop career, education, hobbies, sport and pastimes; family members feeling 'trapped' by circumstance
- **stigma** – the family unit participates in any stigma that attaches to the disease that 'resides' within their home.

> The quality of life of carers who live with patients, especially for female carers, is diminished almost regardless of the severity of the patient's disability.[33]

The experience of chronic illness blurs the boundaries of patient, spouse and family; they become a new functional (and, possibly, dysfunctional) unit, sharing out the caring tasks of daily living and illness management. This gives rise to questions of *agency*, such as confidentiality, testamentary capacity, and doctor–patient contract (who is the patient? and who can speak for the patient?). A further dimension relates to responsibility and hierarchy among the carers. There can be competition – for example, between a chief carer and next of kin in decision-making. The locus of control often moves away from the patient, with loss of autonomy, self-efficacy and sense of worth. Where both spouses suffer chronic illnesses and disability competition may arise that is attention seeking ('I'm sicker than you!').

The role of carers is explored in more detail in Chapter 4, along with social care.

The sick role: the person and illness behaviour

> For the chronically ill the sick role can be a permanent state.[34]

The negative connotations attached to being a patient can be traced back to ancient literature. The biblical Book of Ecclesiastes (38:5) has the aphorism: 'He that sinneth before his Maker, let him fall into the hands of the physician.' The seventeenth-century English *Book of Common Prayer* confesses: 'We have left undone those things which we ought to have done; and we have done those things which we ought not to have done. And there is no health in us.' The implications are clear – unhealthiness, sickness and needing to receive treatment have been perceived as indicators of moral failure, of self-harming through life choices, of not behaving responsibly, or of punishment for prior wrongdoing. The growing contemporary awareness of *'lifestyle diseases'* is curiously in keeping with these ancient precepts. There is a rich field for sociologists, as well as moralists, in exploring the sickness role.

Illness is by definition an undesirable state. Therefore, so also is patient-hood. Since the 1950s a school of sociological thought led by Parsons[35] has defined illness as *deviance* from the norm of health; thus to be ill is to experience *stigma*.[36] It should not be forgotten, however, that negative experiences and states can be turned to good effect. Without such it is doubtful whether we should undergo much personal growth or maturing of character, or whether we would develop capacities such as empathy. Like the immune system, we develop largely through challenge.

The concept of *patient*, like the experience of illness, is not simple and straightforward and it deserves a bit of 'unwrapping'. The word 'patient' derives from the Latin word for one who is suffering (*patiens*). As we move beyond the demand-led roots of medical practice towards more prevention and anticipatory care, the word patient becomes extended beyond its root meaning. It now encompasses all, ill or otherwise, who attend a clinician or doctor for whatever reason, or who are likely to do so by virtue of custom or registration. In a nationalised health system, such as in the UK, every citizen is thus a patient of some GP or other, whether or not he or she ever takes up the service provided. This recent historical development has attenuated the stigma attached to the term patient. Nevertheless, there is a quest for suitable, alternative terminology. Recent emphasis on rights and a consumer perspective have led to the use of other terms, such as client, customer and service user, borrowed from other contexts. The use of these terms is sometimes challenged.

EXAMPLE 2

Passengers on a transport system are now referred to as customers, implying that they are active participants in a transaction of services rather than just sitting in a vehicle that would be running in any case; their pattern of uptake constitutes demand in a market sense and this ought to be a determining factor in how the transport network functions.

A further example is those higher education institutes that now regard their clientele as customers rather than students. This may, perhaps, imply that their primary activity is no longer that of studying, but one of payment for use of the facilities provided.

Terms like this have influence on the philosophy and values at work beneath the surface of society. They suggest a shift of power relationship and a commoditisation of services. As dentistry moves towards an emphasis on 'the smile' and cosmetic interventions, it is not unusual to hear it described in the media as an industry.

Medical professionals, especially GPs, seem determined to retain the term 'patient'. This is despite their clinical work being dominated by an increasing emphasis on wellness, health promotion, surveillance and disease prevention. This stance is not purely semantic, but asserts that the doctor–patient relationship is, and will continue to be, a therapeutic one rather than an economic one. We have seen the growth of the word *transaction* to describe what is going on during the GP consultation process and this has been deemed appropriate since it expresses a patient-centred stance and the active participation of the patient in a two-way exchange of something valuable. The GP consultation has been described as '*a meeting between experts*'.[37]

Although the term 'patient' has value and dignity in the view of clinicians, it is a word that most people regard with ambivalence. They accept and endorse it as long as it applies to other people. Few seem happy to embrace it themselves, even those who are frequent attendees. It conjures up images of being in bed, clothed in nightwear (the uniform of infirmity), losing autonomy over their person and bodily functions, and adopting a humiliating position of dependency. In Parson's terms such abnormality of social function is expressed as deviance, and it bears a sense of stigma.

The role that relates to being a patient is not easy, even for those whose nervousness about their health leads them to internalise every perceived threat, ruminate on the significance of each sensation and 'run to the doctor'. There are many ways for people to express their resentment of the patient role:

- people who want their blood pressure checked at frequent intervals but do not take their anti-hypertensive medications
- those who weep copiously and yet are appalled at the suggestion of an antidepressant
- heavy users of tobacco or alcohol who will not 'pollute their system' with an antibiotic.
- demand for an urgent appointment but then not attending.

Ambivalence is not the preserve of patients only. Doctors become alarmed and defensive when a person enthusiastically embraces the sick role, suggests an array of treatments to be tried and produces a wad of Internet print-out.

There has to be a gain or a substantial reason for any adult to overcome the obstacles and to enter the state of patient-hood, however partial or temporary. It may be in response to a pressing symptom, or as a rational risk–benefit calculation. Public health campaigns offer a subtle balance of information and threat to motivate people to overcome the barriers to attending. They attempt to persuade the well person that he or she owes it to him- or herself to undertake a health-related action. Even health-enhancing activities that reinforce the autonomy of the person, such as change in diet or taking exercise, require persuasion. The external agent of change is resisted unless there is an element of fear or a reasoned assessment of threat. This is perhaps why healthy people nonetheless come to doctors to have screening tests, vaccinations, health checks and smoking-cessation help. *Be a patient in a small way now or you will become one later, big time!*

Alternatively, many well people demand their 'MOT' (routine check, like the annual vehicle inspection) with evident complacency which suggests a form of 'bargaining', the relief of existential anxiety, warding off for a time the threat of misfortune, even though the only established benefit is to private practitioners as a funding stream. The great popularity of alternative or complementary therapies may be seen as another form of bargaining against the sick role (though they may have benefits of other kinds).

Health-seeking behaviour is closely bound up with cognitive dissonance, that uncomfortable feeling that the way you are is not the way you would like to be, so you will make an appointment to have it fixed. Anxiety, unwelcome body shape, the loneliness of the smoker outside the pub on a wet night, the only one in the office who does not know their cholesterol number … all these allow people to cross the boundary from wellness into the realm of the sick, the clinic waiting room (and there you may have to be really patient!). Bit by bit people adjust to the patient role through minor, non-threatening episodes that relieve their cognitive dissonance. They feel better for it – dissonance resolved. They are pronounced well, screened, immunised and helped towards positive lifestyle change ('I'll see you again in three years …'), and the autonomy of feeling invincible and immortal is resumed and reinforced.

But not always:

> 'I'm glad you phoned for your result, the doctor wants to see you again; … no, I can't tell you any more than that …'

Whatever emphasis is placed on the lack of urgency of this message the recipient will insist on an emergency slot, and tomorrow is not good enough. The currency of screening, health promotion and prevention is fear of the Grim Reaper, that patient-hood is about to happen any time, for real.

The high road to patient-hood, however, is the onset of serious illness. Most of the common ones are self-limiting and mostly people doctor themselves. Severe, recurring, persistent or threatening sensations override the bargaining power or resistance to adopting the patient role. For most people such patient-hood is occasional, transient and limited. It can soon be forgotten, however unwelcome at the time. When significant illness becomes prolonged, severe or recurrent the role of the patient can become an identity that dominates the person's existence and distorts and complicates their other social roles.

Health, disease and illness

Health is a homeostatic mechanism – the continuing interaction of physical, psychological, social and environmental determinants, and not simply the absence of disease. Good health is compatible with encounters with illness. Very many people (40%) with established conditions describe their health as good; 72% of over-75s describe their health as good or fairly good, even though it is known that about 70% of over-75s suffer long-term conditions.[38] This is perhaps because they feel they are functioning as well as they can possibly expect, given their age and peer perceptions, and they have an optimistic frame of mind. The eminent American social psychologist Anselm Strauss is quoted by Cockerham[39] as stating that the chief business of the chronic sick is to live as normally as possible despite the effects of their disease, and this is not a bad definition of health for many people. Health can be defined negatively as the absence of disease, functionally as the ability to cope with everyday activities, or positively as fitness and wellbeing. Health also has commercial connotations: body maintenance associated with new trends in marketing ('Looking good is feeling good'), and transvaluation – that is, creating a commodity market promoted as health benefit around products, clothing, machines for jogging, slimming and so forth in what amounts to a fitness industry.[40]

With regard to disease in its various guises, there are a few terms where definitions represent significant differences.

- *Illness* is the experience of disease. It is subjective and defined by the patient (irrespective of whether or not there is defined pathology) and it normally results in changed behaviour on the part of the patient.
- *Disease*, on the other hand, is medically defined, as a patho-physiological dysfunction affecting an individual person, such as a tumour or a metabolic error.
- Sociologists, therefore, regard illness as a form of *deviant behaviour*, whereas the medical view of illness is of a *deviation from a physiological norm* of health and well-being.[41]
- *Sickness* is a social state signifying an *impaired social role* for those who are ill – for example, unfitness for work and confinement to bed.
- *Illness behaviour* is the expectation and normative behaviour that wider society has of people who are defined as *sick* by some authority (they 'should not be out enjoying themselves').

Illness as deviance: Parson's sick role

Illness has been defined by Parsons as a form of deviance by virtue of the expectations of altered social role and behaviour. These, the *sick role* and *illness behaviour*, can be legitimised through *medicalisation* as *disease*. This lends importance to the *labelling of the illness* as endorsement by physicians, and legitimising a set of otherwise deviant behaviours that then become acceptable, if not even compulsory.

Mostly society expects this to be a temporary state and there has to be very good reason for it to be prolonged or permanent. Sickness then, being a form of deviance, means that medicine is an institution for *social control* of this 'deviant behaviour'. The physician's role can thus be seen as one endorsed by society through rites of passage (training) and validation (by qualification and certification) to manage illness on behalf of society. The GP is seen as the gatekeeper, not only of the NHS but of the sick role, out of it as well as in, and having the power to 'medicalise society', a power that Friedson[42] saw as subversive. With regard to the exercise of medical powers, like writing certificates or ordering procedures, it has been suggested that doctors in some way create and ratify illness. This may be caricatured as, '*I went to the doctor about my problem. He didn't throw me out; in fact he ordered blood tests. I must be ill.*'

Illness as stigma

The sick role, as described by Parsons' model, is characterised by rights and obligations.[43]

> *The rights*:   exempt from performing normal social roles
>
>   exempt from responsibility for their own state
>
> *The obligations*: to want to get well as soon as possible
>
>   to consult and cooperate with medical experts whenever the
>
>   severity of their condition warrants it.

These definitions minimise the *stigma* that accompanies any behaviour that is regarded as socially deviant. However, stigma is not so easily avoided. It applies unevenly to people and their conditions depending on the element of *moral judgement* that is applied or experienced. An illness, such as HIV/AIDS, that may be *medicalised as disease* may be *moralised as stigma*.[44] Thus, alcohol dependency may be seen as disease (medical model) or as moral failure (deviant behaviour model). Goffman's[45] widely quoted definition of the stigmatised identity states:

> The stigmatised are a pejorative category of people who are devalued or otherwise lessened in their life chances and in access to the humanising benefits of free and unfettered social intercourse.

Stigma, then, is not simply about adverse moral judgement by society but an *experience* of deprivation or exclusion from full social freedom. Thus people who are in a wheelchair may pass unnoticed in a social gathering, feel excluded from conversations and unable to access public spaces. Their sense of their own personhood or dignity is accordingly diminished. They may feel the need to respond to this with assertiveness and invoking defined rights.

Behaviour in illness

People with long-term conditions face three particular challenging tasks, identified by Corbin and Strauss[46] as follows.

1. *Medical management*: this relates to monitoring symptoms, changing health behaviour, working with the therapeutic team.
2. *Emotional management*: dealing with the consequences of having a long-term condition – for example, anger, guilt, hopelessness or irritability.
3. *Role management*: some significant changes in social position or functioning – healthy to sick, breadwinner to unemployed, provider to burden, strongman to invalid.

In the light of these it is possible to appreciate reasons that might underlie some problematic behaviour, such as:

- the *paradoxical patient*, those who seem to use health services more than average but with perversely less than expected progress or change
- help-seeking behaviour that is entirely crisis-driven
- those who repeatedly default on medical appointments
- problems of compliance with prescribed treatments.

Some such problem behaviours correlate with the quality of communication in the doctor–patient relationship, the degree of partnership and mutual engagement achieved.[47] These qualities are of particular importance in the management of chronic illness and long-term conditions.

Disability and handicap

> It is a classic misconception that impairment causes disability – therefore the worse the impairment the greater the disability.[48]

The impact of disability depends on what is important to you. A recurring tennis elbow may spell unemployment for a bricklayer but a minor irritant for a teacher. Impairment of speech fluency may be incompatible with a career as a politician but not for his or her researcher. A few more definitions are therefore called for. Those provided by Wood[49] have stood the test of time and correctness, and are endorsed by the WHO – they are as follows.

- *Impairment* is *any loss or abnormality of psychological, physiological or anatomical structure or function*; that is, the extent to which a person's body is different from that of a person in perfect health. This approximately equates to a lesion or consequence of disease.
- *Disability* is *any restriction or lack (resulting from impairment) of ability to perform*

an activity in the manner or within the range considered normal for a human being. Thus, rather than being a disease it is a disturbance of function at the level of the person, the loss of functional integrity.

- *Handicap* is *a disadvantage for a given individual, resulting from an impairment or a disability, that limits or prevents the fulfilment of a role that is normal for that individual.* This reflects a societal imposition on people rather than what they can do to manage their condition (i.e. consequent disadvantage).[50] The simplest model of possible connection between disease, impairment, disability and handicap is shown in Figure 3.4. In reality, of course, their connectedness is much more complex, with loops and reciprocal lines of influence.

---

disease → impairment → disability → handicap

FIGURE 3.4 A linear model of disease and its consequences (after Locker[51])

These statements of definition, though useful, should be held up to some further scrutiny. Impairment, it is clear, is not always a consequence of disease or a cause of disability. Sensory impairment may be a concomitant of ageing and therefore be developmental and compatible with normal function in activities of daily living. Although there is a relationship between impairment and disability it may not be linear, but can be compensated to avoid or minimise disability (normalising). The term handicap has acquired pejorative connotations and is falling into disfavour,

---

Social Model:
Disabled people are disadvantaged by Society's failure to accommodate everybody's abilities.
Disabled people are oppressed by current social and economic institutions.
Disadvantage is best overcome by society adapting itself to everybody's abilities.

Medical Model:
Disabled people are disadvantaged by their impairment.
Disabled people are pitied as the victims of personal tragedy, disease or accident.
Disadvantage is best overcome through medical treatment or rehabilitation.

FIGURE 3.5 Disability: medical and social models compared (*source*: Aylward and Sawney[52])

and disability has emerged as the more commonly used due to acceptability as expressed by service users' groups. This reflects an uneasy dialogue between medical and sociological perspectives. Some comparisons between these are shown in Figure 3.5.

These two models and their components are not mutually exclusive or comprehensive. They are greatly influenced by context, perspective or intention on the part of individuals or groups since they address both causation and consequence implicitly. They do, however, illustrate one of the great divides in chronic care, between the medical and social care perspectives, and these have consequences for multidisciplinary approaches. All team participants bring to the table their respective cultural, ideological and sociological baggage wrapped up in their respective vocabularies (and each is tempted to dismiss the others' vocabularies as 'jargon').

THE HEALER ROLE

> Just as doctors have professional referral systems so potential patients have lay referral systems. The whole process of seeking help involves a network of potential consultants from the intimate confines of the nuclear family through successively more select, distant and authoritative laymen until the professional is reached.[53]

Klineman[54] suggested that professionalism has a tendency to distance practitioners from patients and to lead to a focus on disease (medically defined) as opposed to illness (patient defined). He delineated three areas of healthcare:
1. popular care, consisting of self-help and self-medication
2. folk care, seeking help from non-professionals
3. professional care, presenting to biomedical professionals.

> It is crucial to understand that whether or not people consult their doctors does not depend only on the presence of disease but also on how they, or others, respond to symptoms.[55]

These are reminiscent of 'the Iceberg Model of Health' as described by Last,[56] whereby professional health services treat only the tip of the sum total of ill health. There is a mismatch, a gap of unmet need, between the need for healthcare and the demand. Scambler[57] quotes a figure of one consultation for every 18 symptoms reported in one study. It is clear that the interface of presentation to medical services is far from simple. Much self-care goes on along with alternative, folk-model or non-orthodox therapies. There is evidence that one in three of the population go to alternative practitioners. This may partly reflect disillusionment with conventional medicine.

Help-seeking behaviour is complex and frequently inconsistent. Mechanic[58] listed as many as ten variables that influence illness and help-seeking behaviour that may be clustered as:

- perceptual salience of symptoms and their perceived seriousness
- disruptive symptoms; frequency, recurrence or persistence of symptoms
- culture, information level or understanding of significance; tolerance threshold; capacity for denial
- competing interpretations of symptoms; competing needs that inhibit illness response
- availability and access to treatment resources.

All clinicians know how complex their roles and their relationships with their patients can be. One of the first sociologists to study the physician role was Parsons in his major work, *The Social System*,[59] and whose model is still widely accepted. He constructed the basic paradigm of the *Patient and the Sick Role*, alongside the corollary, *the Doctor and the Professional Role*. Much of this is self-explanatory, and its similarity to current definitions of professionalism is striking. The doctor's professional role may be summarised as:

Obligations:	apply a high degree of skill and knowledge
	act for the welfare of the patient rather than own self-interest
	be objective and emotionally detached, non-judgemental from own value system
	guided by rules of professional practice
Rights:	granted right to examine patients and enquire into intimate areas of life, personal and physical
	granted considerable professional autonomy
	occupy a position of authority in relation to the patient.

Transactional analysis and the healer role

In a further development of role relationship models, Eric Byrne's *Transactional Analysis Model* reduced all social roles to three: the *parent*, the *adult* and the *child*.[60] He hypothesised that in every social situation we adopt one or more of these personae. These three modes are reminiscent of Freud's ego states, the Super-ego, Ego and Id; they are not age related but abstract. The Parent state is characterised as controlling, authoritarian and directive; the Child state is playful, spontaneous and instinct-driven, manipulative, and perhaps attention-seeking, dependent or complaining. The Adult state, on the other hand, is detached, autonomous, non-directive, reality-based and logical. When people address one another from different modalities, stresses and conflict are liable to enter; when from equivalent modes there is likely to be congruence only in adult-to-adult mode; otherwise there is conflict (parent-to-parent) or play (child-to-child).

The relevance of this relates to how individuals communicate, as in the consultation (or in meetings), and especially where it goes wrong. In adult-to-adult mode issues get discussed, agreements made and things achieved. The aim of promoting communication is to attempt to shift the discourse into adult-to-adult mode, wherever it starts out. The construct can be a useful analytic tool for addressing issues of social interaction, especially conflict. Models of role do not need to be literal to be useful as descriptors; they may serve a useful symbolic purpose. They are not judgemental.

EXAMPLE 3

For a very long time the doctor role, in interactions with patients, has been compared with that of father to child (paternalism). He is endowed with authority, a body of specialised knowledge that people need, validated by a title, qualifications, accreditation and regulated obligations. Additionally, there is the power to provide resources. Accordingly he is trusted, bound by a code of professionalism and ethics with a vocational, altruistic foundation. Therefore he behaves responsibly and for the good of his patients. Like a 'parent' (idealised!). Patients, on the other hand, are free to be whoever they are or wish to be. They can approach the doctor at any time and about any matter. In adopting the sick role they relinquish some of the adult characteristics; they may act out their distress, be attention-seeking, manipulative or dependent and expect to be understood and accepted. Like a 'child'. In developmental terms regression takes place; as Cockerham tells us, 'illness can result in a child-like state of dependency'.[61]

Small wonder, then, that doctors are subject to criticism in terms such as bossy, authoritarian, paternalistic, never listening. In transactional analysis terms the doctor may also subconsciously react to the regression of the patient and mirror it by embracing childish behaviour, such as complaining, self-pity, hurt or aggression; alternatively, he or she may misuse the parent style and become controlling, reproachful, directive and even coercive. The game theory suggests resolution of conflict through consciously adopting adult mode: calm, rational, negotiating, and facilitating the patient to accomplish a similar shift.

Implications for practice: clinical leadership

Undoubtedly the physician role is one of authority and responsibility. The power balance is a constant factor and has to be modulated actively rather than denied or asserted. Greenhalgh[62] eloquently expresses it thus:

An unequal power relationship between doctor and patient is inevitable. Clinical
Leadership is about how we handle this inequity for the benefit of the patient … it
is the illness itself, not medical paternalism, that makes the patient vulnerable and
the clinical relationship necessarily unequal … Doctors are invested with symbolic
authority – the socially sanctioned witness to suffering … **Clinical leadership is
maximising the power to heal while minimising the risk of abusing this power.**
(Emphasis added)

It is the professional who has to be the skilled communicator and have the interpersonal accomplishments creatively to cope with whichever ego state the patient
presents. Hence the centrality of consultation and communication skills in training for all health professionals. When chronic disease presents its marathon,
crisis-ridden course, role relationships are severely tested through prolonged and
repeated contact. Successful management requires establishing and maintaining
adult-to-adult mode in as far as possible. This implies that the clinician relate to the
patient in an attitude of equity and respect, with empathy and mutuality, to establish a cooperative, whereby participation in decision-making is the norm and the
patient is actively *empowered* towards *autonomy*, *responsibility* and *self-care*. This
is a recurring demand expressed by people with long-term conditions and their
peer advocates, and it is validated by the self-help organisations. If successful this
correlates with improved clinical outcomes.[63] The role of primary care physician is
particularly that of interpreter and navigator. He or she knows the labyrinthine corners of services in health and social care, the language and symbolism of disease, and
this is an area of vital importance to people. It is the professional's responsibility to
ensure quality of care provision, not to be derailed by the disease or the suffering of
the patient.

Our role is a complex one. We lurk in the murky waters between health and illness,
frequently with little in the way of guidelines that help us. When we do offer help,
that act can become part of the justification of the problem. If I wasn't ill the doctor wouldn't have helped, so it must have been an illness.[64]

Quality of care as a sociological construct

The sociologist Graham Scambler holds that quality of care encompasses more than
biomedical thoroughness. He goes on to list criteria for good care as:
- co-participation in care (emphasising autonomy and decision-making)
- open agenda in encounters
- holistic rather than merely disease management
- counselling skills to complement technical skills.[65]

All of these address and redress the power imbalance between physician and patient. In sociological terms quality of care is closely associated with quality of life. Health-related quality of life is concerned with the effects of an illness, including its treatments as seen from the person's viewpoint, their experience of symptom burden, and perception of well-being.[66]

All the social determinants of health interact continuously with quality of care. In poor neighbourhoods services are likely to be strained. Those most in need of healthcare are less likely to present for or receive it. GPs see more patients, work harder and achieve lower income than those in more privileged settings. They are liable to occupy poorer premises, with fewer staff members and are less likely to be training practices (these score more highly on indices of care quality).[67] Notwithstanding this, some of the outstanding examples of general practice provision are to be found in the most deprived areas. Quality in clinical care will be explored in Chapter 5.

> Everybody says that proper medicine is holistic medicine. And surely this is right. A proper doctor does not just treat a problem; he treats a person who happens to have a problem. He treats a mind-body-spirit unity. In this respect doctors are unique among professionals.[68]

Adherence and the treatment burden

Adherence is a major issue for patients' welfare, especially in their self-care. A few facts may illustrate this. One-third to one-half of medications prescribed for long-term conditions are not taken as prescribed.[69] A study for the Royal Pharmaceutical Society of Great Britain found that 15% of patients do not have their prescription dispensed; of those who do, 20% comply almost perfectly; 40% comply well enough to derive some benefit; 40% comply so poorly as to get no benefit; 92% of all transplant register deaths were due to non-compliance.[70] Medicines wastage and associated costs amount to £150 million in the UK.[71] In serious mental illness, 55%–60% of hospital readmissions result from non-compliance with prescribed medications[72] and in bipolar disorder 60% of annual mental health costs are due to hospitalisation, at an average cost of £12 000 per admission. The clinical consequences of non-adherence among mental health patients include increased risk of readmission, poorer long-term prognosis, impaired response to treatments and delay in achieving remission.[73]

Three related terms are often used synonymously, although they are not synonymous.

1. *Compliance* is the degree to which a course of prescribed treatment is actually consumed.

2. *Concordance* is the implementation by the patient of a plan of treatment that has been *negotiated and agreed* between patient and doctor.
3. *Adherence* is the continuing observance by the patient of a prospective plan of action.

These distinctions may be subtle but they imply degrees of duration, acceptability and participation in the process. Compliance is passive, concordance means involvement whereas adherence is persistence.

It is widely recognised that chronic disease sufferers are overburdened with treatment regimens, partly as a result of our healthcare systems. There have been calls for '*minimally disruptive medicine*', which takes account of the realities of patients' lives and tailors treatments accordingly.

> To the burden of illness is added the expanding burden of treatment regimens.[74]

This is not the only factor. Patients find onerous the organisation of visits to clinics for treatments, laboratory tests and other investigations, and communicating with different professionals from a variety of agencies. Added to this, in many healthcare systems, is managing the requirements of medical insurance and welfare agencies. These considerations by May *et al.*[75] suggest that clinicians should pay attention to:

- ways of identifying the overburdened patient
- ways of improving coordination of care
- development of guidelines for managing multiple conditions simultaneously
- involving patients and carers in streamlining processes.

> Thinking seriously about the burden of treatment may help us to think about minimally disruptive medicine – the form of effective treatments and service provision that are designed to reduce the burden of treatments on their users.

THE SOCIAL DETERMINANTS OF HEALTH AND DISEASE

It appears that almost every conceivable sociological phenomenon has an influence on health status, which must make sociology a fundamental health science. They are particularly influential in chronic disease. Those generally considered to be most influential are:

- social stratification and wealth
- work and occupation
- age
- ethnicity (especially minority status)
- gender
- housing, living conditions, locality, homelessness

- socialisation – adverse life events (bereavement, isolation and other stressors)
- lifestyle (nutrition, exercise, substance dependencies).

The epidemiological triangle expresses the causation of disease in terms of three components that influence one another: the agent, the host and the environment. The social determinants of health impinge on all three. Examples of these are, respectively, exposure to noxious agents (germs, toxins and air pollution), the host susceptibility (nutritional state, immunity) and environmental (ecological issues, socialisation, wealth and other resources).

> The WHO describes the social determinants of health as those conditions in which people are born, grow, live, work and age, including the health system. These circumstances are shaped by the distribution of money, power and resources at global, national and local levels which are themselves influenced by policy choices .... The social determinants of health are mostly responsible for health inequalities – the unfair and avoidable differences in health status seen between and within countries.[76]

Social stratification and wealth

The *inverse care law*,[77] first expressed by Julian Tudor Hart, postulates that the uptake of healthcare provision is inversely proportional to need. This implies that those who suffer least deprivation are best placed to access and make use of available services. The WHO[78] refers to *the path from chronic disease to poverty and the path from poverty to chronic conditions*. Elsewhere it states that inequalities are politically, socially and economically unacceptable.[79] People who are lower in the social scale (however defined) are likely to suffer disproportionately from all mortality, accidents, poor maternal and child indices (low birthweight and late antenatal booking – both correlate with higher perinatal mortality), and suboptimal uptake of immunisations, cervical screening and dental services.

These observations have changed little since 1981 when they were first recorded in the Black Report, published in Townsend and Davidson,[80] and reaffirmed by the Acheson Report 16 years later.[81] UK primary healthcare in deprived areas (notably inner city) has been characterised by deficiencies such as inadequate premises (due partly to high unit cost), problems in recruitment and retention of doctors and other staff, and a high proportion of single-handed and non-training practices. Rural areas have their own parallel set of deprivation indices. Contractual changes in the UK in 1994 and 2004 designed to redress '*the postcode lottery effect*' have had relatively little success. Overall services have improved but the deprivation gap remains resolutely evident. Recent UK government policy has committed to *equity* as a fundamental value in the NHS. Equity means the redress of these imbalances, first defined by Whitehead[82] (in 1990 and endorsed by the WHO) as *health inequalities* – differences in health that are unnecessary, avoidable, unfair and unjust. As Sir Michael Marriott, president of the British Medical Association said:

> We should have two main aims. One to improve health for everybody including the worst off. The second is to narrow the gap. We've done one but not the other.[83]

Work

Issues of impairment, disability and handicap are closely related to the ability to seek, gain and retain employment. It is no accident, therefore, that 50% of disabled people live in poverty.[84] Work as a determinant of health has profound implications for the person and society. Worklessness correlates strongly with higher morbidity and social disadvantage. According to figures from the Department of Work and Pensions,[85] in 2007 in the UK:

- 175 million working days were lost due to sickness absence in 2006 (or about 7 days per worker)
- 2.6 million people, about 7% of the working-age population, were in receipt of incapacity benefit (costing the taxpayer over £60 billion)
- at a total cost to the economy of £100 billion per year, which was more than the total cost of the NHS in England in 2008 (the time of reporting).

There is a strong correlation between unemployment and poor health, both physical and mental. People who work recover more rapidly from illness and, compared with those in work, people who experience redundancy are twice as likely to die.[86] There is strong evidence that unemployment leads to poorer physical health, with increased all-cause mortality, cardiovascular mortality and suicide.[87]

In the light of this influence of worklessness on health it is interesting to note that the influence of medical measures on work rehabilitation is relatively small. Hampton[88] reported the findings of the Leicestershire Fit for Work Scheme that 22% of those helped to return to work cited medical interventions, while 78% cited non-medical interventions such as mediation, personal support or help with new employment; he indicated the importance of de-medicalising people's problems.

Frequently, however, work itself can be a problem area. The Dunedin Longitudinal Study found that work-related stress is a major non-environmental contributor that doubles the risk of major depression.[89] Crude mortality rates are highest in heavy manual workers. The Whitehall Studies showed a gradient of health indices, lowest-grade civil servants having a mortality rate three times that of those with higher positions. Reports in 2012 showed up to half of GPs in the UK suffering from stress-related problems (*see* Chapter 8).

> Work and health are symbiotically intertwined.[90]

Age

To the sociologist age is a social determinant of health, not just a biological one. Life expectancy at birth is increasing steadily; infant death is a rare catastrophe; school days go on longer, adolescence begins earlier, around 50% go on to third-level education, childbirth is postponed to the brink of middle age. The goal posts are shifting. As the 'post-war baby boomers' reach pensionable age the concept of old age is being reviewed. They reach retirement on the whole well fed, well housed and medically supported, and many carry considerable affluence into 'the third age'. Substantial pension accumulation enables many to retire prematurely with the intention of enjoying prolonged and leisurely 'golden years', doing all the things they had not time to do before. This has been referred to as SKIING – 'spending the kids' inheritance'. By contrast, recent economic austerity is hitting the living standards of their children with effects that will be, for them, long-lasting. There is the prospect of a shrinking base of wealth production supporting a growing population of high-maintenance elders who have high expectations.

Among the retired there appear to be two distinct sets. Healthy life expectancy and disability-free life expectancy have increased, but so has the length of life with disability and illness. In the over-75 population, 72% suffer from a significant disability or chronic disease. The elderly have the highest rates of hospital admission, length of stay, polypharmacy and consultation rates. The single elderly are particularly vulnerable to poverty, especially women.

So, when does old age begin? The Theory of Disengagement describes voluntary withdrawal from normal social roles, occupational and family, in favour of the quiet life, making space for the younger generation to enter these roles. The Theory of Structured Dependency states that this is imposed by public policy with designated retirement ages (regardless of capability) and poverty-level pensions, leading to *the redundancy of the elders*. Third Age Theory suggests a new life of self-discovery and self-expression, as exemplified by the concept of a University of the Third Age. Perhaps these theories express coexisting realities related to a wealth gradient.

Whether wealthy or poor, this is expensive to society. The dependency ratio refers to the number of those aged under 16 and over 65, compared with those who are economically productive. Society is becoming top-heavy with dependent elders. In response the age of retirement is being pushed up even though discrimination at work on the grounds of age (ageism) continues to be felt.

So, age as a social determinant is not just about old age. In Chapter 2 we encountered the teen-transition problem in secondary care. Ask any 16-year-old with a hospital-dependent condition; age matters. It also matters to people aged 65–70 who are no longer 'normal' patients; they suddenly become geriatric. Age-bound silos are as divisive as any other kind.

Ethnicity

In the wealthy economies minority status correlates with disadvantage. Advantage appears to correlate with being a white, male, employed, middle-aged national. Immigrants, non-Caucasian nationals and travellers make up the main ethnic minorities. However vital they may be in economic terms, they experience disadvantage for reasons that are not just due to racial prejudice, although this is historically a major contributory factor. Social factors include:

- culture, especially in relation to family, family size and structure, and isolation
- educational attainment and linguistic capability
- confidence, assertiveness and mobility; feeling marginalised
- access to, and uptake of, high-quality healthcare and the need for interpreters, both cultural and linguistic
- lack of role models of success for young people
- the practice of remitting wealth to family and place of origin elsewhere
- housing, including the tendency for minorities to cluster in urban localities for mutual support, or for economic migrants and asylum seekers to be housed in undesirable estates far from the means of social support, recreation and integration.

While women are by no means a minority they share many of the characteristics of disadvantage that pertains to minority status. A black woman in the 1980s expressed the 'double minority' perspective, as shown in the following quotation (perhaps the recent increase in numbers of female medics has redressed her sense of grievance):

> When we approach the health services, as clients, we are confronted with a set-up which is both directed and controlled by white, middle-class men. This means that we can expect to face a barrage of assumptions about our race, class and sex by a profession which has no interest in the maintenance of our health, and little genuine insight into the factors in our lives which cause us to fall ill.[91]

Gender

Women are less likely than men to be high earners, employed or run businesses. They provide the bulk of domestic caring duties especially in relation to the elderly, the sick or disabled, and the extended family. They are more likely than men to be abandoned or widowed, to suffer domestic violence or to live as lone parents. In particular, in cultural minorities they experience restrictions on social integration and participation in the wider society. Childbearing, child rearing and other care duties interfere with employment and progress in the workplace. Women experience a persisting pay gap despite gender equality legislation – quoted frequently as 83% of average male wage. Thus, lifetime income is impaired and on retirement they receive smaller occupational pensions than men and are particularly liable to experience great poverty in old age. These factors combine to create what has been called 'the feminisation of poverty'.[92]

Patterns of marriage have changed considerably over the past two generations across Europe and the United States. In the UK 15% of families are lone-parent units and of these almost 90% are female-headed; 24% of children are raised in single-parent units, 90% by their mothers.[93] There is an overall reduction in fertility rates, first conception at increased age, increasing numbers of women do not bear children, and childbirth has become overwhelmingly medicalised. These gender-specific issues have health implications that are complex.

Women have greater life expectancy despite a generally poorer health experience. Relative deprivation and disempowerment correlate with poorer overall health and high risk of domestic violence. Nevertheless, women's health has improved greatly through advanced gynaecology and obstetrics. Life expectancy at birth and healthy life expectancy exceed those of men and suicide rates remain lower. These patterns are changing as women tend to adopt more masculine risk profiles through lifestyle changes, such as smoking and alcohol use. Disorders of body image and appetite disorders continue to be largely female concerns and all of these may be intensified by social consumerist and marketing trends. An excellent account of women and health may be found in an essay by sociologist Annette Scambler.[94]

Housing

Quality of housing is an important social determinant. It both reflects and creates social stratification. Residential areas of greater wealth are characterised by high quality housing, more and better social amenities for recreation and healthy living, access to educational, health and social care facilities, transport and other infrastructure, cleaner air, lower population density and better indices of public order. At the other end of the scale, homelessness has features of a chronic disease. The homeless have higher morbidity and mortality rates, poor nutrition and fragmentary healthcare, that is, lacking consistency and continuity. The life expectancy of a homeless man in one urban study in Leicester was 40 years and a national study from Sheffield University reported the average age of death as 47 years.[95] In times of economic recession, with reduced household income and rising unemployment, there is a rapid social sedimentation effect with increased homelessness irrespective of other factors. Unsuitable housing is a factor that affects people who suffer disabilities, especially in respect of accessibility. Rendering a family home suitable to accommodate a family member who becomes chronically ill or severely disabled can be problematic. There is a major problem area in social care placement for frail elderly or dependent patients following hospital discharge. This has created back-pressure on acute healthcare sectors. There is an overall shortage of social housing in the UK, largely attributable to the free market policies of successive governments since the 1980s. Isolation may result from housing issues such as placement of vulnerable people and lone parents far from family support and familiar social structures with consequences for their mental health and well-being, and for the care of children. The same is true of the so-called 'sink estates', which combine high-density housing, marginalised location, deficient social amenities and transport infrastructure, and poor access to employment. Such areas show high levels of illness and long-term conditions, high use of primary care and acute care, and social services that are stretched. Fluctuations in public expenditure have disproportionate impact on such neighbourhoods. They tend to be the last to benefit and the first to suffer. Living in a better area may not give you better neighbours, just better health.

Socialisation

Loneliness and isolation are bad for your health. Those who find difficulty with social integration are prone to depression, addictions and associated physical health problems. These further intensify isolation. Sudden dislocation of social circumstances such as widowhood, loss of partner, loss of mobility, unemployment, imprisonment and change of location for any reason are among the causes of isolation. So also is the experience of chronic disease, especially mental illness and disability. Increased levels of social coherence, the sense of belonging, create enhanced resilience in the face of the stress of life events. This *social capital*, as defined by the OECD, describes the pattern and intensity of networks among people and the shared values which arise from those networks, and is a measure of *social cohesion*, that is, *connectedness and solidarity among groups.*[96]

Health is tied to our sense of connection to community.[97]

Lifestyle

Life choices that people make have a major bearing on their health status. Indeed, these include the big five risk factors that underlie many non-communicable diseases and this is a recurring theme throughout other chapters of this book. They are obesity, lack of physical exercise, smoking, hypertension and elevated cholesterol level. Along with other addiction behaviour and trauma, these correlate highly with deprivation and marginalisation, that is, with poverty, poor housing, unemployment, isolation, low social participation and chronic mental illness. This is not to say that these factors are freely adopted and self-inflicted, or even to suggest that they are purely styles of living. There are chemical and genetic factors implicated in obesity, lipid level and addictions but the elements of these risk factors that are least amenable to control appear to be the behavioural ones. There is an interesting correlation between such lifestyle disorders and a history of traumatic experiences in childhood.[98]

SCENARIO: a reflective learning diary – patients, their carers and advocates

The e-mail popped up announcing a government-sponsored consultative day-conference entitled 'Developing Services for People with Long-Term Conditions'. Chronic disease is what GPs do; this looks good for the CPD portfolio, it's a day out and it's free. (I'll suggest to the new trainee that she should consider coming too, if we can sort out the rota.)

It turned out not to be what I expected. I was the only GP there and there was not a single clinical thought all day. In true civil service style it was multidisciplinary and inclusive across the natural boundaries of health and social care: managers and policymakers, patient groups and community organisations. There was an independent chair, minute takers, catered breaks and lots of *break out into your small groups and report back on ...'* To my surprise I learned much, and came away with copious notes and the outline of a Reflective Learning Diary concerning things I had little prior appreciation of, such as community work and self-help organisations.

Government and health authorities place much emphasis on the 'voice of the consumer'. They show the kind of attentive respect that provoked wistful thoughts in this GP. In turn, the bodies that represent the interests of patients demonstrate a grasp of the politics of service provision and a commitment to their 'community of interest' despite their mutual competitiveness. I was impressed with the depth of work that is going on at community level. The constellation of disease-specific organisations for self-help had found that forming a federation gave them a voice, an informed and informative network that filtered every public document for implication, threat and opportunity. This Long Term Conditions Alliance links with other bodies at a national level that network information and experience about what works elsewhere. The consequent depth of their analysis showed some sensitivity to the challenges faced by practitioners across the range of health and social services.

They draw on a wide skill-base of people who live with long-term conditions: business people, politicians, media personalities, teachers, academics, community developers and articulate individuals of no particular professional background. They came with confidence gained from knowing what they are talking about, that their experience has validity ('we are experts by experience'). They were not afraid of plain speaking.

Yet vulnerabilities were demonstrable in their sensitivities about use of language in discourse: 'people, not patients', long-term conditions rather than diseases; illness rather than disease; service-users rather than clients; disability rather than handicap; medications rather than drugs. At the same time there were hints of consultative fatigue, expressed as *'... another talking shop and still no mention of a strategy; ... but there is no new money; ... they expect us to find ways to work smarter as well as harder with what there is'.*

They had gone beyond the point of discovery that all long-term conditions share common ground. It is clear to those who attend day-centres and self-help courses that the other attendees have different diagnoses but that they share concerns over the majority of issues. They quote a figure of 80% of common ground in the care pathways of all chronic conditions. This leads them to conclude that services and programmes of care must be generic, although with flexibility to take account of specifics and complex need. 'Specialists may be special, but all patients are generalists', as one said. They have moved from a base that is condition-specific towards the generic understanding of long-term conditions, at the same time as shifting their strategy from competition to cooperation between voluntary organisations and beyond, towards the federation model. Naturally they have not abandoned or coalesced their individual power base, which is the local, disease-specific support group. That would serve to weaken the voice and validity they have gained. They know the dangers of fragmentation of effort and they know what it is like to receive fragmentary care.

Underneath a veneer of assertiveness, the professional patina that representatives need to adopt, an array of emotions were detectable ranging from a diplomatic conciliatory voice to anger that verged on aggression. They acknowledge and 'own' the full range of expressions from negotiation and advocacy to denunciation. They freely admit that people with illness are not always at their best (who is?), and often not easy to satisfy. They cannot afford to bask in a glow of complacency that progress is being made. Their membership will not for long tolerate a passive, time-serving representative. In this sense they are political, sceptical about 'progress without change' and consultation without product.

Oscar Wilde defined cynics as those who know the price of everything but the value of nothing. Representatives of patient organisations are not cynics. Costs they understand; values are at the core of what they do. With no profit incentives, their goal is to bring a sense of normality to groups of individuals, many of whom feel stigmatised, alienated and marginalised. They appear to be highly motivated to promote their community of interest.

People with long-term conditions want to feel normal, to live ordinary lives and to participate in family life and the life of their community. Clearly their respective long-term conditions (mainly cardiovascular, respiratory or neurological diseases, diabetes, cancers, sensory disability and mental illness) impinge on life in characteristic ways. That is the 20% or so of their agenda that is disease-specific, the remainder being the common ground.

Among the challenges they face are:

- persisting, recurring problems of symptom control: pain, breathlessness, weakness and fatigue
- uncertainty about the future that ranges from life expectancy to the timing of a weekend break
- lifestyle restriction: the limitation imposed by their condition, such as the difficulties with moving around their home, dietary restrictions, timing and use of drugs, and communication problems
- impact on family life through relationship stress, impaired sexual performance, contraction of the social circle, participation in family roles and activities that were once taken for granted
- the sense of dependency on caregivers, primarily the family and kinship circle
- care needs that stretch the patience of the patient: the patient experiences convoluted clinical pathways (especially where there is co-morbid disease); the patient spends a lot of time waiting ... for appointments, for the district nurse to turn up, for the spouse to come back from work
- guilt at loss of ability to carry out productive roles as bread-winner, parent or employee
- impoverishment: more than half of all those with significant disability live below the average household income because of loss of earning capacity and the increased living costs associated with their condition, such as heating and laundry
- stigma: the feeling or perception that they are seen as different or to be pitied, and thus deprived of respect, opportunity and inclusion
- despondency: the diminished sense of hope, actual mood disorders like anxiety and depression
- non-disease complaints include sleep disorder, diminished energy, accident proneness and constipation
- loss of self-esteem: self-efficacy, self-worth, impaired body image; loss of respect and privacy, especially regarding hygiene and intimate bodily functions.

Disempowerment results from many of these factors. When all sorts of things get done to you, with regimens prescribed for you, your world begins to shrink. From this emerges the 'Big Birthday Present List' (see Figure 3.3) of attitudes, activities and services that those with long-term conditions would like to receive from a compassionate and supportive society.

At the end of the workshop as we went our separate ways, all the words having ebbed away, I was left with strong images of what it is like to be a patient, of stories told and of living experiences shared. It was the first time in a career of over 30 years as a GP that I had given space in a focused way to this area. There was no rocket science, but I had learned much. Lasting impressions were encapsulated in a few whimsical sayings, a folk-wisdom that kept re-emerging mantra-like through the day and whose truth shone through any apparent triteness:

'Added life to years rather than added years to life.'

'We are people not patients.'

'I just live one day at a time.'

'Today is the first day of the rest of your life.'

'I may not have any degrees but I do know about sore joints and disjointed clinics.'

'The best time to plant a tree is 20 years ago; the second best is now.'

To which I mentally added a few lines, perhaps as a 'memo to self':

'If you don't really want to know, don't ask; if you don't want to listen, don't sympathise; if you don't want to do something, don't make promises and don't promise things unless you intend to deliver.'

(*Source*: McEvoy,[99] reproduced with permission of the *British Journal of General Practice*)

CONCLUSION AND REFLECTION

How can the journey through chronic disease be summarised? Something so individual and personal to people as their illness and their lived lives requires more than listening to their story. It also requires knowledge and the discerning of recognisable patterns. Much of this chapter has dwelt on pattern creation because that is the sum of the stories – making models that can help us to understand, interpret and draw conclusions. The patient complex, trajectory model and sociology all derive from the stories of countless individuals, distilled and condensed. To let the models throw light on what is happening we have to attend to the patient's story. However, we must not try to make the story fit the model.

Chronic disease may be agonising in physical, mental and social terms, boring, demoralising, full of fear, stigma or guilt, substance dependency, apathy and loss of adherence to treatment regimens. In reality, however, most people with long term conditions feel reasonably well much of the time. It is the crises that attract attention and interventions. The trajectory reminds us that the disease is going on even beneath the plateau surface. During the quieter passages denial and non-compliance tend to occur, with loss of preventive opportunities.

The full trajectory, the story and the sociology all deserve our attention.

REFERENCES

1. Sontag S. *Illness as Metaphor*. New York, NY: Farrar, Straus & Giroux; 1978.
2. Strauss A. *Chronic Illness and Quality of life*. 2nd ed. Chicago: Mosby; 1984. Cited in: Cockerham WC. *Medical Sociology*. 10th ed. Upper Saddle River, NJ: Pearson; 2007. p. 167.
3. Belfield G, Colin-Thomé. *Improving Chronic Disease Management*. Available at: www.natpact.info/uploads/ChronicDiseaseDHNotes.pdf (accessed 10 April 2014).
4. Locker D. Living with chronic illness. In: Scambler G, editor. *Sociology as Applied to Medicine*. 6th ed. Edinburgh: Saunders Elsevier; 2008.
5. Harris M, Klein R, Welborn T, *et al*. Onset of NIDDM occurs at least 4–7 yr before clinical diagnosis. *Diabetes Care*. 1992; **15**(7): 815–19.
6. Robinson I. Re-constructing lives: negotiating the meaning of multiple sclerosis. In: Anderson R, Bury M, editors. *Living with Chronic Illness: the experience of patients and their families*. London: Hyman Unwin; 1988.
7. Cockerham WC. *Medical Sociology*. Upper Saddle River, NJ: Pearson; 2007.
8. Gerada C. A tale of three practices. *Br J Gen Pract*. 2008; **58**(554): 653.
9. Chesterton GK. *Illustrated London News*. 10 August 1929.
10. Hamilton W. Cancer diagnosis in primary care. *Br J Gen Pract*. 2010; **60**: 121–8.
11. Kübler-Ross E. *On Death and Dying*. London: Tavistock; 1969.
12. Charmaz K. Struggling for a self: identity levels of the chronically ill. *Res Sociol Health Care*. 1987; **6**: 283–321.
13. Robinson, op. cit.
14. Prochaska JO, DiClemente CC. Stages and processes of self-change of smoking: toward an integrative model of change. *J Consult Clin Psychol*. 1983; **51**(3): 390–5.
15. Tuckman BW. Developmental sequences in small groups. *Psychol Bull*. 1965; **63**: 384–99.
16. Locker, op. cit.
17. Maslow A. A theory of human motivation. *Psychol Rev*. 1943; **50**(4): 370–96.
18. McEvoy PJ. Patients with long-term conditions, their carers, and advocates. *Br J Gen Pract*. 2013; **63**(608): 148–9.
19. Ibid.
20. Hjortdahl P. What do patients value? *Fam Pract*. 2006; **23**: 210–19.
21. Kelleher D. Self-help groups and their relationship to medicine. In: Gabe J, Kelleher D, Williams G, editors. *Challenging Medicine*. London: Routledge; 1994.
22. Bate P, Bevan H, Robert G; NHS Modernisation Agency. *Towards a Million Change Agents:*

a review of the social movements literature; implications for large scale change in the NHS. London: The Stationery Office; 2004.

23. Anderson R, Bury M. Conclusion. In: Anderson R, Bury M, editors. *Living With Chronic Illness: the experiences of patients and their families.* London: Unwin Hyman; 1988. p. 246.

24. Chinthapalli K. The birth and death of the Liverpool care pathway. *BMJ.* 2013; **374**: f4669.

25. Neuberger J. *Review of Liverpool Care Pathway: independent report.* London: Department of Health; 2013.

26. *European Certificate in Essential Palliative Care.* 9th ed. Esher, Surrey: Princess Alice Hospice; 2010.

27. Corbin JM, Strauss A. *Unending Work and Care: managing chronic illness at home.* San Francisco, CA: Jossey-Bass; 1988.

28. Mitchell S. (translator). Rilke RM. *Letters to a Young Poet.* London: Random House; 1984. pp. 85–6.

29. McEvoy, op. cit.

30. Locker, op. cit.

31. Anderson R. The quality of life of stroke patients and their carers. In: Anderson R, Bury M, editors. *Living With Chronic Illness: the experiences of patients and their families.* London: Unwin Hyman; 1988.

32. Ibid.

33. Ibid.

34. Cockerham WC. *Medical Sociology.* 10th ed. Upper Saddle River, NJ: Pearson/Prentice Hall; 2007.

35. Parsons T. *The Social System.* Glencoe, IL: Free Press; 1951.

36. Scambler G. Deviance, sick role and stigma. In: Scambler G, editor. *Sociology as Applied to Medicine.* 4th ed. London: Saunders; 1997.

37. Tuckett D, Boulton M, Oban C, *et al. Meetings Between Experts: an approach to sharing ideas in medical consultations.* London: Tavistock; 1985.

38. Scambler G. Health and illness behaviour. In: Scambler G. *Sociology as Applied to Medicine.* 4th ed. London: Saunders; 1997.

39. Strauss, op. cit.

40. Scambler G, Health and illness behaviour. In, Scambler G (editor), op. cit. p. 36.

41. Parsons, op. cit.

42. Scambler G. Deviance, sick role and stigma, op. cit. p. 172.

43. Morgan M. The doctor-patient relationship. In: Scambler G, editor. *Sociology as Applied to Medicine.* 4th ed. London: Saunders; 1997. p. 48.

44. Scambler G. Deviance, sick role and stigma, op. cit.

45. Goffman E. *Stigma: notes on the management of spoiled identity.* Englewood Cliffs, NJ: Prentice-Hall; 1963.

46. Corbin and Strauss, op. cit.

47. Loxterkamp D. Humanism in the time of metrics. *BMJ.* 2013; **347**: f5539.

48. Furze G, Donnison J, Lewin R. *The Clinician's Guide to Chronic Disease Management for Long Term Conditions: a cognitive behaviour approach.* Keswick, Cumbria: M&K Publishing; 2008.

49. Wood P. *International Classification of Impairments, Disabilities and Handicaps.* Geneva: World Health Organization; 1980.

50. Badley EM. An introduction to the concepts and classification of the International

Classification of Impairments, Disabilities, and Handicaps. *Disabil Rehabil.* 1993; **15**(4): 161–78.

51. Locker, op. cit.
52. Aylward M, Sawney P. Disability assessment medicine. *BMJ.* 1999. **318**: 2–3.
53. Freidson E. *Profession of Medicine.* New York, NY: Dodds Mead; 1970. Cited in: Scambler G. Sociology as Applied to Medicine. 4th ed. London: Saunders; 1997. p. 42.
54. Klineman A. Indigenous systems of healing: questions for professional, popular and folk care. In: Salmon J, editor. *Alternative Medicine: popular and policy perspectives.* London: Tavistock; 1985.
55. Scambler G. Health and illness behaviour. In: Scambler G, editor. *Sociology as Applied to Medicine.* 6th ed. Edinburgh: Elsevier; 2008. p. 46.
56. Last JM. The iceberg: completing the clinical picture in general practice. *Lancet.* 1963; **7297**: 28–31.
57. Scambler G, Health and illness behaviour. In: Scambler G. 1997, op. cit. p. 38.
58. Mechanic D. *Medical Sociology.* 2nd ed. New York, NY: Free Press; 1978.
59. Parsons, op. cit.
60. Byrne E. *Games People Play.* Harmondsworth: Penguin; 1964.
61. Cockerham, op. cit.
62. Greenhalgh T. Leadership reframed. *Br J Gen Pract.* 2012; **62**(601): 431.
63. Murray E. Providing information for patients is insufficient on its own to improve clinical outcomes. *BMJ.* 2008; **337**(7665): Article a280.
64. Haslam D. It's a fine line between health and disease. *Practitioner.* 2011; **255**(1746): 30.
65. Scambler G, Deviance, sick role and stigma, op. cit. p. 179.
66. Furze J, Donnison J, Lewin R. *The Clinician's Guide to Chronic Disease Management for Long Term Conditions: a cognitive behaviour approach.* Keswick, Cumbria: M&K Publishing; 2008.
67. Russell M, Lough M. Deprived areas: deprived of training? *Br J Gen Pract.* 2010; **60**(580): 846–8.
68. Foster C. Why doctors should get a life. *J R Soc Med.* 2009; **102**(12): 519–20.
69. National Institute for Clinical Excellence. *Medicines Adherence: NICE clinical guideline 76.* London: NICE; 2009.
70. McGavock H. *A Review of the Literature on Drug Adherence.* London: Royal Pharmaceutical Society of Great Britain; 1996.
71. Department of Health. *Making the Best Use of Medicines.* Report of a Department of Health round-table event hosted by the King's Fund. London: The King's Fund; 2011.
72. Young A, Copp P, Jerram P, *et al. Improving Treatment Adherence to Improve Patient Outcomes in Severe Mental Illness: increasing quality and addressing unnecessary NHS costs.* London: Astra-Zeneca; 2012.
73. Ibid.
74. May C, Mair F, Montori V. We need minimally disruptive medicine. *BMJ.* 2009; **339**: b2803.
75. Ibid.
76. Chief Medical Officer for Northern Ireland. *Annual Report 2008.* Belfast: Department of Health, Social Services and Public Safety; 2008.
77. Hart JT. The inverse care law. *Lancet.* 1971; **1**(7696): 405–12.
78. World Health Organization. *Innovative Care for Chronic Conditions: building blocks for action.* Global Report. Geneva: WHO; 2002.

79. World Health Organization. *The World Health Report: primary health care now more than ever.* Geneva: WHO; 2008.

80. Townsend P, Davidson N. Inequalities in Health: the Black report. Harmondsworth: Penguin; 1982.

81. *Independent Inquiry into Inequalities in Health Report.* Acheson Report. London: The Stationery Office; 1998.

82. Whitehead M. The concepts and principles of equity in health. *Int J Health Serv.* 1992; **22**(3): 429–45.

83. Marriott M. Presidential Address to BMA Conference 2012.

84. Organisation for Economic Co-operation and Development. *Sickness, Disability and Work: breaking the barriers.* Vol. 3. Denmark: OECD Publishing. 2010.

85. Black C. *Working for a Healthier Tomorrow; Dame Carol Black's review of the health of Britain's working age population.* London: The Stationery Office; 2008.

86. Chief Medical Officer for Northern Ireland, op. cit.

87. Bland P. Helping patients back to work. *Practitioner.* 2010; **254**(1729): 7.

88. Hampton R. Fitness for work – time to say goodbye to fit notes? *Medeconomics.* 11 Jan 2012.

89. Melchior M, Caspi A, Danese A, *et al.* Work stress precipitates depression and anxiety in young, working men and women. *Psychol Med.* 2007; **37**(8): 1119–29.

90. Bradshaw SE. Life's work: occupational health – the wealth of the nation. *Br J Gen Pract.* 2008; **58**(554): 605–6.

91. Bryan B, Dadzie S, Scarfe S. *The Heart of the Race: black women's lives in Britain.* London: Virago; 1985.

92. Pearce D. The feminisation of poverty: women, work and welfare. *Urban Soc Change Rev.* 1978; **11**: 28–36.

93. Office for National Statistics. *Social Trends.* Basingstoke: Palgrave Macmillan; 2011. pp. 7–11.

94. Scambler A. Women and health. In: Scambler G, editor. *Sociology as Applied to Medicine.* 6th ed. Edinburgh: Saunders Elsevier; 2008.

95. Thomas B. *Homelessness Kills: an analysis of the mortality of homeless people in early twenty-first century England.* London: Crisis; 2012. Available at: www.crisis.org.uk/pages/homelessness-kills.html (accessed 21 April 2014).

96. What is Social Capital? Organisation for Economic Co-operation and Development. Available at: www.oecd.org/insights/37966934.pdf (accessed 20 April 2014).

97. Loxterkamp, op. cit.

98. Ibid.

99. McEvoy, op. cit.

CHAPTER 4

Care of the chronic sick: the community complex

Contents

CHAPTER OVERVIEW

This chapter on the care of people with chronic diseases will look at what goes on outside the professionally led zones of care. It will examine the self-management role of the person who is afflicted with chronic disease, in prevention and in continuing self-care, supported by the carers who are the extension of that individual's own capacities, and then the social care provision of the community in its voluntary and statutory sectors. It concludes with a historical snapshot of how the NHS and social services evolved in the UK.

Chronic disease, as we have seen, is a familiar experience for a great and growing proportion of the population. It affects all age groups and is increasing in prevalence; its effects are cumulative over a protracted time span; it is complicated by other health issues; it affects the household and family of the victim; frequently it involves complex treatment pathways; the demands for, and costs of, care make it a social and political issue. Those who suffer from chronic disease find that what they require from society and the community is largely common to the range of long-term conditions. This suggests that care services should be structured around the needs of the long-term sick in ways that promote effective, personalised, continuing care – that is, *person-centred* care. Enhancing self-management is important in preventing deterioration and promoting health. Carers and families make remarkable contributions in these areas. Within the chronic disease paradigm (*see* Appendix 2) the *community complex* overlaps with the *patient complex* and carries the work of caring beyond the household. Since it describes the responses of society to the needs of carers and patients, Chapter 4 is of relevance to all clinical professionals, and especially to community workers and providers of social care services.

WHO CARES?

> Research based solely on the functional disabilities of people with the disease, on the one hand, or their individual psychological status on the other hand, cannot document the complexity and effects of social interaction on how people, their spouses and their families experience and manage their lives.[1]

The provision of care for people who have disabilities and the long-term sick is like a minefield. It is one of the greatest unsolved problems in the whole field of chronic disease management. We pour resources into the health services and get tangible clinical outputs and clinical quality, and we know what the costs are – around 10% of GDP. Battalions of people – volunteers, professionals and non-governmental organisations labour in the field of social care but what are the outputs, the costs and the quality? No one seems to know. Are they unquantified because they are unquantifiable? Does not the community simply absorb the bulk of caring responsibilities, with the assistance of the health services that take charge of medical matters? How robust is this dualism, how real is the partnership between healthcare and social care, or do we just operate dual standards? And where, in all of this, is the voice of the patients? What are the costs to them and how are they to pay for the escalating expenses that accrue with frailty and dependency?

SCENARIO: the village

Once upon a time there was a village in a valley. Everybody knew everybody else and all their business too. Those who had some 'get up and go' got up and went. They were the young, upwardly mobile people. They looked back on their village as bleak and dull, an inward-looking cultural wasteland. They called it 'the valley of the squinting windows' because they found it oppressive and intrusive. In the city they enjoy the salaries, smart apartments, wine bars, the liberated society and retail therapy. They form partnerships and have a child at the age of 35; they get a mortgage and begin to pay crèche fees. As the child grows they spend every leisure moment taking her to improving events and activities. Life is busy, good and expensive. They make their own wholemeal bread, home-brew beer, eat organic, hike the forest, vote green and take the child to the petting farm at the weekend. They have not forgotten the village. It was quaint. At half-term they visit the elders in the village.

But the child develops asthma (how could she, the house is so clean?). There are regular crises when she brings home a cold and begins to wheeze mightily, and the nursery school refuses to have her in that day, or the next. The boss at work grows hostile to sudden absenteeism; the GP does not open at 7.30 a.m. so they can't get child seen before work. Granny from the village has to parachute in to solve a crisis from time to time.

Later, granny gets ill back in the village and is slow to recover. It is out of the question to take her to live in the city; there's no room and she wouldn't fit in. Besides, younger sister is still single and she could move back home to look after granny. But no. She too likes the Chablis wine bar, the other girls at the office and the disco. And there's no point in asking brother to do it.

Fortunately, back in the village there is a young mum with several kids who lives around the corner from granny. She has known granny since she was a child and she pops in several time a day to keep an eye, count the pills, and bring the shopping … and a bit of casserole for granny's dinner. The GP and vicar have visited, and the social services are setting up some home help and meals on wheels from the local Red Cross. The good neighbour still comes around for a cup of tea and chat and keeps the young ones in the city informed. Problem solved. Even so, what is going to happen to granny when she gets worse? There is an old peoples' home in the next town, but there are rumours that it will be shut down. Something about money, or was it standards of care?

The multigenerational household is an endangered species. Now, with urbanisation and mobility, people have to look out for themselves; after all, most care is self-care;

but what are the limits? Our compact way of life means that there is no space for another dependent person to move into when circumstances change. It takes two incomes to pay the bills and there is no slack in the home situation. Why should women be expected to mend the loose ends of caring needs when men expect to be free of responsibilities in the home? When there is a child with a disability (as around 10% of them have) or frail elders, how do our expectations of personal fulfilment and family life accommodate this? Should there not be better services to take this load off the over-busy nuclear family? After all, they pay their taxes.

The robust family of the mythical village is giving way to the fragile, less stereotypical, urbanised one. Both have qualities and drawbacks. There have been undeniable gains, especially for the roles of women. But there is a price, and this is paid at the level of the community, through disjointed, fragmentary, expensive services that do not deliver neat solutions. We may plan for seamless, integrated medical services because there is a workforce of professionals which is coherent. The community is not like that. The phrase 'herding cats' comes to mind. One problem is the plasticity of our understanding of the overused word *community*. What is this community that all this care is supposed to reside in? Our mythical village embodies one image of community where people help one another out of messes because they belong and do not expect a market transaction return. The currency is interconnectedness, which is one of the sociologist's determinants of health. But the media speak of notional communities, the various ethnic, immigrant, religious, gay or homeless populations as 'communities', as if these were big, happy, extended families when what they mean is subsets of society. Furthermore, 'care in the community' means anything that does not involve occupying a hospital bed. This allows society to shrink inpatient services of all kinds because these are expensive, in favour of care in the abstract (and homely sounding) 'community', as if this were cheap. And it is, if we don't care or we don't care to pay for it. This is where the minefield has been sown and it is thick with explosive devices – downsizing public expenditure, women's rights, men's obligations, human rights, social mobility, child protection, family values, 'the big society', welfare dependency, the free market, workforce mobility – to name a few.

Somebody ought to do something!

So, who cares? Society is not a community and community is not the same thing as 'the community', which is shorthand for non-hospital structures that subsist in society. An awful lot of caring does go on, some of it structured, remunerated and formalised, but most of it informal and unnoticed. The last thing this informal economy of voluntary care needs is to have structures and regulation imposed on it to tidy it up. Regulation strangles community work. It is chaotic, and this should be respected because this chaos means complexity, autonomous forces impinging and interacting in unpredictable ways that, nevertheless, create patterns that have meaning. These patterns and meanings are the essence of care in, and by, the community.

The retreat from care in the bosom of the family and from institutional alternatives has created tensions in the caring function. Three metaphors may illustrate this:

1. the 'Pontius Pilate attitude', whereby we 'wash our hands of' responsibilities and consequences
2. the 'no room at the inn' realities at our places of refuge, hospitals and homes
3. the 'Bermuda Triangle effect' – that mysterious disappearance off the radar by some who stray into certain territory, even in calm conditions.

EXAMPLE

'We can't cope with grandpa's mood, dribbling and memory loss, he can't cope on his own and he fell out of bed last night; the GP will have to do something – get him into hospital.' [*Sorry, there's no room and he's not actually sick.*] 'OK, Dr, so we're calling an ambulance to take him to A&E; they'll get him in …'

[weeks later …] 'Your father is ready to go home now and he will be discharged at the start of next week, to give you time to make some arrangements.'

'Sorry, Nurse. I would take him home but there's no room and nobody to look after him during the day; you'll have to find a place for him somewhere – in a home …'

[*days/weeks later …*]

'We have found a very good place for him and it's only fifteen miles away and he will get some care from the district nurse there … yes, there probably will be charges for his residential care. The social worker will be able to tell you more.'

'But Nurse, he's a sick old man! He's not well enough to leave the hospital.'

'We understand your difficulties but he's not sick enough to need a hospital bed and we have a backlog of admissions waiting for a bed in this ward; we'll get the hospital social worker to talk to you; so, next Monday then, OK?'

Since 1979 in the UK the number of acute hospital beds has been reduced by 43% and length of stay has reduced from 9.4 to 3 days. This has been concentrated in particular sectors: geriatric beds have declined by 65%; for mental illness by 70%, and learning disability 96%.[2] The hospital sector has beaten a retreat from chronic illness care, especially those areas that involve extended stay and multiple impairments. No wonder it is now referred to as 'the acute sector'.

CARE IN THE COMMUNITY

Where is the patient's voice in the dialogue? The Bermuda Triangle of care is bounded by a rectangle – bounded by the hospital, the family, the community infrastructure and primary care. Under stress it is not long before these end up in mutual conflict, each for understandable reasons. What gets lost in the box is the vulnerable patient. His voice gets drowned out by the surrounding chatter and other issues that defy resolution. What does he want? Where does he wish to live? Can we facilitate this?

Have you ideas about how to resolve issues of 'bed-blocking' (now more politely called *discharge delay*), overloaded A&E departments and emergency services, undersupply of sheltered housing and residential care, insufficient domiciliary care workers or failures in integrated pathways? But we must not be negative. Tough cases make bad laws and utopia is a dream. As Schön said, we manage messes. The elderly and frail are not the cause of these problems and the caring challenges arising in sickness and disability extend far beyond the 'geriatric giants' and fragile families. Imperfect as society is there is a vast reservoir of resource, idealism, heroism and energy at work in it, and there is still a lot of community about.

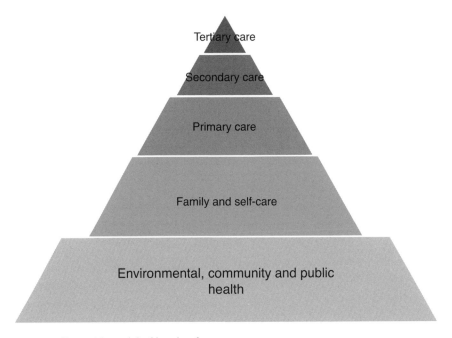

FIGURE 4.1 Pyramid model of levels of care

The care of the sick and people who suffer disability, especially those with chronic disease is a collaborative exercise and to be effective it has to involve all the stakeholders in a coordinated fashion. There is a well-known pyramidal paradigm of healthcare that places the most specialised at the apex and less specialised progressively further down (*see* Figure 4.1). The broadly based bulk of the pyramid is self-care. What is missing from this simple model is *the bedrock* upon which the pyramid is constructed. To extend this metaphor, it is the stability of the Giza Plateau that supports the pharaonic pyramid over the millennia. For our purposes the bedrock represents the contribution of the social units of the family system, community and society. A further development of the pyramid model would show an oblique sector of self-help running right through all levels of care, from the broad base that is self-care (where it represents the adoption of health-conscious behaviours and lifestyles), right to the pinnacle of tertiary care (where it might represent self-managed home dialysis while awaiting renal transplantation) (*see* Appendix 3).

LEVELS OF CARE: HOW MUCH, WHO CARES, WHERE AND AT WHAT COST?

The core of health and social care remains, as it always has been, self-care but there is a continuum of self-care that ranges from complete autonomy to total institutionalised dependency. Self-care represents the bulk of our pyramid below the stratified upper levels of professional care. When something goes wrong people look to those around them for advice, insights and help in solving problems. Self-care includes the use of complementary and alternative treatment sectors where self-referral applies. Scambler[3] describes these informal referral pathways and explains that just as doctors have a professional referral system, so do potential patients have lay referral systems.

Maslow's well-known hierarchy of needs describes the foundational building blocks of self-care. Alderfer[4] refined this as a three-level model (Alderfer's ERG theory):

level 1: **E**xistence – physiological and security needs
level 2: **R**elatedness – social interaction, contribution
level 3: **G**rowth – self-esteem, self-actualisation.

All three levels contribute to health, well-being and prevention of disorder and have to be sustained. Alderfer proposed that the less a high-level need (growth) is satisfied, the greater the importance that attaches to the lower-level needs (relatedness and existence). Serious illness threatens the capacity for personal growth (level 3) unless the patient discovers and develops compensatory capacities, such as social involvement and contribution (level 2), which support the patient and enable him or her to continue to function at the higher level despite the difficulties. People who succeed in this become the backbone of voluntary organisations and expert patient programmes.

The patient complex is the collective term used in Chapter 3 for the person within his or her nuclear and extended family, and this is embedded in the *community complex*. Family surrounds the individual like a survival suit, sharing the burden, the successes, failures, stigma and other consequences of the ill member's illness. The patient and family participate also in the benefits and resources that go with belonging in a community. Relatedness can compensate for loss of the higher 'growth' functions and the family system is paramount in this. Failing this, formal structures of social care can act as a backstop by guaranteeing the most basic level of Alderfer's needs hierarchy, the means of survival. Community and society further support the existence of the family unit to varying degrees related to socialisation, social capital and state welfare provision. In adversity, such as serious or long-term illness, caring is a function of all these strata of society. Breakdown in health at the level of the individual person leads to calling on resources from successively higher strata. Thus when illness leads to the individual adopting the sick role, their impaired self-care is supplemented by the nuclear family, then wider family.

Where this is deficient, neighbours and friends are co-opted as proxies. Reinforcement from the wider community may be called upon. Primary healthcare and social care bring further resources (such as district nurse or home help) and the voluntary sector may be activated (welfare rights advice, meals on wheels, etc.) (*see* Figure 4.2). Behind this many-layered capacity for response there has to be an organising principal in order to avoid chaotic and overblown responses, or indeed, stasis. People need help to learn how to carry out this collaborative function. This is a major component of chronic care, involving patient education, support and behaviour change. It is called *supported self-care*. As Friedson observed:

> The whole process of seeking help involves a network of potential consultants from the intimate confines of the nuclear family through successively more select, distant and authoritative laymen until the professional is reached.[5]

Professional interventions are formalised within a community care plan to coordinate the respective contributions. At the national level, society underpins all of this with financial resources, benefits, systems, policies and enabling legislation. In terms of the chronic disease paradigm, the patient complex merges into the community complex and both link into the clinical and policy complexes (*see* Appendix 1).

Family system: spouse, children, siblings and beyond

Community system: friends, neighbours, colleagues, community self-help

Social care system: care workers, social workers

Health system: district nurse, GP and beyond

FIGURE 4.2 The range of caring resources in the community

Provision of care may be categorised as:

- informal care – unpaid caregivers within the patient complex
- formal care – care workers, those paid to provide personal care services to the patient at home (or elsewhere)
- community self-help – the third sector, those support groups or voluntary organisations providing programmes of care
- statutory and social services – social workers and associates, implementing 'care in the community' policies.

Care: how much?

> The effect of caring on carers can be immense, both in physical and financial terms.[6]

An occasional review of my patients indicated that some were in contact with as many as 10 different agencies providing health, social and community support. The real, cumulative extent of social care is unquantified. This is partly because we have been relying heavily on the efforts of the extended family system, and society has forgotten to pay them. The lack of attention accorded to the contribution made by voluntary, informal carers has been attributed to 'state collusion'. This infers that the state consciously provides minimalist support and that this is designed to protect the system from liability for massive expenditure, and to prevent breakdown of informal caring rather than relief of distress. 'Care in the community' then becomes 'care by the community'. Informal caring relies on personal ties, those of kinship, friendship and neighbourliness.[7] Public policy concerning care in the community is based on the expectation that formal care arrangements will be thus routinely and informally supplemented, notably by women. This raises a question as to whether self-care and family care should be remunerated, and within what limits. The dimensions of the informal care scene may be gauged from a few descriptors (the website of Carers Trust is a rich source of data on carers[8]):

- the estimated number in the UK with long-term conditions is 15 million
- there are reckoned to be six and a half million carers in 2011
- this amounts to one in seven workers, or 11% of all those aged more than five

- 75% of carers are looking after an elderly person, 80% caring for a relative, providing physical or emotional support or both
- 70% are financially worse off after becoming a carer and 24% provide 50 hours per week or more
- women predominate as formal care workers, as informal caregivers under the age of 65, and outnumber men as carers until the age of 75, when the balance becomes even
- 58% of informal carers are female; women have a 50% chance of becoming a carer before the age of 60, men a 5% chance by age 64
- the peak age for caring is 50–59, and rising[9]
- the value of all of this to the economy has been estimated as outstripping the cost of the NHS at £119 billion; of the 65 and over population 11.5% provide some kind of care.

With increasing life expectancy, men are taking up a greater share of the care burden.[10] Among spouse carers, the gender balance is even. Although both men and women of all social classes are providers, women in lower social classes are disproportionately involved. Women provide more personal care, while men provide more 'instrumental' care (that is, 'hands-off', such as shopping, money management or heavy housework). Women provide the bulk of care for children with disability; studies show that around 12% of children have one or more disability.[11]

Carers become defined by the social context of the situation in which they find themselves and not necessarily through personal choice. Some coercion may lie behind this. It is not uncommon to find reluctant but guilt-ridden carers looking after a relative who, in turn, may exhibit hostile dependency. This tends to result in insecurity and fragility of care, which may lead to breakdown of care arrangements. Relationships are almost inevitably changed through provision of care. Equality in friendships, partnerships or sexual relationships gives way to dependency and loss of emotional reciprocity (*see* also Chapter 3, 'Relationship complexity'). A substantial contribution to caring activity is provided by the very young. It can be difficult to identify who the carers are – they are often reluctant to self-identify. Stevenson, recommends that

> GPs should create a register of carers, endorse their medical notes … identify them, listen and ask their opinions, and provide information, that is, treat them as a part of the care team.[12]

CASE REPORT: JOSEPH

Joseph is a 40-year-old company representative who enjoys the social contact and driving that his work entails. He is married, with two teen children and has a mortgage on his modern home. As a result of a serious road accident and head injury he develops personality change, headaches that become chronic and he begins to suffer grand mal episodes. As the sole wage earner he soon finds the sudden loss of income unsustainable. The house has to be sold, but he is fortunate to be allocated a small house by the local authority. His wife learns to drive for the first time and seeks employment, having no particular qualifications. Joseph becomes depressed, increasingly dependent, avoids taking responsibilities and begins to use increasing doses of analgesics and psychotropics in addition to his anticonvulsants. A series of legal disputes, including the aetiology and time of onset of his epilepsy, delays and reduces his compensation award. When it comes through, his wife, unable to find employment, decides to invest it in a small florist business. The daughters help out in the shop after school, willingly at first. New levels of responsibility combined with caring needs result in Joseph's wife becoming anxious, then deeply depressed. The business fails. The youngsters, though intelligent, are unable to prolong their education. The elder daughter takes on a caring role for her parents and her younger sister, who eventually finds a job as a shop assistant. Apart from state benefits and continuing prescriptions, there is little support demanded or received by Joseph and his family. They continue to live as a unit though increasingly isolated and despondent.

Informal carers

> provide unpaid support to family or friends who could not manage without this help. This could be caring for a relative, partner or friend who is ill, frail, disabled or has mental health or substance misuse problems.[13]

Some of the issues and concerns that arise for carers are exemplified in the Scenario in Chapter 3 entitled 'a case study').The many possible descriptors of a carer might include some of the following:

- most likely to be a woman in her fifties
- a dual ('sandwich') carer, with childcare duties in addition to elder care
- a spouse, family member, relation or live-in partner, next of kin
- a lone carer, unmarried daughter, socially isolated
- a young person of school age, a person in employment, an old-age pensioner
- in a decision-making capacity
- in an unfit state of health to do the job
- not doing it willingly and voluntarily.

Their position does have some safeguards and recognition. In 2008 the European Court of Justice ruled that laws that protect disabled people against discrimination apply also to their carer.[14] All carers are entitled to a *Carer Assessment*, which is carried out by social services and aims to:

- recognise and value the work of carers and support them in their role
- quantify care and its impact on them
- identify and support their needs – for example, respite
- identify means and sources of support for them.

This procedure may work better in theory than in practice, since it may not carry a designated budget. The duties of caregiving are bound to conflict with other life priorities. A crucial one is paid employment outside the home. Work is frequently a lifeline for the carer in terms of socialisation, mental well-being and family income. The demands of long-term care tend to increase with time, but the positive effects of employment are perhaps more crucial than ever when the domestic caring pressures are high. There comes a point of decision-making when the balance between the dual roles and obligations becomes problematic. A carer thinking of giving up work should get advice about all options (from, for example, their trades union, personnel manager, Citizens Advice Bureau, health and social care trust). Possibilities may include:

- a career break
- compassionate leave, carers' leave or leave of absence (no pay, but job protection)
- reduction in working hours
- flexible working
- work from home
- redeployment
- welfare rights advice.

Hints for doctors

- Accord carers as much dignity and respect as you do to patients
- Record who is the chief carer (as you would next of kin – they are often different)
- Consider inquiring about carers' health and personal issues; they carry burdens of their own in addition to their caring role; breakdown of caring arrangement hurts everyone
- Request or arrange a carers' assessment by social worker
- Inform about respite possibilities
- Be alert for juvenile carers and those with depression, fatigue, burnout or other risk factors.

If the carer leaves the surgery feeling more confident, that their role has been understood and acknowledged, they will be better able to avoid health risks that are due to the stress of feeling alone.

Anonymous caring relative

Children as carers

The hidden army of young carers.[15]

Saul Becker

There is a little-researched cadre of youthful care providers that had been estimated at 1% of the under-16s. A survey in 2011 by the British Broadcasting Corporation of 4000 secondary school pupils revealed that one in twelve said they carried out care duties such as dressing, washing or bathing. If representative of the UK population, this indicates 700 000, rather than the official estimate of 175 000.[16] There are estimated to be a quarter of a million young carers under the age of 19.[17]

Becker reported that young carers commonly showed characteristics summarised in Figure 4.3.

Carer assessment in this special group is aimed at:
- supporting the childhood of the child
- school support, education and training
- after-school clubs
- emotional and developmental support
- respite, leisure and personal development.

- Restricted opportunities for social networking and peer friendships
- Health problems and emotional difficulties
- Widespread educational problems; limited horizons/aspirations
- Sense of 'stigma by association' (especially if parents have alcohol or drug misuse, mental illness or HIV/AIDS); lack of understanding by peers
- Fear of what professionals might do to them
- Keeping silence and secrets through fear (of attitudes of professionals or the public)
- Significant difficulties in making the transition from childhood to adulthood

---

FIGURE 4.3 Young carers: characteristics and outcomes (*source*: based on Becker *et al.*[18])

Formal carers

Care workers (or care assistants and 'home helps') are employed to provide basic assistance with personal care and the activities of daily living at home. They are often employed through private sector agencies or by social services, and may work exclusively within supported accommodation or nursing homes. Their terms of employment are often characterised by part-time or short-term contracts, low levels of training and status, payment at minimum wage level and absence of career structure, so that retention rates are poor. Recruitment is largely from among deprived groups, notably migrant workers or social minorities, women and school leavers. In hospitals intimate patient care is increasingly delegated to unqualified staff. Following reports in 2013 of instances of poor standards of care in some English hospitals, the Cavendish Review recommended that all healthcare assistants (in hospitals, care homes and domiciliary care) should undergo training and certification before they can care for people unsupervised.[19]

There has been much criticism of the service provided by care workers, for reasons that are mostly beyond their control:

- rigid, inappropriate or unrealistic allocation of time
- lack of continuity – you may not know which care worker is going to arrive in next
- erratic timekeeping, delays and lack of punctuality
- cultural and linguistic incompatibilities with the recipient.

Issues such as these may be addressed through *the Direct Payments Scheme*, which permits the individual to employ directly on their own terms, the personal attendant of their choice, within an allocated budget (v.i.). People in the UK may receive other benefits that may enable them to purchase or commission additional resources by themselves.

> If you do not treat care workers well how can you expect them to treat well those for whom they are caring?[20]
>
> Baroness Julia Neuberger

Care: where?

The care system – that is, the collective resources and processes that are concerned with the provision of community care – aims to sustain and enhance the dignity, well-being and self-sufficiency of the person through supporting his or her existence at its optimal level *in the situation of least intensity*. The default situation is in the person's own home, with appropriate levels of support. Financial arrangements through the *Direct Payments Scheme* (also known as personal budgets) permit, as we have seen, the individual to purchase directly elements of their own care, perhaps by employing the care workers of their own choice. This is supported through an advisory service that assists with employment technicalities. Compared with usual funding arrangements, the personal budget is intended to be cost-neutral and to 'allow me to be the expert on me'.

Personal care plans are packages of care that are individual, formulated by the social services, usually at a multidisciplinary case conference of all stakeholders. Based on a needs assessment, this takes account of the person's care requirements, financial means and the degree of informal care available. A named care manager and key worker are appointed to implement and oversee the process. Such a plan may include:

- allocation of 'home help hours' to support daily living at home
- a care assistant to help with dressing, bathing, mobilising from bed to chair, and so forth
- welfare rights assessment and advice
- voluntary sector involvement (e.g. mobility and transport assistance, meals on wheels, day centre attendance, support group)
- essential home-nursing care, such as managing a stoma, catheter or dressings
- occupational therapy assessment of needs, for mobility aids, domestic appliances and other *assistive technology* or even house alterations to promote disability access or sanitary facilities
- periodic review of progress and needs.

The principle of *care in the location of least intensity* implies that there is a variety of levels of supported living. Within the home, much clinical care can be provided through intermediate care processes such as hospital-at-home, virtual ward, connected healthcare and telemedicine (*see* Chapter 5). Where home-based care is no longer a viable option, admission to *supported living* may be necessary. This is designed for autonomous living, with supports and safeguards:

- a resident warden in a supervisory role
- basic support for activities of daily living
- basic personal security measures
- social support through communal living options (e.g. a recreation room, facilities for socialising and provision of meals).

Access to supported living is under the control of the social services. Providers are mostly in the charitable, private or commercial sector since in parts of the UK half of state-run residential homes have been closed. Costs may be financed from social care budgets, depending on means-assessed eligibility. Service quality is the responsibility of the Care Quality Commission. Healthcare is provided through the person's own general practitioners.

This merges into the institutional territory of *residential care homes* where comprehensive, social care is provided, indefinitely if necessary, and *nursing homes* where the degree of need requires the full range of nursing care, including administration of medication. Admission to institutional care should take place when home care or supported living arrangements cease to be compatible with optimum care. It should be for the shortest period of time that is effective in restoring patients to living at home, but may need to be long-term. This should not be a merely financial calculation, although cost will be a consideration. The patient's wishes should be respected and protected, in so far as their testamentary capacity and personal safety can be assured.

Care: at what cost? Funding social care

Social care is one of the great unresolved issues of our time.

> A method for funding long term social care costs needs to be agreed urgently to cope with the demographic bombshell.
>
> Helena McKeown, chair of the British Medical Association's
> Committee on Community Care

Social care policy is controversial in the UK, as elsewhere. It has a restricted meaning in policy terms – the need to undertake for people who are no longer able to live independently even with the support of their informal care network; when their care needs require a degree of formal care support. Faced with the population time bomb resulting from the post-war 'baby boom' (among other factors), the prospect of writing blank cheques recurrently into the future is anxiety-provoking for government. Individuals, however, encounter mounting expenditure in relation to their real needs, since residential care is not covered by the free NHS but means-tested as a benefit. Potentially crippling charges cause problems especially for the frail elderly when they are deemed fit for discharge from hospital care but, unfit to live autonomously in the community, they require expensive social care provision. The back pressure that results from consequent discharge-delay is experienced in hospitals in the form of prolonged hospital stay, slow turnover and delays to admissions through congested A&E departments; and in primary care in the form of lengthening waiting lists as hospital services become saturated.

CASE REPORT: PATRICK

Patrick is a 76-year-old Alzheimer's sufferer who is physically strong but whose confused and aggressive behaviour has required admission to a specialist unit for assessment and symptom control. He gradually improves through stabilisation of his diabetes, treatment of a urinary infection and rationalisation of his medication. Eventually he is declared fit for discharge home. His relatives object on the grounds that they could not manage to care for him at home. An alternative offer of a place in a residential home with community mental health team support is rejected because the cost of the social component of care would affect the finances of the family. He remains an inpatient pending resolution of an appeal to the Clinical Commissioning Group.

There is a high degree of concern about the implications for public policy of an ageing society where there is enhanced life expectancy with disability. The Commission on Funding of Care and Support (Dilnot Commission)[21] was established in the UK with the remit to make recommendations to government on means of funding the demand for social care. A variety of options were considered, including:

- *social care insurance* – through compulsory income contributions
- *equity release* – a kind of mortgage on property assets
- *deferred payment* – to be realised from the estate of the individual following demise
- *co-payment* – shared payment by the State and the individual according to his or her circumstances
- *payment ceiling* – a guaranteed upper limit to personal liability (Dilnot recommended £35 000)
- *advance payment* – a lump sum paid at commencement irrespective of duration of survival within the care system.

The UK government has accepted the lifetime payment ceiling option, but the Treasury insisted on raising this ceiling to £75 000 per person.

The welfare system is the big public service spender in the UK. A constant preoccupation of government is to reduce this and punish any fraudulent claimants. The historical accumulation of separate benefits and allowances was pruned and consolidated in 2013 as part of the ever-changing kaleidoscope of social security. Patients and carers who necessarily rely on benefits experience stress, an increased sense of stigma and constant uncertainty in the face of frequent changes. Benefits may be means tested and taxable.

Disability is complex and individual, and benefits ought to match degrees of need. However, simplifying the benefits system risks unfairness and one-size-fits-all solutions belittle disability. Frequently the stress that results creeps into the consultation in general practice and GPs are poorly equipped to manage this. People need expert advisers on entitlement to act as advocates and assist them in navigating the forms and websites. An independent Citizens Advice Bureau is an essential feature of civil society. Few people live the high life on social security. There is a balance to be struck that avoids the extreme of a system that 'washes its hands of responsibilities'.

> We don't want the nanny State, but we don't want the Pontius Pilate State either.
>
> John Reid, former UK Health Secretary

ISSUES IN CARE: AUTONOMY, ADVOCACY AND AGENCY

Respect for the autonomy of the individual is one of the four conventions of medical ethics, the others being beneficence, non-maleficence and justice (or fairness and equity).[22] Without resorting to rights-based arguments (which tend to be problematic), there is widespread support for these as fundamental professional values. Autonomy is usually expressed as preferences and decisions, and mental capacity is vital for these functions. *Testamentary capacity* informs all decisions that relate to care and treatment, especially where there is significant mental illness, physical vulnerability, at the end-of-life trajectory phase and in situations where the person has to be protected from exploitation, fraud and manipulation. This involves an evidence-based judgement reached by a competent authority (such as a psychogeriatric specialist) as to whether the person is capable of informed consent. An example of a highly emotive situation, for those who are experiencing increasing dependency, is the decision to relinquish their home, since this is vested with deep significance. Various parties are involved in this, in addition to the patient – their next of kin, principal carer, and medical and social work professionals. The guardians of the patient's rights include all of these and, ultimately, the courts of law. Various legal instruments play a part – *power of attorney* (recorded by the patient while mentally competent, this enables a nominee to act on his or her behalf), *living will* (advance directive), the Mental Health Act 1983 and court orders. These govern difficult and extreme circumstances such as end-of-life issues or where compulsory treatment is contemplated.

Much debate surrounds decisions by people to bring about the end of their own life ('voluntary euthanasia'), especially where it is seen to be possible only through the complicity of others ('assisted suicide'). This raises profound issues relating to ethics, law, custom and precedent, especially where it may involve action by medical professionals to terminate life. Then the principle of autonomy is in direct conflict with the millennia-old medical ethic of nurturing and sustaining life until its natural end. This profound conflict of values challenges the caring professions to develop alternatives, such as to maximise the full range of palliative skills and measures. There is no fundamental conflict between ethical principles and considerations of empathy or humaneness. For example, the principle of *the act of double effect* foresees that if increases in the required levels of medications were to compromise the terminally ill person's viability this would not infringe the principle of respect for life, since the primary intention is to relieve distress.[23] There is much evidence of historical underuse of opioid pain relief in palliative care and little evidence that high doses used in relief of severe pain curtail life.[24]

THE EXPERT PATIENT AND SELF-MANAGEMENT

> Expert patients are those who take responsibility for the day-to-day decisions about their health and who work with healthcare providers as collaborators and partners to produce the best possible health given the resources at hand. Expert patients are not only consumers of healthcare, they are also producers of healthcare.[25]

Expert input is most useful where there are matters that are complicated, such as needing judgement, knowledge, information and communication skills or special expertise. But professional expertise has limitations, creates dependency, is expensive to provide and only intermittently available. People, on the whole, wish to take responsibility for their own illnesses, especially for the everyday aspects. Self-management programmes (SMPs) strive to achieve the elements of both personal responsibility and expert input. The best known of these is the *Chronic Disease Self-Management Programme*, or the *Stanford Model*, which in the UK gave rise to *the Expert Patient Programme* (EPP).[26] There are many kinds of self-help group-based models, but the EPP is the most highly developed one in the UK.

> Self-management is the responsibility of the individual. However, this does not mean people doing it alone. Successful self-management relies upon people having access to the right information, education, support and services. It also depends upon professionals understanding and embracing a person-centred, empowering approach in which the individual is the leading partner in managing their own life and conditions.[27]

The chronic disease self-management programme

> Self-management of long term conditions is not a luxury but a necessity.
>
> **Sir John Oldham**

SMPs date back to 1970 in the United States, to the collaboration between Kate Lorig and Albert Bandura at Stanford University, which combined her pioneering work on practical self-management with his social learning theory on self-efficacy. The initial courses addressed the needs of arthritis sufferers and the resulting programme was successfully introduced to the UK by Arthritis Care as the Arthritis Self-Care Programme.[28] Under the auspices of the Long Term Conditions Alliance it was found to be easily adaptable to other chronic illness situations and groups. When implemented as a generic course, across a range of lay-led SMPs, supplementary disease-specific modules were incorporated, with additional benefit.

The Stanford course is based on a structure of six weekly sessions serving 10–15 people. It utilises trained leaders, one peer leader with perhaps, in addition, a health professional as second leader. Its UK variant, the EPP, covers topics such as the aims of self-management, symptom management, medicines management, resources available, taking control, exercise, nutrition and communication. Clearly, these topics reflect the common challenges encountered by all those living with chronic diseases. The group process provides social support, combats isolation, promotes self-sufficiency and empowerment through peer-learning and pooling of experience. There is an emphasis on problem-solving and goal-setting.

Among the limitations of the method are the highly structured nature of the programme, which requires attendance throughout the course duration, and the restriction on numbers of those who can attend the group. Furthermore, programmes that require group adherence may not be suitable for people who are uncomfortable with group work because of cognitive style or other cause, or for groups of people who are likely to have problems in attending meetings – for example, those with restricted mobility, the housebound, full-time employed workers and young people.

Evidence for the effectiveness of SMPs is mixed, despite enthusiastic adoption of the EPP in England. A systematic review of 17 randomised controlled trials found that benefits included enhanced self-efficacy, self-rated health, cognitive symptom management and reduced health distress.[29] However, there was no benefit in healthcare utilisation, health-related quality of life, psychological well-being or levels of pain, disability, fatigue, depression, dyspnoea or measured HbA_{1c}. It concluded that there is insufficient evidence at present to justify widespread implementation of lay-led SMPs if the aim is to reduce healthcare resource use.[30] As in many areas of healthcare it is difficult to demonstrate benefit in terms of savings however beneficial the participants may feel them to be. Well-informed and motivated patients may actually make greater use of services on offer because of their increase in awareness and uptake; and that is, after all, what services are about.

Peer support interventions are less formalised than SMPs. They do not structure the content in advance, may not necessarily place limits on course size or duration, and they may import and incorporate elements of other 'groupie' activities. Because of their generally more relaxed, supportive aims they may have greater appeal while still being effective in promoting and facilitating exchange of information, sharing of experiences, and provision of mutual, emotional and social support.

Self-help groups are mainly independent of the formal healthcare sector, although health professionals have initiated many of them. The sociologist Scambler[31] questions their validity. He poses the question whether they are a basic component of primary care, supplementing the specific, technical, organisational or expert assistance of the professional health services; or may they represent a poor substitute for 'real care' when there is a deficiency of real services a lack of understanding, care, treatment or support from health professionals?

Similar questions may be asked in relation to health promotion and health education (*see* Chapter 5). Either way, and bearing in mind the generic nature of needs expressed by people with chronic illness, it is important that there is a diversity of vehicles for the broad agenda of support and help that such people deserve, with 'different strokes for different folks'. The self-help or community-development model of service provision is not intended to be free-standing or comprehensive. Rather, it is an integral part of a broadly based strategy for managing chronic illness and disability.

> Improving clinical outcomes needs more than just information and support – it requires partnership between patients and their health professionals with the patient actively involved in self-care.[32]

A further development has been the use of trained lay link workers whose role is to connect patients and practices with community resources for help.

As reported in Chapter 2, people with long-term conditions face three challenges:
1. medical management – monitoring symptoms, changing health behaviour
2. emotional management – dealing with the consequences
3. role management – a shift in social role, as in healthy to sick, or provider to 'burden'.

Self-help and support groups and SMPs contribute much to all three of these.

Personal and public involvement (PPI)

> Rhetorical slogans like 'no decisions about us without us' appeal to widely shared norms and values of transparency and patient-centredness ... but PPI in rationing decisions is both practically and ethically complex and may or may not be in the best interests of the sick or dying patient.[33]

This statement delineates both the values and limitations of PPI – transparency, patient centredness, and participation in shared decision-making at policy level, but it may become adversarial or even rebound on the individual patient's interests when applied to difficult or sensitive decisions. The Alma-Ata Declaration made it a fundamental right of citizenship, and almost a duty, to participate in healthcare provision, but what does participation mean? Macdonald, in his radical book *Primary Health Care*,[34] provides an analysis of participation at a variety of levels.

- *De-participation* describes those whose level of participation is sub-zero. Marginalised, deprived and alienated minorities are incapable of participatory action because of powerlessness – the absence of self-efficacy. This clearly impinges on, and complicates, the self-management of illness, and is consistent with the correlation between chronic disease and high levels of deprivation.
- *Participation in benefit* means positive involvement in a programme or organisation, perhaps being motivated towards enhanced involvement and playing a responsible role in an organisation; for example many patients enjoy becoming volunteers, with benefits both for themselves and others.
- *Participation in implementation* is a high degree of active involvement in carrying out social aims. Importantly, this does not rule out exploitation, for example, of unskilled workers or volunteers whose contribution can be taken for granted. Many health and social care ancillary workers occupy this level, having a key role without necessarily having a voice. As pressures within health systems increase there are many clinicians who are beginning to identify with this descriptor.
- *Participation in evaluation*: having the ability to shape an organisation or service, like shareholders at the AGM of a business.
- *Participation in decision-making*: taking responsibility or ownership in the organisation and of its impact on the individual – for example, by joining the management board.

Clearly, in the management of chronic illness, in order to promote participation and self-management, it is important to find ways of shifting people along this gradient. This relies on a community development approach, that of informing, conscientising (raising awareness), mobilising opinion, motivating and organising.

> In a democratic society service users should have the right to influence decisions and activities that affect them.[35]

PPI operates on many levels. In the UK there is an active research scene sponsored by the Department of Health. Here PPI operates at three levels: (1) consultation, (2) collaboration and (3) user control of the research agenda.[36] In service delivery there is no widespread agreement as to how this should apply, beyond the present statutory lay representation (in the UK) on decision-making and regulatory bodies. It is less clear how PPI should express itself closer to the level of the individual, how representation might be optimised and what part service users should play in crunch decisions, such as in rationing care. By the nature of general practice, which places great value on patient centredness and continuity, much feedback and personal involvement on the part of patients are implicit, even in the absence of formal structures of PPI. In many places individual practices have instituted *patient participation groups* with ad hoc terms of reference that might include rights of comment on service quality and current issues, such as access, complaints, advocacy or mediation. Public bodies are obliged to ensure lay representation at board level and policymakers must consult on a wide front. PPI in decision-making is a central part of the NHS mission and it is a statutory responsibility for commissioners of care. For example, government places high value on advice from elected public bodies and third sector organisations, such as long-term conditions alliances, Age Concern, Mind or Diabetes UK.

Advocacy is an important function of PPI and third sector organisations, where it takes a variety of forms:

- collective – concerning service provision and policy (lobbying)
- individual – supporting and representing concerns and perceived grievance in particular cases
- campaigning – the use of media and publicity to advance the welfare of their constituency via public forums.

Peer advocacy is another model of the expert patient, whereby a patient undertakes special training to carry out a *mentorship* role in relation to other service users who need information, support or interpretation concerning pathways of treatment. The peer advocate is prepared to act on behalf of the patient to seek redress from the service provider up to the level of formal complaint, or even public denunciation through the media. The term '*expert by experience*' is often used in this context.

THE CARING PROFESSIONS

No account of providers of care would be complete without reference to the formal providers, the community social services and the primary healthcare team (the latter is discussed in detail in Chapter 5). Much long term support, mostly ambulant, is also provided by hospital specialists and their teams. In the UK there are moves to integrate healthcare and social services at both policy and provider levels in the interests of integration of care.

Social services teams tend to be organised around four main task groups: (1) care of the elderly, (2) child and family welfare, (3) disability and (4) mental health.

Clearly, most of these relate to people with long-term conditions. Their methodology is based on social casework and they have become increasingly distanced from the archaic 'do-gooder' image. Social workers became increasingly professionalised following the Seebohm Report from 1968, which brought together a fragmented collection of social providers (many of them in the voluntary sector), making social workers professionally qualified, generic and community based. Interestingly, Seebohm also recommended social worker secondment to general practice. Social services in the UK assumed an enhanced role in the 1990s through the introduction of *the care in the community policy*. This entailed running down provision of long-stay care in geriatric wards, mental hospitals and mental disability units, with transfer of resources from institutional, inpatient capacity towards enhanced community-located social care. This introduced a methodological shift towards care programmes, based on individual *care packages*, to support autonomous living or alternative placement in community-based 'halfway houses' and specialised residential units, most of them provided in the private sector. The social services retain a quality inspection involvement in these.

The elements of such placement and care packages are administered through a managed care model based on the *multidisciplinary case conference*, convened and chaired by a senior social worker and involving all necessary stakeholders, including the patient (or representative). The GP is normally invited to participate and should consider doing so (although workload pressures mean he or she often has to delegate this to a team member, such as the district nurse). A *case manager* is appointed, to implement and oversee the personal care plan, and nominates a *key worker* from among those most intimately involved with the recipient to act as point of contact liaison with all agencies involved. The availability of resources, such as skills, personnel, funding and appliances, is an ever-present problem in implementing services. A neat transfer of funds released from the run-down of institutional care does not directly translate into enhanced community social provision. Any reciprocal relationship between institutional shrinkage and community expansion is liable to be notional, and this has implications for those who are now commissioning services for people with long-term conditions and disabilities. The money does not easily follow the patient.

The primary healthcare team is considered at length in Chapter 5. As originally understood in the 1970s in the UK it included a social worker, to great effect in service integration. Following the demise of the Seebohm model, gradual fragmentation resulted in the task-force model already described. The chasm between healthcare and social care in the community remains to be bridged. One necessary preliminary to redressing this is reinforcement of the role, recruitment and morale of the social services workforce.

A HISTORICAL NOTE ON UK SYSTEMS OF HEALTH AND SOCIAL CARE

In the British Isles, as in much of Europe, the systems of healthcare and social care have performed a 'pas de deux' that is centuries old. In mediaeval Europe a model emerged that was based on provision by religious orders and the charitable institutions they founded. These provided terminology that is familiar to this day in the vocabulary of caring; concepts such as hospital, hostel, hospice, asylum, sanctuary, almshouse, infirmary and almoner. These still echo with meaning universally as institutions that provide accommodation for the needy, places of respite for the homeless or wayfarer, places where the sick, the stigmatised and outcasts of society could find protection and healing. Shortly after the sixteenth-century destruction of the monastic system in northern Europe it was found to be necessary to introduce systems to replace such services. England introduced measures (*the Elizabethan Poor Law*) that made local communities (parish councils) responsible for the relief of the poor and 'indigent sick'. The parishes could pool their resources (forming Unions) to create workhouses with attached infirmaries and dispensaries. Many district hospitals in the UK to this day retain at their core the characteristic, sombre, stone-built edifice with long corridors. Within my memory the local hospital was referred to, by the older generations, as the Old Union, and shunned as the place where people go, never to be seen again. These local authority-run institutions, initially charitable foundations, were incorporated into the NHS at its inception in 1948, and progressively removed from local or county council control, along with a host of independent philanthropic hospitals large and small, that represented a fragmented, informal network of healthcare institutions.

Social care remained the responsibility of the local authority and the social work profession emerged from an earlier cadre of welfare workers, some of whom I recall still bearing the mediaeval title of almoner. Following the 1990 Care in the Community reforms the current pattern described earlier was put in place.

GPs emerged from a fusion of medical practitioners and apothecaries who plied their trade wherever they could. In each area one GP would be appointed as 'medical officer of health' – the beginnings of the system of public health medicine. Some GPs were employed by emerging trades unions and, through reforms brought about by Lloyd George early in the twentieth century, had responsibilities for the care of the 'panel' of workers. Until recently the GP was sometimes referred to as 'the panel doctor' and the standard manual record was based on the 'Lloyd George Envelope'. Mid-nineteenth-century attempts to professionalise family practitioners were blocked by the aristocratic Royal College of Physicians, and did not organise professionally until the College of General Practitioners was founded in 1952. There was thus a long-established class division between GPs and Consultants that survived the formation of the NHS, when community-practising doctors were forced to elect to be either hospital doctors or family doctors. Echoes of this 'institutionalised 'inferiority' remain in public perceptions of the GP and are a limiting factor on the emergence of true medical partnership across the secondary–primary interface.

SCENARIO: a practice policy on carers

A bitter and disruptive breakdown in one family's care arrangement led to the GP having to seek emergency admission of a frail elderly lady to respite care through the social services elderly care team. It was a Monday morning in winter and it had not been easy or quick. The crisis had been brewing over the weekend when the chief carer, an unemployed bachelor son, had once again left his mother unattended and gone out drinking. He had been found to be still drunk the next day when his sister called in to see why their mother was answering the phone in a distressed and incoherent state. The old lady had gotten out of bed and fallen. Later in the day when family members had gathered together they called the out-of-hours service and were advised to contact the GP first thing in the morning if she was still in pain. The GP was able to rule out a significant trauma but found the family in a state of uproar about the old lady's care arrangements. The son was normally reliable but had been drinking a lot recently and probably was depressed. This was to be followed up through an urgent appointment. The story came up at coffee time and gave rise to other stories about families coping with chronic conditions. One proposal was that we should give some thought to how carers cope and why they come to the point of failing to cope. The trainee volunteered to do a bit of web-search on the needs of carers; the nurse practitioner agreed to gather the views of the district nurses and health visitors; at the next team training meeting these would be discussed and collated by the practice manager, to formulate an outline practice policy on carers. This eventually resulted in a brief document for discussion, as follows.

Proposed practice policy on carers
Background:
1 This Practice recognises, esteems and supports the work done by carers as a key contribution to the well-being, management and recovery of our patients.
2 Carers are those who look after family, partners, friends or neighbours who are in need of help because they are ill, frail or have a disability; it does not include those who are paid care providers.
3 There are over six million carers in the UK, or about 8% of the population.
4 Many carers have health needs themselves; physical and mental illness can be exacerbated by care duties; their risk of substantial sickness or disability is twice that of the general population.

5 Some carers need particular support, e.g. elderly or under-age carers, students and lone parents.

6 Carers frequently have other responsibilities in family life, education or employment.

7 Carers often feel isolated and may not know what help is available, either for the person for whom they care or for themselves.

8 Carers are not always next-of-kin; it can be difficult to know who is in charge or can make decisions.

9 Where prolonged or substantial domiciliary treatment is required the practice team is in a position to:

    a. ascertain who are the key figures and, with consent, record this on file

    b. show concern for the welfare of key carers

    c. provide support, information about self-help and guidance concerning available services

    d. liaise with key carers concerning management of the patient

    e. request social services to carry out a carers' assessment.

10 Of paramount importance is respect for the well-being, dignity and autonomy of the patient.

The Protocol

Where a patient needs care at home due to chronic illness, disability or frailty he or she will be asked to indicate who are the key carer and next-of-kin; contact data will be recorded in the patient's file.

Subject to consent, and when appropriate, the team will liaise with key carers.

Carers will be treated with respect and consideration; their views regarding the health needs and care of the patient will taken into account where possible.

Personal health needs of key carers will be addressed wherever this is appropriate; the Team will be alert to those carers who are in special need through age, youth, disability or poor health.

The Team will seek to support carers in the important work they do through:

a. information on notice boards, waiting rooms and the practice web-site

b. indicating the existence of self-help and support groups

c. involving or referring to other agencies in the community

d. requesting carers' assessment by the social services where appropriate

e. providing documentation in support of welfare claims

f. liaising with social services concerning care packages.

This policy will be reviewed and updated in 6 months, initially.

CONCLUSION AND REFLECTION

The influential *medical model of healthcare* has enjoyed international currency and its 'paternalism' relegated the patient and family to a relatively passive role on the sidelines. The paradigm shift, as proposed by the World Health Organization, is designed to rearrange clinical, public health and lay roles in order to bring about person-centred integration of care and the emergence of policies that will be more suitable for responding to the growing threats and challenges that patients with chronic conditions encounter. Patients are empowered and given a voice through self-help, supported self-management and representation through PPI. Third sector organisations play important roles in community care. The recognition of the essential contribution of family and other carers has grown with the awareness of the need for chronic care in the community. This has raised awareness of the needs of carers. Hospitals have been forced by policy trends to beat a tactical retreat from the front line of chronic care and this is being passed progressively to the primary care sector. The great inherited interface divides, between doctor and patient, medical and social care, and between classes of doctors, are being challenged at the most fundamental levels. The steady rise in the chronic disease burden is the catalyst that will change all of these, as will become apparent in the next chapters.

POINTS FOR REFLECTION

Identify a seriously ill or disabled patient; interview their chief carer in depth, noting:

- the impact of the caring role on the carer's way of life, health and family life
- economic and work consequences
- the extent of unmet needs.

How does your practice support the contribution that carers make?
How do you promote and support:

- the autonomy of the patient?
- patient self-management?
- patient involvement?

Refer back to the case report on Joseph earlier in this chapter: what interventions by health or social care might have helped make a difference for this family?

REFERENCES

1. Robinson I. Reconstructing lives: negotiating the meaning of multiple sclerosis. In: Anderson R, Bury M. *Living With Chronic Disease*. London: Hyman Unwin; 1988.
2. Appleby J. The hospital bed: on its way out? *BMJ*. 2013; **346**: f1563.
3. Scambler G. Health and illness behaviour. In: Scambler G, editor. *Sociology as Applied to Medicine*. 4th ed. London: Saunders; 1997. p. 42.
4. Alderfer CP. *Existence, Relatedness and Growth: human needs in organisational settings*. New York, NY: Free Press; 1972.
5. Friedson E. *The Profession of Medicine*. New York, NY: Dodds Mead; 1970. Cited in: Scambler G, op. cit. p. 42.
6. Higgs P. Later life, health and society. In: Scambler G, editor. *Sociology as Applied to Medicine*. 6th ed. Edinburgh: Saunders; 2008. p. 185.
7. Ibid.
8. Carers UK website. Available at: www.carers.org/key-facts-about-carers (accessed 21 April 2014).
9. Ibid.
10. Ibid.
11. Hogan P, Rogers M, Msall M. Functional limitations and key indicators of well-being in children with disabilities. *Arch Pediat Adolesc Med*. 2000; **154**(10): 1042–1048.
12. Stevenson F. Community care and informal caring. In: Scambler G, editor. *Sociology as Applied to Medicine*. 6th ed. Edinburgh: Saunders; 2008. p. 266.
13. Carers Trust. *What is a Carer?* Available at: www.carers.org/what-carer (accessed 20 April 2014).
14. Western Health and Social Care Trust. Carers get protection at work following landmark European Court of Justice case. *Carers Newsletter*. 2008; **7**: 2.
15. Becker S, Aldridge J, Dearden C. *Young Carers and Their Families*. Oxford: Blackwell Science; 1998.
16. British Broadcasting Corporation. *'Hidden Army' of Young Carers could be Four Times as High as Official Figures*. Press Release. London: Young Carers Survey; 16 November 2010. Available at: www.bbc.co.uk/pressoffice/pressreleases/stories/2010/11_november/16/carers.shtml (accessed 20 April 2013).
17. *Young Carers: quarter of a million children provide care for others*. London: BBC; 2013. Available at: www.bbc.co.uk/news/education-22529237 (accessed 20 April 2014).
18. Becker, Aldridge, Dearden, op. cit.
19. Cavendish C. *The Cavendish Review: an independent review into healthcare assistants and support workers in the NHS and social care settings*. London: Department of Health; 2013.
20. Neuberger J. Interview on RTÉ Radio 1; 7 July 2008.
21. www.dilnotcommission.dh.gov.uk
22. Beauchamp TL, Childress J. *Principles of Biomedical Ethics*. 6th ed. Oxford: Oxford University Press; 2009.
23. Segan JC. *Concise Dictionary of Modern Medicine*. New York, NY: McGraw-Hill; 2006.
24. Watson M. *European Certificate in Essential Palliative Care*. 10th ed. Esher, Surrey: Princess Alice Hospice; 2012.
25. Lorig K. Partnerships between expert patients and physicians. *Lancet*. 2002; **359**: 814–15.
26. Expert Patient Task Force. *A New Approach to Chronic Disease Management for the 21st Century*. London: Department of Health; 2001.

27. Long Term Conditions Alliance Scotland. In: *Long Term Conditions: working together*. Belfast: Long Term Conditions Alliance Northern Ireland with the Department of Health, Social Services and Public Safety; 2008.

28. www.expertpatients.co.uk (accessed 27 April 2014).

29. Foster G, Taylor SJC, Eldridge S, *et al.* Self-management education programmes by lay leaders for people with chronic conditions. *Cochrane Database Syst Rev.* 2009; (4): CD005108.

30. Ibid.

31. Scambler G. Health and illness behaviour. In: Scambler G, editor. *Sociology as Applied to Medicine*. 4th ed. London: Saunders; 1997. p. 43.

32. Murray E. Internet-delivered treatments for long-term conditions: strategies, efficacy and cost-effectiveness. *Expert Rev Pharmacoecon Outcomes Res.* 2008; **8**(3): 261–72.

33. Russell J, Greenhalgh T, Burnett A, *et al.* Individual healthcare rationing in a fiscal ice age. *BMJ.* **342**; d3279.

34. Macdonald JJ. *Primary Health Care: medicine in its place*. London: Earthscan; 2000.

35. Iliffe S, Willcock J Manthorpe J, *et al.* Can clinicians benefit from patient satisfaction surveys? Evaluating the National Service Framework for Older People. 2005–2006. *J R Soc Med.* 2008; **101**: 598–604.

36. Research and Design Service Yorkshire and Humber. Patient and Public Involvement. Available at: www.rds-yh.nihr.ac.uk/ppi/ (accessed 20 April 2014).

CHAPTER 5

The clinical complex: the general practitioner and chronic care

Contents

CHAPTER OVERVIEW

The clinical complex is the engine room of chronic illness care. It encompasses all clinicians, allied health professionals (AHPs), clinical teams and their enabling managers, whether in hospitals or community based, who contribute to the care of people with long-term conditions. The World Health Organization (WHO) paradigm change has highlighted the key contribution of primary care and that is why this chapter begins with the role and methodology of general practice and how it relates to the acute (hospital) sector. Clinicians within the NHS will know much of this, having survived through the policy developments of the past decade. Students and trainees, and clinicians from elsewhere, may welcome the quasi-textbook approach that emphasises explanation and definition of terms, with some international comparisons. However, the chief reason behind this description of general practice is to demonstrate its relevance, track record and potential in chronic care. For ease of navigation by readers this chapter is divided into two parts. The narrative is in Part One. Part Two presents developments in service delivery, notably in IT, integration and commissioning of care. It concludes with some key universal themes that all clinicians will recognise: quality, governance, safety and evidence-based practice.

Part One: general practice as the focus of chronic disease management

It is by no means self-evident that the UK-style general medical practice is the most credible provider in chronic care. Wagner[1] (of the well-known chronic care model) expressed the view of sceptics this way:

> Many [case management programmes] seem to operate on four major premises:
> 1. Reduction in the costs of chronic illness is the major goal and is assumed to be associated with improvements in health
> 2. The best way to achieve reduction is to focus on the highest cost patients in the chronically ill population
> 3. Primary care is not up to the task of chronic illness care
> 4. Patients will do better if their chronic disease management is largely removed from primary care and is delegated to a case manager.
>
> These premises need to be examined.

There is widespread consensus that, in countries that have progressive health services, the home of management of chronic diseases is the community-based generalist physician (in the United States they even describe the primary care health centre as *the medical home*). There are several reasons for this.

- WHO policy documents on chronic care are predicated on the primary care model ever since the Alma-Ata Declaration of 1979.
- As medical graduates with specialist-level training, GPs are capable of the range

of skills and knowledge necessary for an informed engagement with the range of long-term conditions that are likely to afflict, and coexist in, their patients.

- Suitably equipped and resourced, within multidisciplinary teams backed up with IT systems, they can provide the continuity and expertise without which adequate long-term management will often be impossible.
- There is evidence that the cost and complexity of addressing chronic conditions can be managed most effectively where there is a strong, continuing doctor–patient relationship, as in general practice.
- Many patients with chronic conditions receive their long term support substantially through outpatient clinics (ambulatory care). However, in those countries where healthcare provision is dominated by disease-specific, hospital-based specialists, the care of people with long-term conditions is fragmented or costly or both; in chronic care the necessary function of hospital specialists is best exercised in supportive, consultative and expert advisory capacities.
- Although self-management is a crucial factor in long-term conditions there is no evidence of patient-led initiatives being successful in the clinical management of serious chronic and co-morbid disease.
- The third sector organisations that represent patients have a strong track record in supporting, rather than as providers of, comprehensive clinical services, although they do provide and commission a variety of specific services.
- Professions allied to medicine, as currently constituted, function best in specific skill areas within coordinated team-based strategies; under the US system, specialist nurses have a claim to be providers of chronic care in their own right.

Autonomous commercial organisations delivering targeted programmes of healthcare have an increasing profile as service providers (even bidding to take over general practice contracts in the UK). Healthcare in the United States is commonly provided through non-state corporations that deliver *managed care programmes*; these are circumscribed by contracts and, except where they employ generalists, lack open access and comprehensive functions that encompass the full disease trajectory from prevention and premorbid stages through to palliative and terminal care for a whole population denominator. The US model of managed care is the most credible alternative to general practice for provision of chronic care and is being carefully studied by UK authorities for their possible cost benefits (*see* Chapter 6).

It would probably come as a great relief to many GPs if some other sector were to step up and assume responsibility for all chronic care. They would then have a lot less stress and still plenty to do on the acute side. Such a radical amputation, however, would fundamentally disrupt the highly evolved identity of the GP in the NHS and in other similar systems. General practice would then resemble a drop-in centre or A&E substitute for the locality (a view that actually seems to pervade the thinking of many hospital-based doctors and managers as well as press and politicians). This, however, is an improbable alternative scenario, but it might just become conceivable if GPs in the UK were required to resume their former contractual responsibility for 24-hour continuity of personal care as prevailed prior to 1998, in an era when general practice was not far removed from being a cottage industry.

It is crucial to bear in mind that the centrality of general practice is not being asserted to the detriment of the specialist clinical and hospital sector. Good primary care is a prerequisite for an effective and affordable hospital system. The converse is also true, that without the backup of comprehensive and accessible specialist services, general practice would resemble an expensive counselling service in a first-aid post. The *interface* is a term that represents both the barrier and the bond between primary and specialist clinical services. The two are closely symbiotic.

The management of chronic disease is like a continuous thread that links the diverse activities of modern primary care medicine. Aspects of management may be examined in terms of agency (who does what?), method (what is processed and what are the procedures?), quality (how good is it and can it improve?) and governance (how are values enshrined in the structure?). These will be examined in some detail.

WHAT GPs DO: FISHING OR FILTERING?

> Primary care is a low-risk setting for patients … however, the sheer volume of patients seen, the inherent difficulty of picking out the sick from the well, the range of illness tackled and the unenviable position within a complex, but not always efficiently functioning healthcare system, make it inevitable that sub-optimal care can and does occur.[2]

Any discourse on general practice must recognise that while continuing and chronic care is a salient feature, the GP's job is dominated by the risk of catastrophic events. It is essential to safety-net against their occurrence and to ensure prompt effective intervention when they arise. This may be imagined as an angler standing in a fast-flowing stream who pulls out the occasional big fish (but what about the ones that got away?). A more realistic image is of the GP at the intake point of the clinical service pipeline, acting as *a high-volume filter* with adjustable mesh size; if too fine primary care gets 'congestive failure', resulting in excessive onward referrals; too wide and significant cues and signals pass undetected. Small adjustments in the gauge of the filter result in large fluctuations in the load passed on to the specialist sectors. The GP has to pick up the signs of impending crises such as, strokes, coronaries, respiratory failure, acute abdominal crises, obstetric haemorrhage, meningitis and avoidable suicide. Few other events have such definitive outcome if missed at early presentation. The risk of sudden, avoidable death lurks within the mass of undifferentiated presenting complaints and is a major preoccupation for every GP. All else has to serve this priority.

Properly calibrated in terms of risk and managed uncertainty, the clinical workload is sorted through the filter. A small proportion is diverted for referral or follow-up. Much is processed as self-limiting or minor illness, mostly for palliation. Many of such complaints are non-disease-specific conditions such as disordered sleep, anxiety and depression, stress, pain syndromes or digestive tract upsets. Among these there may be harbingers of serious and long-term conditions, but time will tell, especially if there is an effective channel for them to return if … (safety-netting).

It is a truism, but worth repeating, that early detection of serious and long-term illness improves prognosis and outcomes. Indeed, the aim is to convert the threat of fatal progression into a manageable longer-term condition. Effective acute care enables the patient to survive long enough for secondary preventive measures to click in and support continuing life. Thus, fewer young people need die of asthma, epilepsy or rapid-onset type 1 diabetes. This is the dramatic end of the spectrum of clinical intervention, where great satisfaction can, paradoxically, be derived for both doctor and patient in the midst of what is really not good news. An early diagnosis can be life enhancing, even if it has formidable consequences. There is the prospect of life with asthma, cancer, diabetes or arthritis. Not so bad, perhaps, when you think of the alternatives. As we have seen, many people die with, rather than from, chronic disease. **Life-saving technology seeks to convert the crisis into a process whose timeline enables the doctor and patient to strive to reconstruct a way of life that approximates to normality.**

Prevention is better than cure, so runs the folk wisdom. This may give GPs some consolation, faced with the rarity of cure compared with the vast quantity of preventive work that is addressed daily. Prevention has been considered in Chapter 2, but it bears some repetition here since prevention is one of the busiest areas of chronic disease management for the GP.

Successful primary prevention of long term conditions is most evident in the immunisation of infants against erstwhile common infections; also in nutrition, lifestyle modification and neonatal screening, which detects metabolic errors and aborts the onset of irreversible developmental problems – for example, those consequent on thyroid failure and phenylketonuria.

Secondary prevention, as a term, has achieved common currency in relatively recent years. The invention of effective, well-tolerated drugs that reduce risk has transformed the progression of diseases beyond the initial event crisis. Following the acute stenting of an atheromatous coronary vessel, a cocktail of four drugs is commonly imposed for lifetime use by the perplexed neophyte patient, who never really felt ill in the first place, 'just a wee niggle in the chest'. And what an agenda that triggers for the GP! Repeat prescribing protocols and reviews, biomonitoring, cardiac rehabilitation, lifestyle changes to embed … permanently. The magic of secondary prevention is undeniable, but at high cost to the patient's way of life and the GP's workload. There are no free rides in the healthcare industry.

And then there is tertiary prevention, those 'downstream' actions, in the further reaches of the disease trajectory, where physical, psychological and social functioning become impaired. It aims to limit collateral damage associated with the disease, to maintain mental health, preserve joint function, prevent contractures, reduce fall frequency, facilitate return to work, and much more. It has much in common with rehabilitation. Damage limitation and 'keeping the show on the road' is the province of some of our most valued colleagues in primary care – the nurse, physiotherapist, occupational therapist, podiatrist and nutritionist.

The *premises* that house and provide the operational base for the GP influence healthcare delivery greatly. Crucial factors include their location in relation to their catchment community, transport links, disability access, capacity, the range of services available, atmosphere and user-friendliness. Attention to the industrial triad is essential: *plant, personnel and equipment* – that is, the premises, the team and the processes that produce the goods. All three merit continuing maintenance and periodic overhaul (*see* Chapter 8).

One vital process characteristic of general practice is *continuing care*. This is not the same as continuity of care. No individual doctor could guarantee the necessary availability and memory capacity to manage effectively the long-term illnesses of his or her patient list. In chronic care it is the *group practice*, the multidisciplinary and information-connected team that is the guarantor of continuity, and this will be examined in more detail later.

Why group practice? I tend to think in terms of practices of, say, six GPs serving a denominator of 10 000 registered people, since this represents my career experience in three urban areas over 35 years. Although the range in sizes of practices is wide, the trend is towards increasing size. There are policy reasons for fostering the growth of practices towards a 'critical mass', where economies of scale and diversity of skill-mix would achieve equilibrium with manageability and geographic cohesion. Such policies would see the small, single-handed practice as obsolete. This may be somewhat presumptuous, because there are many GPs who are contentedly single-handed. In rural areas this small, nuclear practice model is congruent with low population density. They benefit from short lines of communication with their staff and patients. To address the range of essential tasks in small practices, much responsibility is devolved to nurses, additional skills being brought in as needed and resources shared with neighbouring units. There is no simple correlation between practice size and quality.[3] In many countries in central and southern Europe this small practice model is the norm. From my observations they are challenged by the demands inherent in managing chronic disease effectively. They tend to flourish where there is a ready supply of community-practising specialists – notably, paediatricians and gynaecologists. The GP under such systems then approximates to a community-based specialist in (adult) internal medicine.

Whatever the size of practice or premises, general practice requires *teamwork*. The core team surrounds the GP with nurses of a range of degrees of specialism and grade, and an administrative team. AHPs, such as physiotherapist, occupational therapist, nutritionist, podiatrist or pharmacist, are recruited as necessary, perhaps on a sessional basis; social workers, formerly seen as core team, are accessed through referral and care management procedures (*see* 'Primary care and multidisciplinary teamwork').

In corporate terms group general practices are (typically) small organisations that are self-contained units of healthcare resource, close to the patient and in touch with the community they serve. In the UK system they are also self-governing and distributed throughout the nation in approximate accordance with population density. This fortunate distribution did not arise accidentally. It reflects two crucial concepts:

1. *Universal coverage*: in keeping with the WHO dogma that healthcare is a right of citizenship, the NHS ensures that every citizen has access to healthcare that is free of charge at the point of uptake (funded from taxation and National Insurance contributions). This is achieved through *universal registration*. Thus, every citizen knows who his or her GP is, and the practice knows them. It maintains an up-to-date registry of patients that contains the personal, continuing, cumulative and comprehensive record of all health encounters. The extreme value of this was impressed on me when working in the Third World with undefined catchment, postal addresses that were arbitrary and an infrastructure of communications that was rudimentary. Healthcare was, accordingly, episodic, disease centred and crisis driven. Chronic care was virtually impossible.

2. *Regulatory control* is exercised by health trusts, or clinical commissioning groups (CCGs), which can decline to recognise or enter into contract with any proposed new practice formation, unless there is a local deficiency of service coverage. The trust or CCG is obligated to ensure adequate and fair provision of local primary care services. It holds the contracts of the practitioners in its area and holds them to account through a variety of governance measures. Unfortunately, until now the even distribution of general practice has been confused with fair distribution. Equal does not mean equitable. Where deprived communities experience up to a fourfold increase in relative risk there ought to be increased manpower, with task forces and services to redress the balance if fairness is to become a reality.

GENERAL PRACTICE: CONCEPT AND METHOD

Is primary healthcare the same as general practice?

In a reflective and thought-provoking study on the Alma-Ata Declaration, Macdonald[4] quotes the WHO 1979 document as follows:

> PHC [primary healthcare] is essential health care … made universally accessible …
> at a cost [to] the community that the country can afford and is the first level of con-
> tact of individuals, the family and the community with the national health system,
> bringing health care as close as possible to where people live and work.

Is primary healthcare the same as general practice? Yes and no. GPs operate *primary medical services* in a community setting. Some hospital services, especially A&E, are utilised by the public as a primary healthcare resource, especially in the United States, where the emergency room may be the sole provider for a substantial proportion of citizens. A further area of primary healthcare lies with public health medicine, which is intimately concerned with the health of the community as a whole. Public and environmental health bridges the gap between health policy and local service sectors such as statistical analysis, emergency planning, public safety, hygiene, health promotion, and addressing the social antecedents of disease through intersectoral action and epidemiological surveillance. Since *self-help* is regarded as a vital strand of management of long-term conditions, patients themselves play important roles in primary care, along with third sector organisations. Community social services have a strong claim to be partners in the overall picture. But there is much more to primary healthcare than even these. Much health promotion work is carried out in schools and places of employment, where health and safety structures add a further dimension. Zola's[5] influential metaphor of *the river of health and illness* imagines a torrent of disease into which the physician plunges to fish out those afflicted without having time to understand and do anything about those factors that are pushing people into the river in the first place. These lie 'upstream' in the form of social determinants of health, environmental conditions, culture, risk factors and other health hazards. Macdonald[6] likens the doctor-rescuer to the 'microscope' of medical view, as compared with the more inclusive 'macroscope': PHC is much more than an addition to existing health services. It is a reorientation of all health services towards the health needs of communities, both local and national.

The primary healthcare model has three pillars: participation, intersectoral collaboration and equity. There is more to be said on these later (*see* Chapter 6). There is an underlying theme here, which is *quality of care*. While much of this broader primary healthcare agenda lies outside the scope of most GPs (although those involved in commissioning will need to get out their macroscope), quality is a vital area in the management and provision of care services. Quality and clinical effectiveness will be discussed at length towards the end of this chapter.

Defining general practice

There are many definitions of general practice – the European (Leeuwenhorst 1974),[7] the WONCA Europe[8] and the American Academy of Family Physicians[9] definitions, to name a few. They are worth looking at. Since definitions vary somewhat, and we are concerned here with chronic disease, for the purposes of this narrative it is sufficient to look at those characteristics of general practice that relate most to long term condition management.

The general medical practitioner in the community is the hub of clinical care for individuals and families, committed to a holistic, continuing therapeutic relationship with his or her patients:

- a local accessible interface with the full health system
- a high-volume filter and sorter for all presenting problems
- advocate on behalf of the patients; their navigator through illness and service pathways
- gatekeeper to the NHS, promoting safe, rational and economical use of resources
- leader and coordinator of a multidisciplinary team providing primary services and linking with other sectors
- expresses professional values of patient centredness, teamwork, quality of care and process, and provision of continuing care, both ambulatory and domiciliary
- the closest thing to a scientist most people know; trained in communication skills and chronic illness care; able to explain risk and interpret data, present the bio-psychosocial context of health and disease, provide perspective and impart informed advice; these attributes should also enrich the resource base of the wider community.

The remainder of Part One will explore a variety of key areas of practice: continuity, teamwork, clinics, interface with hospitals and health promotion.

Continuity of care

Continuity of care is a product of consistent, personalised, quality-assured teamwork, rather than simply 'the same old face' always being around and available. People with long-term conditions place great value on continuity of care; of all our patients they are the ones who stand to gain most from it. Their definition of it will differ from that of the GP and hospital doctor, whose diverse duties dilute their capacity to provide personal continuing attention.

The institution, the team and data linkage guarantee the essence of continuity. Safety and quality of attention must be balanced with the wish to see the same individual every time. Hospitals encounter particular difficulties in providing continuity due to reducing length of in-patient stay, transience within large teams and the diversity of responsibilities. The patient will have to be content with being 'under the care of Dr X' even though he or she may seldom see Dr X, who, as the named responsible clinician, is the guarantor of clinical quality. In reality, it is the nursing staff who provide the continuity presence within hospitals.

In general practice there is less of a problem, being smaller, more local and with commitment to patient-centred practice. However, out-of-hours cover arrangements and the trend towards larger practice size are challenges to the continuity offered by GPs. These larger units hope for benefits of scale, enhanced skill-mix, sharing of resources and amenities, and centralising of functions such as management of 'human resources', finance, quality assurance and other systems. Adopting managed care or task force-based approaches may improve continuity for selected patients but detract from it with regard to the organisation overall. A partial solution is to have *a named responsible person* for each patient who requires more active management. Tasks may be devolved while retaining, for patient and practice, the knowledge of who holds the reins and should be contactable as issues arise. As the urgency, complexity or threat level for the patient increases, the importance of the nominated key worker becomes greater. The named specialist or GP, and assigned key worker (nurse or social worker), are fundamental to care planning. Periodic *case review* at team meetings ensures continuing awareness, newly identified cases are evaluated, significant events discussed, care plans adopted, tasks and responsibilities allocated to nominated staff, and continuing workload monitored.

A more intense level of continuity is achieved through the 'virtual ward' concept. For the duration of a crisis the patient is 'admitted' to a notional category that attracts a more intense and focused level of care with frequent contact, enhanced intervention, observation and recording of status, and close communication. As the crisis abates, the patient is 'discharged' to resume usual service levels. The archetype of this is terminal care managed through a hospice home-care team.

Thus it is that the quality conscious, multi-skilled, e-connected team with designated leads delivers continuity of care.

Continuity and out-of-hours care

Provision of clinical care during unsocial hours is probably the most controversial issue in continuity, at least in the UK. Unfortunately, the acute needs of the chronic sick become confused with other issues, such as the valid need by the occasionally unwell for access to episodic care, and demands by people who have jobs that normal services should operate extended service hours. People need access to essential clinical care at all times but there are frequent complaints of feeling confused about who is responsible outside office hours. A&E departments feel besieged by demand, much of it deemed inappropriate. Variations on models of delivery of out-of-hours care come and go. In the UK there is a mixture of advisory call-centres, nurse-led telephone triage, GP-led treatment centres with mobile outreach, and minor treatment drop-in centres. An effective and affordable system remains elusive.

One priority aim in chronic care is to modify the disease trajectory to reduce relapses, exacerbations and crises. There has been progress. Effective systems of intermediate care and telehealth reduce emergency admissions, improve expectant care and reduce crisis-driven responses. Two decades of improving primary chronic care mean that control of childhood asthma has improved and recurring calls at 3 a.m. for cardiac asthma are history. Care planning takes account of foreseeable risks and make provision for them. These require 24-hour backup with interventional capability. Both prevention and responsiveness must be built into chronic care.

The primary care team and multidisciplinary teamwork

> A team is an energetic group of people who are committed to achieving common objectives, who work well together and enjoy doing so and who produce high quality results.[10]

The primary healthcare team, as we have seen, is the platform that supports chronic disease management. It is GP led and includes the associated nursing and AHPs, and the organisational support that enables them to deliver their expertise directly to patients and their families. The primary care team, as it originated in the UK in the 1960s, consisted of the GP, district nurse, health visitor and social worker. This concept has undergone much modification over the years with both fragmentation and extension.

Fragmentation is most obvious in the loss of the practice-based social worker, whose role and presence I recall as a valuable ready resource. Public policy has dictated that social workers be managed within a profession-specific framework and operate through task forces for discrete social priorities. Community nursing services are a further area of fragmentation. In many places the district nurse has been withdrawn from the GP practice base (which is defined by patient registration) in favour of a locality 'patch' base (geographically defined), to form their own team unit under nurse management.

Extension of the team, on the other hand, has been considerable with the growth in chronic care as a priority. Practice-based nursing teams make a major and growing contribution, based on the familiar *treatment room nurse* and specialised *nurse practitioners*. The latter undertake higher qualifications that enable them to practise with greater autonomy and to develop areas of special expertise. Specialist nurses provide skilled services in tissue viability, continence problems, intermediate care and in various disease-specific areas, including epilepsy, cardiac failure, respiratory support and diabetes. They greatly enhance the skill-mix of the group, especially when nurses can devolve more routine tasks to other, less specialised grades of staff – for example, using nursing assistants and phlebotomists to undertake the time-consuming but vital routines of basic measurements and blood sampling. Frequently the practice-based clinics are nurse run, in conjunction with AHPs who are brought in to staff these clinics on a sessional or contractual basis. These perform essential roles in prevention and health promotion for diabetic and vascular clinics. Thus, the diabetic clinic is a convenient, reliable and integrated 'one-stop shop'. Pharmacists are finding an increasing role in managing and advising on complex regimens of medications, as typified by the average diabetic or other patient beset by co-morbidities. Physiotherapist expertise is accessed through patient referral according to need. Where the size of the practice unit is suitable these may all be permanent team members. The clinic system lends itself to providing designated 'packages of care', which may be conveniently 'bundled' for the purposes of primary care commissioning.

The role of the community psychiatric nurse has been strengthened greatly by growing emphasis on community mental healthcare. This has brought whole psychiatric teams out of their traditional base in the Victorian-style mental hospitals to adapt their modus operandi to a context closer to the patient and congruent with supporting primary care needs. This is reflected also in community addiction treatment services.

McDerment[11] summarises factors that influence teamwork beneficially as:
- clear objectives and agreed goals
- openness and confrontation
- support and trust
- cooperation and conflict resolution
- sound procedures
- leadership
- regular review
- individual development
- sound inter-group relations.

> The quality of teamwork is directly and positively related to quality of patient care and innovation in healthcare.[12]

The *practice manager* deserves special mention as team leader of the administrative staff, and more. Skill-mix requires coordination. Our notional practice of 10 000 patients and 6 doctors is a complex organism with a nursing staff of perhaps 8 to 10, around 15 ancillary workers and notional budgets amounting to several million pounds. Whatever external support services are available there is a formidable role for a manager. Financial management is crucial since the practice is responsible for payroll and other recurring expenditure. A wide variety of legislation has to be observed, particularly in areas such as employment law, health and safety in the workplace and civil liability. Arrangements related to quality in practice need to be implemented, and team meetings serviced. 'Front of house' and administrative services (reception, communications, IT and 'housekeeping' infrastructures) need to be supervised and rostered. Alongside this, the practice manager is the first point of contact for matters in public relations, problem-solving and responding to complaints.

He or she performs a central role in chronic disease management, since this depends on a sophisticated IT and communications system, and systems that support the organisation of clinics, the throughflow of patients and processing their maintenance requirements in a smooth stream (e.g. for repeat prescription requests). This is a major workload factor for administrative staff. Without them the diabetic patient runs out of insulin, the asthma clinic does not happen, the vaccines remain in the fridge and the lights go out.

Chronic care means multidisciplinary teamwork

> Good teamwork makes a critical contribution in health care delivery, and also contributes to the team member's well-being.[13]

Meetings, meetings, meetings! Why can't we just get on with doing what we do best – seeing patients? Clinicians of all kinds frequently express the tension between their clinical care and service management roles. Perhaps it is because they think of meetings as wasting clinical time or a necessary bolt-on to be tolerated. Perhaps they feel that the work involved in coordinating and administering is of secondary value to that of patient care. Perhaps they lack training in 'meeting-ology', or are uncomfortable with the group dynamics involved in teamwork. When it comes to working together in small groups a little knowledge is a dangerous thing; but some knowledge is also a dangerous thing to be without, and well-run meetings can turn a toil into a pleasure.

The total healthcare infrastructure is nourished and sustained by meetings. At an earlier evolutionary stage, when general practice was more demand led and acute care oriented, meetings were occasional if at all. The range of services that have accumulated over recent decades has brought complexity. The diverse tasks and objectives require coordination and continuing professional training to deliver the whole team's potential. Aliquots of time need to be ring-fenced within the weekly schedule of clinical work, but to what end? Regular encounters between professionals contribute to delivery of a quality service by addressing recurring issues, disseminating information, problem-solving, case management, discussion of significant events, new policy briefings, feedback and complaints, reviewing goals, in-service training plans, reporting and handover arrangements, and liaison with the out-of-hours service.

Informal chats over coffee are no substitute for team-based exchanges. However, they fulfil a crucial function in combating professional isolation. Trainees miss a major component of their former life in hospitals – the buzz of a large institution, the camaraderie of the common room, the stimulus of clinical discussion and peer support. They find general practice lonely, an endless procession of individual encounters, confined to the one room, followed by hours at the same desk deep in conversation with the computer terminal. Without regular meetings professional isolation, unrelieved stress, diminishing satisfaction and waning enthusiasm are sure to result.

Chronic care means *multidisciplinary care*, and this is a term that recurs throughout the voluminous literature on the management of chronic disease, almost always without clarification or definition. It is easy to assume that we know what it means, but do we? Do we know how to do it, and do we do it? What do we need to know to do it effectively? The reasons behind the need for multi-professional approaches in chronic care will by now by apparent from this and previous chapters, and this account will be confined to setting out aspects of it that define the practicalities.

Multidisciplinary working is not new. Hospitals have been doing it ever since operating theatres were invented. Integrated clinical teams came into being, particularly with the rise of organ transplantation services that involve a whole chain of command bridging multiple settings. The introduction in the 1990s of integrated cancer services was a further leap forward. Paediatrics began to branch into the community, forming the specialty of the community paediatrician. This evolved along the lines of multi-professional teamwork, essential for the coordination of services for children with complex needs and their families – notably, those afflicted with congenital abnormalities, cerebral palsy, developmental delay or neurological syndromes. In primary care in the UK the Family Doctors' Charter of 1966 put in place supports for group practice, with administrative backup, the primary care team, postgraduate education and purpose-built health centre premises. The new task for GPs is to harness the capacities of a diverse team and apply them across the trajectory and range of long term conditions. This is challenging, given the 'Lone Ranger style' of much of general practice in the past.

The difficulties of interprofessional working are well known:

> Separate lines of control, different payment systems leading to suspicion over motives, diverse objectives, professional barriers and perceived inequalities in

status, all play a part in limiting the potential of multi-professional, multi-agency teamwork ... for those working under such circumstances efficient teamwork remains elusive.[14]

Sounds familiar? Especially when Borrill also speaks of, *rudimentary organisational systems and resources for supporting and managing teams*. Many GPs' surgeries lack basic amenities such as space for a conference room, audiovisual equipment, a chronic care team management system or even parking space for visiting participants. **It is important not to build an edifice of chronic care around the community generalist physician when key sectors of its infrastructure have not been put in place.**

However, multi-professional developments in general practice have taken root and begun to flourish. The most obvious examples are the practice-based diabetic clinic and the palliative care meeting that implements the gold standard guidelines in conjunction with the hospice team. Generalising from such templates to the wider case-mix of general practice may be a key to multidisciplinary chronic care in the community. Multi-professional working, therefore, is not new to UK general practice. We have become accustomed to working within the group practice of doctors with a diverse skill-mix, a team of nurses with a variety of qualifications, grades and specialisms, AHPs and managers. Effective chronic illness programmes determine and utilise the team skill-mix.

So we are doing it, but do we know how to do it? Within general practice it tends to happen organically, through small team relationships, almost like a family atmosphere of cosy chats, and with ad hoc procedures. We need to learn to systematise and professionalise it, to evolve approaches that create a vehicle which will carry the demands of chronic care into the future.

On consulting websites on multidisciplinary working, one is left with two strong impressions.

1. They mostly relate to cancer care, within cancer unit networks. Since this appears to be the brand leader it will merit a closer look for information that might be transferrable.
2. There is a plethora of terminology that can only be described as resembling a matrix of permutations and combinations of frequently used terms that may be mixed and matched almost at will: *multi-* or *inter-*; *professional* or *disciplinary*; *working, learning, training* or *teamwork*; and some additional ones such as *inter-agency work* and *integrated approaches*.

I am sure there are subtle, or perhaps obvious, distinctions between, for example, MDT and interprofessional working, backed by valid academic insights, but there appears to be no simple formulation that governs preferences in this. For the sake of practicality the term 'multidisciplinary teamwork' is used here to represent all of these.

One special case that does not fit into this is *interagency working*, where representatives of separate public bodies or non-governmental organisations collaborate as part of their methodology. An example of this is in the justice system where police, probation service, education and youth service, social services, addiction treatment and mental health organisations pool their respective expertise through a standing committee for dealing with offenders who are subject to probation orders. They have statutory powers and diverse approaches and they have to negotiate how their mandates may be merged to solve problems or manage cases. Each individual brings to the table a baggage of lines of authority, powers, legal responsibilities and public accountability. This is resolved through agreed standing orders and procedure. All of these issues apply in MDT in healthcare, but somewhat less starkly demarcated, since our respective 'silos' of clinical interest and identity are more congruent and there exists the strong bonding cement of patient centredness.

To return to the subject of MDT in cancer services, the constitution of the National Cancer Action Team[15] describes a useful structure that has evolved over 20 years. The headlines of a specification for such a team appear in Figure 5.1. This list of headings may be sufficient in itself to provide a template for practices to elaborate their own approaches to MDT.

The cancer care team works well because it has been constituted:

- on a task-force model, coherent and focused
- as a special project mandated by a government report and the political will to 'defeat cancer'
- on a nationally agreed model with a clear constitution and operational blueprint
- with provision for generous resourcing and infrastructure, and backed up with cancer centres
- aimed at a specified population with predictable caseload, clear outcome measures and definable end points
- with a finite range of clinical pathways.

Feasibility of the multidisciplinary team in general practice

Transferring this template from the specialised zone of the cancer programme into the high-volume, diverse setting of general practice would require some transformational groundwork. This would need to take account of the limiting factors that restrict the growth of existing levels of teamwork in practices – limitations such as scale, capacity, time, competing tasks and priorities, space, finance and amenities. Programmes such as those for cancer or palliative and terminal care are inspiring, but they exemplify the issues raised by services that are packaged as programmes of care. Demarcated, and with special sectoral funding according to priorities that may

The team

Membership: core/fixed, plus case variable; by co-option

Attendance and deputising guidelines; protected time

Leadership: manage disruptive personalities and conflict; consensual decision-making; roles of chair and team (administrative) leader

Team working and culture; acceptable team behaviour guidelines

Personal and team development; skills training; role in teaching

Infrastructure for meeting

Physical environment of meeting venue

Technology and equipment – availability and use

Protected time

Meeting organisation and logistics

Scheduling of meeting

Preparation prior to MDT meeting

Organisation and administration

Post-MDT meeting – coordination of services

Communication, implementation, tracking patients' pathways

Patient-centred clinical decision-making

Who to discuss

Patient-centred care

Clinical decision-making process

Team governance

Organisational support

Data collection, analysis and audit of processes and outcomes

Clinical governance

FIGURE 5.1 Outline headings for multidisciplinary teamwork (MDT) structure and function (*source*: adapted from National Cancer Action Team)[15]

be politically determined, they create beacons of excellence that contrast with the other areas of 'normal' service, which can never hope to achieve the same levels of service provision. The special achievements of such programmes, to a degree, come at the expense of more general sectors through diversion of resources. So what can be done in general practice, bearing in mind that we are focusing on the needs of the chronically ill?

There should be an awareness of the basic requirements of MDT:
- it should not take up a disproportionate percentage of professional time
- aim for simplicity, minimal bureaucracy, economy of effort and resource use
- strike a balance between heavy formalism and ineffectual informality
- have some guidelines on procedure, group-work process, recording and decision-making
- specify the kinds of patients for whom this team management approach is required (case selection, risk stratification)
- have entry and exit guidelines so that the active list of patients is kept to a manageable size – the revolving door model
- create illness pathway management templates and other decision supports
- value chairing and administrative skills
- value the respective skill sets and potential training function of all attendees.

The options that are available within general practice include:
- organic growth, building on existing practices of team working
- programmed growth, working towards task-force models in cancer, diabetes and respiratory disease; developing further the existing model of practice-based clinics
- new structures, based on the Kaiser Model, identifying and actively managing the top-risk 5% only
- formal structure – a chronic care task force resembling the cancer action team format
- clinical governance model – addressing and managing identified hazards, critical events or patient crises.

Significant MDT has been achieved in the past through simplicity and informality. The trend towards increasing scale and federations of practices will require new structures that reflect the diverse skill-mix of the larger institution. Along with this, the increasing burden of chronic disease will require advances in interprofessional cooperation. Teamwork requires processes of governance since it is not just the personal diligence and competence of one therapist that is at stake, but the quality of the many links in the chain of service delivery. Let us hope that this does not create a further web of complexity, political correctness and time-wasting box-ticking. Perhaps, rather than waiting for formal structures to be imposed along civil service lines, we should just focus on organic, in-house, creative, autonomous development of communication and cooperation within the small practice team. After all, much of the effective collaborative work in general practice is achieved by empowering and mandating fellow professionals to get on with what they do best. For example, there is evidence that nurses perform twice as well as doctors in implementing lipid management protocols. Optimising the use of the team's skill-mix may not necessarily require a cumbersome superstructure of meetings and minutes. A lengthy multi-author report commissioned by the Department of Health concluded, among other things, that 'NHS organisations have to develop as team-based, rather than hierarchical'.[16]

There is a relative lack of literature on **multi-professional learning** in this area, except at undergraduate level. The trend in diversifying medical faculties into schools of biomedical sciences has enabled much shared teaching across boundaries of discipline at the level of basic clinical sciences before the respective groups of students diverge. True multi-professional learning begins when students encounter clinical practice through placements and attachments where teamwork is modelled. Training programmes should draw attention to this area through their curricula – for example, by 'fieldwork' attendances at case conferences and programmed contributions by tutors from other disciplines to broaden the learners' perspective and sensitise them to MDT. However, it is when they commence practising their respective crafts in the clinical setting that young professionals really encounter the learning opportunities in MDT. Every team meeting ought to be educative and this should be one of the aims of leadership in teams. Continuing professional development is an aspect of chronic disease management that should be individual or discipline specific only when necessary.

> The best and most cost-effective outcomes for patients and clients are achieved when professionals work together, learn together, engage in clinical audit of outcomes together, and generate innovation to ensure progress in practice and service.[17]

SCENARIO: a multidisciplinary learning exercise

Our new trainee's day release course group were discussing MDT. They suggested that a brief joint module with social work students from the local university might be useful. Later in the term this was convened, in conjunction with the head of social work. It was based largely on discussion of cases and dilemmas selected for their psychosocial content. The social work students were vocal and confident. The GP trainees were reticent and appeared to be out of their comfort zone, being recently out of hospital-based training. In feedback it appeared that preconceptions on the part of aspirant social workers were confirmed – that medics are haughty, aloof and patronising. The doctors expressed their reticence as not wanting to 'blind the others with science'. It brought up the age-old stereotypes: the social work students had stories about doctors they had encountered; they regard doctors as narrow technicians; none of the GP trainees had been a social worker's client and they lacked prior experience of encounters; they had little time for 'soft knowledge'. It is difficult to evaluate multidisciplinary learning; there are differences in cognitive style, vocabulary, information stock and job description. Whatever the evaluation tools, doctors tend to fall into linear thinking, to forget the rules and pursue the clinical narrative, ignoring the rest of the patient's biography. At least the feedback discussion was fruitful.

One successful MDT programme is the European Certificate in Essential Palliative Care.[18] The generic course and assessments are aimed at doctors and nurses with a terminal care interest, and it is attracting interest by AHPs. Multidisciplinary learning broadens the agenda and, hopefully, awareness on the part of professionals.

DESIGNATED CLINICS IN GENERAL PRACTICE

The 'GP mini-clinic' is a specific area of successful MDT in primary care. It is a somewhat diminutive but venerable term for a well-established vehicle for delivering aspects of chronic disease management and preventive healthcare in general practice through:

- aggregating patients who have particular long-term conditions or monitoring requirements
- designating clinical sessions that permit the confluence of the relevant skill-mix of team members, their equipment and appropriate clinical space
- providing routine interventions, information and surveillance in accordance with quality-assured protocols of care
- optimising symptom control and biometric management
- supplementing hospital specialist care and promoting shared care.

In the notional general practice, the menu of clinics would include many of the following:

- *diabetic clinic* – mostly for type 2, but also the non-acute care of type 1; shared care with diabetologists or metabolic physician
- *vascular disease clinic* – including hypertension, secondary prevention in ischaemic heart disease, stroke, reno-vascular, peripheral vascular and non-acute cardiac failure; shared care with cardiologist or stroke unit
- *respiratory clinic* – for asthma, chronic obstructive pulmonary disease, pulmonary fibrosis and non-acute respiratory failure; care shared with respiratory physician
- *warfarin clinic*, which, by extension, may monitor other hazardous drugs ('red–amber list drugs', mostly disease-modifying drugs and antipsychotics that need bio-monitoring).

These supplement the more general clinics that include *infant/pre-school/child health and developmental clinic* (does what it says, plus vaccines; health visitor led); *maternity care clinic* (antenatal and postnatal shared care with obstetricians; midwife led); *women's health clinic* (cervical screening, gynaecology and health promotion). All GP clinics are predicated on two factors:

1. *the management tier* for setting-up, call and recall, reception, and the follow-up of aberrant results and defaulted appointments
2. *the IT system* for disease registry processes, call and recall, systems IT handling cumulative biometric data, observations and interventions; this supports the clinic operation and integrates it with the overall practice systems and facilitates shared care with specialist services.

Characteristics of clinics in general practice may be listed as:

- dedicated sessions (regular, rolling)
- multidisciplinary; share care with specialists; optimise MDT; enhanced use of AHPs
- implements protocols that are comprehensive, consistent, validated and agreed by interested parties (e.g. the CCG or health trust, and local disease specialist)
- optimum use of team skill-mix, enhanced use of nurses and AHPs
- skills within the practice team are enhanced; the 'GP with Special Interest' (a relatively novel category of GP, who has advanced training and expertise in a clinical niche)
- provides near patient care, accessible, convenient and familiar; reinforcement of patient self-care
- spare use of the more distant, expensive and specialised hospital-based clinic system
- cumulative biometric database on patients with long-term conditions
- quality of care improved, control of risk factors and smoother control of symptoms through preventive and disease-modifying interventions, health promotion, adherence and problem-solving; reduced exacerbations and admissions
- opportunity for review of total medication list
- measurement of agreed performance markers and accounting or reporting, for funding purposes or statistical returns for use by the commissioning authority; quality assurance facilitated through clinical audit and other governance measures.

On the debit side:

- compete with other priorities for finite practice capacity (space, time, personnel, funding)
- risk reduplicating services, interventions and biometrics carried out elsewhere

- 'secondary-to-primary drift', transfer of workload from hospital to community; import hospital model and disease focus into general practice
- increase workload – require much back-up time for preparation, follow-up and to process the resulting deluge of data
- additional call on patients' time and resources – yet another appointment to keep
- boundary issues for patients (*I've brought wee Johnny with me – he's got nits*)
- not well adapted for rare conditions
- ambulatory care model – needs special provision for housebound.

Much prevention and surveillance can be and is carried out in the course of routine appointments and ordinary consultations, but there are advantages to managing conditions in a collective setting. Clinics function best for major, common, long-term conditions such as those mentioned earlier, where prevalence and impact justify this kind of managed care. IT capacity provides the electronic bridge with the laboratory so that results can download directly into the practice system. Without this facility screening, monitoring and shared care programmes would be nigh impossible on the current scale, and this capacity will need to increase. The limiting factor is human judgement. Data must be interpreted and processed, and this involves serial, small-scale clinical decisions. Hence there is a 1:1 ratio between clinic

---

EXAMPLE 1

Following each attendance by diabetic patients at the hospital diabetic clinic, a spreadsheet of report data is generated and arrives at the surgery as a scanned pro forma, since the hospital IT system does not speak the same language as the practice computers. All the data have to be amalgamated into the practice-based diabetic record manually. Local practices use four different computer software systems and hospital systems cannot all communicate directly with them. IT systems should be compatible across the interfaces, at least locally.

EXAMPLE 2

There is no sharp normal–abnormal boundary for most biochemical and biometric tests. It is fuzzy, and interpretation and action decisions relate to the previous values, trend and context. Raw lab data can be integrated with prior results graphically to show trend rather than plain numerical data; decision support algorithms should be slick, sparing time and effort, rather than being tedious to operate.

time and backup time. **Ways must be found to reduce the systemic stress that is inherent in the process of making large numbers of small-scale judgements in rapid succession.**

The GP clinic is one example of a blurring of boundaries between hospital and general practice that has been occurring, to the point where there is talk of the distinction being abandoned altogether, as evidenced by trends in Kaiser Permanente and use of the phrase 'teams without walls'.[19] Some managed care organisations in the United States are developing partnerships between generalist and specialist, between high- and low-intensity settings, and differing levels of technology. It is difficult to imagine systems without any boundaries. The identities of primary and secondary care will retain at least historical and descriptive validity. The dual role of the GP, as gatekeeper and patients' advocate, has had great value in promoting rational use of specialised resources.

From this profile it is clear that the GP clinic model is the vehicle for a great deal of the chronic disease management in general practice. It provides primary and secondary prevention, information and health promotion, surveillance and screening, medication management and continuing care along with the systems that underpin these. **GP clinics represent integration of care through partnership with the patient, shared care and MDT, utilising the full resources of the health service.** The introduction of the *Quality and Outcomes Framework* in 2004 in the UK highlighted the activities in practice clinics by attaching incentives to performance scales. This has been influential in the organisation of chronic care.

The GP–hospital interface

The *interface* is a term that describes transactions between professional groups in different sectors of care. The most recognisable one is the hospital–community interface – that is, between secondary and primary care settings. Highly regulated by protocol and tradition, there has been in the UK a stark simplicity about it; referral or admission from the GP followed by discharge or return, from specialist care, 'back into the community'. The imperative to reduce hospital costs has led to the development of strategies of outpatient (ambulatory) care, shared or intermediate care, hospital outreach, perhaps based on a polyclinic model, hospital-at-home and virtual ward. These enable, for example, people with advanced cardiac failure to be cared for at home by hospital outreach nurses, with provision for readmission without formality. The archetype of this pattern is derived from the voluntary sector; the hospice home care team is a well-established model whereby a small inpatient unit can maintain a dispersed community service providing high-quality home-based treatment. A further bridge at the interface is the 'terminal care passport' (as piloted by the Royal College of General Practitioners in Northern Ireland) which puts the patient in charge of all necessary data for domiciliary MDT management; this may lead to the introduction of a patient-held smart card as a portable, personal, medical database for all chronic care. The growth of intermediate care measures has generated an increased emphasis on the use of communications technology and telemetry. Such applications of electronic media hold promise for promoting the integrated management of long-term conditions.

The interface is a busy place. It used to be like Checkpoint Charlie – 'count them in and count them out; one at a time, please'. It has come to resemble cyberspace. Sources and settings of care have been network connected rather than having partitions separating the means of care. The 'chatter' that fills this virtual space is getting louder as the traffic generated by complex care pathways increases. GPs struggle to process this stream (or is it a torrent?) of information. Making sensible clinical judgements in conditions of overload is one of the skills that need to be researched, developed, disseminated and applied.

What, then, are hospitals for? The GP, conventionally in the past, used to service the hospital, through rights (or rites and rituals) of referral to specialists, and hospital admission. WHO policy ('the paradigm shift') would suggest that hospitals should redefine their role as one of service to the community, in partnership with the GP as joint providers of the chronic care requirements of patient and community. Both, of course, have responsibilities in acute and emergency care.

GPs look to the hospital sector for:
- resolution of difficult diagnostic problems
- to initiate and deliver specific therapies
- management of acute serious and life-threatening illness
- diagnostic technology
- high-tech interventions (e.g. in cancer, coronary care, renal and stroke units)
- ongoing management of particular conditions requiring specialised expertise or equipment
- second opinion, specialist advice
- shared care of long-term conditions (e.g. diabetes, heart failure, renal failure)
- partnership in intermediate care
- surgical services
- acute neonatal care and intrapartum obstetrics
- resource for crisis management (especially inpatient).

Patients, on the whole, are outcome-oriented irrespective of the details of how services are organised. However, hospitals retain a strong symbolic significance for local communities; there is considerable resistance to any perceived diminution of hospital provision, and politicians reflect these perspectives. There is a great social and financial investment in the *institution*, which reinforces historical medical model values. This is not a criticism of secondary care. There is no place for antagonism.

Indeed, it is to safeguard the effectiveness of secondary care that the primacy of primary care is being asserted. When hospital facilities become log-jammed, through increasing inflow demand, and insufficient community care causes outflow obstruction, GPs face impossible choices in their gatekeeping and patient advocate functions. Waiting lists lengthen, patients and GPs carry increasing burdens of hazard and prolonged stress, and there is back-pressure in the 'high-volume filter' system at the front end of the NHS. They are interdependent. The WHO paradigm shift proposals are more radical than simply adjusting the historical GP–hospital imbalance, as we shall see in later discussion on policy matters (*see* Chapter 6).

A primary care paradigm shift

This health service paradigm shift would seem to require a corresponding realignment on the part of primary healthcare. In many countries this is already well under way – transforming the 'cottage industry' model into a platform that is capable of managing chronic care comprehensively. This, a 'primary care paradigm shift', may be summarised in tabular form to facilitate comparison with the traditional model (*see* Figure 5.2).

Traditional general practice	New paradigm requirements
• Small, local	• Larger group base
• Doctor delivered	• Multidisciplinary, doctor led
• Reactive, demand led	• Proactive
• Disease centred, acute orientation	• Preventive, health promotion
• Manual systems	• Electronic systems based
• Low patient participation	• Patient partnership
• Autonomous	• Connected, accountable, managed
• 'Benign paternalism'	• Quality and governance

FIGURE 5.2 The paradigm shift in primary care: models and methods

HEALTH PROMOTION AND HEALTH EDUCATION

Health promotion is a blanket term for a wide variety of activities, programmes and products whose chief commonality is reliance upon educational approaches; that is, the technology and techniques of transmitting effectively messages and information related to healthcare. It is broadly similar to *health education*, which addresses specific topics in relation to health, lifestyle and disease avoidance. In addition to these specifics, health promotion may include information about institutions and the processes that bear on accessing and utilising services that support healthy living and prevention of disease. It is a major component of the mission of those voluntary and self-help organisations that constitute civil society. In the statutory sector, health trusts have extensive departments specialising in health promotion. The field is diverse. In addition to applying the full range of educational technology, it draws on the media, marketing and advertising expertise, training and research units, and also the relatively new fields of community development and social media. *Health literacy* is a little-studied factor in healthcare. It is defined as the capacity to obtain, communicate, process and understand basic health information and processes to make good health decisions.[20] A leading article in 2012 stated that there was no information about levels of health literacy in England; that studies from the UK, USA and Australia suggest that between one third and one half of people in developed countries have difficulty understanding and engaging with their healthcare, resulting in poorer health outcomes and increased mortality.[21] Health literacy is influenced by many possible factors, such as: level of education, language and reading skills, and ability to comprehend oral, pictorial and written materials.

Health education is an ancient craft. The revered literatures, the scriptures, of the great religions abound in advice, exhortation and direction on what should be done to achieve health, wholeness and well-being. Treatises on healthy living abounded in mediaeval and Renaissance times (Della Casa's *Galateo* and *The Rule of Health of Salerno*, to name but two[22]). Every society has its store of traditional wisdom in which nutrition, hygiene and interpersonal relationships loom large. In Industrial Revolution times individual advances included Dr James Lind and Captain James Cook (with citrus fruit on board to combat scurvy), John Snow with his pump handle campaign against cholera, and Florence Nightingale in her campaign against poor hospital sanitation following the Crimean War. They exemplify the basic triad for health: good nutrition, clean water and efficient sewerage. They illustrate another fundamental: however obvious, simple or beneficial the message, the process is costly. They all had to fight to promulgate the message.

There was, for a long time, the facile belief that health education was what societies provided when they were unable to afford proper medicine – the poor man's health service. The grain of truth in this is reflected in the sophistication of health education research in underprivileged countries while the affluent ones became heavily invested in high-tech medicine. The growing awareness of lifestyle diseases in affluent societies is redressing this imbalance. The challenges that result from disordered appetites of all kinds are proving difficult and costly to overcome. People know the health messages but knowing is not sufficient. Change in behaviour is not easily brought about. Evidence changes nothing, left to itself. Effective health education is complex.

Everything you enjoy is illegal, immoral or unhealthy *(Murphy's Law)*.

However, evidence, skilfully applied at the right time in a personalised setting can change everything. It has long been known that naïf interventions, imparting simple, directive advice are effective in changing behaviour of individuals with up to 10% efficacy. The bald statement, 'you should stop smoking' has been shown to work for some, provided it comes from a trusted, authoritative person and at a time when the patient is receptive to the message, such as during a health crisis. Indeed, people often make autonomous and effective health-enhancing decisions for change without professional intervention. After all, most healthcare is self-care.

> How many health professionals does it take to change a lightbulb?
> None at all, provided the lightbulb is willing to change.

This has been borne out in the case of smoking cessation, (as we have seen in Prochaska and DiClemente's cycle of change out of addiction). It is now accepted that this holds true across the range of addictions, dependency behaviours and lifestyle diseases. Addictions and dependency behaviours in many ways conform to a chronic disease model. Interestingly, there is an epidemiological profile that supports this view: an at-risk population, a chemical pathology of enzyme induction, altered receptor sensitivity, chemical interventions that modify the trajectory, cycles of remittance and relapse, crises and co-morbidities. The cycle of change operates not just in addiction but also more generally in behaviours associated with chronic disease risk.

The Ottawa Charter for Health Promotion[23] identified five key themes of health promotion:
1. building healthy public policy – in all sectors and at all levels of society
2. creating supportive environments – taking health into settings where people work, live and play
3. strengthening community action – developing strategies to assess need and implement programmes
4. developing personal skills – enhancing life skills for social and personal development
5. reorienting the health service towards prevention of illness and promotion of health – in all sectors of healthcare and social services

This model recalls, and is in keeping with, the chronic disease model that describes the elements of chronic disease management. It places health promotion at the core of healthcare for long-term conditions. That, along with the WHO policy on addiction management,[24] places these firmly in primary care. Health promotion must be a central activity of general practice. Every practice, and **all curricula of training for primary care professionals, should include the skills required for health**

promotion and health education, motivational interviewing, behaviour modification and addiction management.

SCENARIO: a review of progress with our once new trainee

Three months into your time here what are your impressions of general practice?

Busy! Anxious all the time, in case I miss something – like early cancer, a coronary, the one child who might be developing meningitis, you know what I mean. But if I investigate every chest pain I'll be there till midnight, with an angry waiting room, or I might make the wrong judgement call and end up in the tabloids. I run over time; the computer throws up flags that have to be assessed; trying to find the information a patient needs; trying to squeeze a quart into a pint pot.

So, what's good about it?

It's interesting and varied. There's a succession of people who come with real issues that overlap and need to be prioritised and sorted. I can provide them with a lot of information and I seem to be able to help most of them. Especially when what they need is reassurance, but that costs me a lot of thought. I haven't come across many who didn't really need to be there.

Is general practice what you had expected?

No! Before this I thought it would be about short encounters for small problems that could be dealt with by a prescription, or a certificate for work or maybe referral to a specialist. But people come to talk over what's on their mind – lots of anxieties and fears. There's often a lot of discussion before it's clear to them (and me) what the problem is, or more often, what they are. Most people have a list of things to cover; ordinary things like another scrip or cert; a blood pressure check; a query about their treatment. And lots of continuing problems like their sleep, weight, pains, energy before they get round to the new stuff. We go all over the place first and I often feel I haven't got to the root of why they're there, so it's hard to know when the consultation is over. Often in the end we find something big and I have to ask them to make another appointment, and that doesn't go down well sometimes. I often think they're testing me out as the new face here.

I used to feel that too, a long time ago! What do you find most difficult about all that?

The things that are all tangled up together, when lots of thing are going on – their joints, indigestion, breathing problems, moods … We often cover all their body systems, including the health system! They're often confused about what's going on at the hospital and don't know what specialists they're seeing, or what investigations or results they're waiting for. They seem to think I should have everything at my fingertips. Then they start talking about what's going on at home – the hubby, jobs or lack of jobs, the kid taking drugs – what an agenda!

There is an agenda there to talk about – managing the consultation. But we have been focusing on chronic disease recently. Are you finding that the ideas apply at all?

It's hard to see it as a whole; it's so mixed in with everything that comes though the door, it doesn't stand out on its own. Except when I do the diabetic or asthma clinic. Then it's clear, but people keep bringing up their other complaints there too, which makes it hard to focus. I suppose that's because they see us as GPs!

True enough. People with chronic conditions get sick too, just like anybody else. We mustn't forget to fit your 'agenda' in. Come back to it in a couple of weeks. OK?

Part Two: developing the clinical complex

Thus far this chapter has dealt mainly with characteristics of primary healthcare. Part Two examines further aspects of healthcare provision that are relevant to the wider clinical professions and settings, and to policy matters. They include the use of electronic media, integrated care, commissioning, quality, governance, guidelines and evidence-based practice.

ELECTRONIC MEDIA AND GENERAL PRACTICE

IT systems that can measure anything that moves … only tell you about the level of activity and not whether the purpose is being achieved.

Simon Caulkin (Press Columnist)

IT underpins every aspect of chronic disease management. **The information era has played a large part in creating the chronic disease era by making it possible to do something effective about long-term condition management.** There is a wide agenda in the use of IT for chronic disease management, beginning with their application to practice-based systems. These include administration, registry, decision support, clinical data and patient records; also networked communications within and reaching out from the practice. Data linkage networks make possible:

- a diverse team that works in a coordinated fashion to communicate with one another, minimise reduplication and maximise coordination of effort
- coordination across interfaces and between settings
- data download and sharing to minimise tedious inputting and reduplication
- multi-user, multifunction, with a variety of portals and portable devices for flexible work location
- intermediate and shared care to operate using shared records, protocols and biometric data
- telemedicine in all its forms, including ambulatory and home-based monitoring
- safer prescription management, especially for complex regimens
- population-based programmes of prevention, screening, surveillance and monitoring
- decision support to be readily available to patients, clinicians and managers
- quality management, governance, performance review and accounting.

However, computers that do not talk to each other are simply word processors and digital archives, and networks that do not talk to each other become information silos. Furthermore:

- information networks are complex, fragile and costly; in the UK there is a 30-year history of IT project failures, at great public expense
- they require capital investment, maintenance and skills training; IT has to be engineered into the design of premises and the organisation of continuing care
- networks leak – confidential information is not easy to manage and data protection is essential
- subject to accident and error; once entered, mistaken data lingers and contaminates the system; cyber-vandalism is common; what do you do in a power cut?
- info-networks are abused; 'load it in and push it around' is a governing principle of clinical intranets based on the fallacy that everyone then will know everything; overload conceals data
- information demands attention and drives the pace; the substitution of information for action; this treadmill effect has been termed 'hamster healthcare'.[25]

The task of tracking large numbers of people with complex disease, and the accompanying treatment regimens, over many years is challenging even for the most automated systems since the element of human judgement has to be integral to the loop. Broadband has not yet reached its speed limits. Human capacity to control and respond will saturate easily. Expectations of instantaneous action create the treadmill effect. This accelerates the pace of multiple sequential small decisions that breeds operator fatigue and the risk of error.[26] But, love them or hate them, you can't do without them.

Any account of IT is likely to be obsolete before it is published. Electronic media are flowing far beyond the functions of data management and archiving. They are extending the reach of the clinical team through the use of smart devices that seem to be taking on a dynamic of their own through the net, the web and the cloud.

Telemedicine is the applied use of e-communications by health professionals to consult together and treat patients using smart technology, such as digital cameras, image transmission, teleconferencing, mobile phone systems, texting and other applications. It is widely used for diagnostic, monitoring and therapeutic purposes. Further developments include *e-connected care*, whereby the status of a patient may be monitored or observed by a remotely placed operator (e.g. a specialist nurse) who has the capacity to intervene as indicated by the patient's condition and informed by telemetry of biomarkers. These media have extended the range of self-care programmes through computer and smartphone applications, and Internet sites.

It is growing in popularity across the world. According to Orange Healthcare, e-health in Europe is one of the fastest growing sectors, where it is growing at 15%–20% annually.[27] A report from New Zealand identified four major areas of application – radiology, dermatology, paediatrics and psychiatry – that use, among other media, digitised image transmission and remote reporting, videoconferencing for peer review and case discussion via Skype.[28] It brings scarce specialist expertise to remote areas for the benefit of doctors for conferring, and to patients for follow-up. These also provide anyone with the capacity to tap into search engines to assess limitless information. In principle it is not new. In the 1970s to my knowledge isolated clinicians in Alaska could routinely consult cardiologists in Seattle via radiotelephone for advice and guidance. Now a 12-lead electrocardiograph can be transmitted via a modem to a cardiology reporting service for instant expert reporting and opinion; there is a one-lead variant that can be worn like a wristwatch and activated by the patient on suspicion of an arrhythmia. There are implantable, *in vivo*, biometric diagnostic devices. The level of sophistication accelerates as devices become smaller and faster. This trend will increase the use of cloud storage. Offering instant access from anywhere, the cloud provides a vast external facility for information backup, 'drop box' function and accessible, active storage. Indeed, all digitised medical records will probably end up there, thus overcoming problems with remote access and active information-sharing between the various sectors in chronic care. The current concerns about security in such data-sharing will be overcome with increasing compartmentalisation. Conceivably, unique personal data may be stored on the person like a barcode using RFID (radio frequency identification).

In the UK, *telehealth* is now part of government policy, and in it is invested much optimism. Systems in current use include:

- NHS Connecting for Health: integrated IT systems and services, including e-health records
- Choose and Book: electronic referral to the specialist of the patient's choice, with the appointment reserved on-line
- the national network providing broadband NHS Internet
- Contact: the standard UK-wide e-mail network for practices
- picture, archival and analysis systems.

Telemedicine aims to achieve three broad outcomes:

1. to reduce hospital admissions and prevent unnecessary referrals and A&E attendance through use of remote monitoring of the patient at home
2. reduce pressure on general practice and other NHS resources through more efficient management and resource allocation
3. improve patient quality of life, through support for independent living, the reduced need for clinical appointments and empowering them to have control over their long-term conditions, and to deliver cost savings accordingly.

EXAMPLE 1

For people with chronic obstructive pulmonary disease or heart failure Telepod will measure at regular intervals throughout the day blood pressure, oxygen saturation, temperature and weight. The lead clinician, usually a specialist nurse equipped with supporting systems, has remote access to the vital signs. A consultation may be prompted, and carried out by telephone. This may suffice, but a variety of possible responses may include a home visit by the intermediate care nursing team or the GP, or direct readmission to hospital. Selection of patients suitable for this kind of integrated multidisciplinary care is based on risk stratification.[29]

In addition to the outcomes already outlined, telehealth systems prompting early detection, rapid responses and prompt intervention are reported to reduce clinical exacerbations, reduce strain on carers, increase uptake of supportive clinical services and enhance workforce satisfaction.[30] This also raises questions of cost, capacity, training and unintended consequences that need to be resolved; there are likely to be false alarms, increased demand on GP domiciliary visits, and increased referrals or readmissions, at least initially, until the entire system calibrates itself within safe, rational limits.

A 2-year pilot of telecardiology in the Manchester area has reported a 60% reduction in referrals to secondary care, saving 200 people-visits to hospital, with potential savings to the NHS calculated at £100 million if rolled out nationally throughout the UK.[31] Systems like these are likely targets for outsourcing to commercial corporations, such as a telecom-type company.

EXAMPLE 2

The MobiHealth System is a vital signs monitoring system based on a body area network of small sensors worn on the body that collect and transmit vital signs using a mobile health service platform. Bluetooth and a mobile phone, via next-generation wireless networks, can link the patient to the care provider or a call centre. It is customised to the patient's needs and measures data such as the electrocardiograph, pulse oximetry, temperature, respiration, motion and level of activity. It is applicable for cardiology (notably arrhythmia), chronic obstructive pulmonary disease, asthma and other long-term conditions.[32]

INTERNET INTERVENTIONS AND PATIENT SELF-HELP

Internet-based applications in chronic care may be summarised as:
- information – the full range from simple to technical, with multimedia, interactive, flexible updating possibilities
- decision support for patients, to help them with making choices on treatments on offer; this may be interactive and includes risk assessment of proposed clinical interventions
- monitoring and feedback on data collected by telemedicine devices
- emotional and social support via bulletin boards, chat rooms and support groups
- behaviour change support, employing self-assessment tools, action plans, goal-setting, facilitation and monitoring of progress in attaining targets.

Benefits for patients include:
- convenient, anonymous, cost-effective, virtual meeting place
- improved self-sufficiency, especially for the non-ambulant
- computer-assisted learning.

One study of systematic reviews by Murray[33] of the impact of Internet interventions was cautiously positive: computerised cognitive behavioural therapy was reported to be as effective as therapist-led cognitive behavioural therapy. However, it has substantial workload implications for the supervising clinician and there is a considerable drop-out rate by patients. Murray concludes that Internet interventions improve user knowledge, self-sufficiency and perceived social support, with better clinical outcomes in depression and anxiety, and improved health behaviour; the Internet provides a virtual meeting space for people with rare conditions, who might otherwise never encounter each other; however, there were no clear benefits in cost-effectiveness and equity. Computer-based encounters may have great value but they are 'glitch-prone' and cause frequent anxiety on the part of non-expert users. Many people with long-term conditions simply do not use the Internet.

E-literate patients are outstripping the capacity of many GPs to respond. The rise of social media facilitates, and raises expectations of, instantaneous communication. While this creates valid channels of communication, especially with 'hard-to-reach' groups such as teenagers, there are problems: patients Internet-search their symptoms and reach conclusions of their own, frequently focusing on a worst-case scenario, before consulting a professional; unfiltered data derived from search engines are unregulated and maybe unsafe; they tend to be anxiety provoking and require interpretation; the term '*cyberchondria*' has been coined to describe the neurosis driven by too much information and too little perspective.

Clinicians find themselves in the midst of an IT and data explosion. It serves real needs but it can overwhelm – frequently data does both. It is necessary to develop cognitive filtering skills, the pattern recognition that spots and extracts the essential point from masses of information, while integrating this with judgement concerning context, deviance, significance, false positive or false negative results. **Data management is becoming one of the most challenging areas of clinical practice.** Learning support should be developed to assist doctors in this.

INTEGRATED CARE

> Optimum outcomes are generated when generalists and specialists collaborate.[34]

Comparison between the two chief healthcare settings, the hospital and the GP, gives rise to what has been called *the paradox of primary care*.[35] Many studies have shown that, compared with generalists, specialists achieve higher standards of care in specific diseases, but this is more expensive. Conversely, primary care delivers better health outcomes for the health system overall and at lower cost. Optimising the respective strengths is a priority. Unravelling the paradox of primary care, Stange and Ferrer[36] suggest, depends on:

> understanding the added value of integrating, prioritizing, contextualizing, and personalizing health care across acute and chronic illness, psychosocial issues and mental health, disease prevention, and optimization of health and meaning.

This sets the agenda for integration and commissioning of care.

The idea of integrated care has been gathering strength during this century as a central goal of health policy. It has three fundamental aims:

1. to improve the patient's experience of the care pathway
2. to improve health outcomes through increased efficiency of services
3. to save money by reducing costly demand on hospital services, especially admissions.

Integrated care has been defined by WHO as:

> a concept that brings together inputs, delivery, management and organisation of services related to diagnosis, treatment, care, rehabilitation and health promotion. Integration is a means to improve services in relation to access, quality, user satisfaction and efficiency.[37]

Rickenbach and Wedderburn[38] use the metaphor '*follow the yellow brick road*' to refer to the process known as *the care pathway*. Like the cinematic original, it is not smooth and straight from the time a patient presents with a disease or episode to its resolution. But at the end of the road is the magic real or illusory? There are gaps and hazards, loops and gradients. **People get lost to systems and within them.** They experience adverse events, insensitivity, delays and difficulties in accessing services. Frequently the process may be almost as bad as the disease. Current literature on integrated care appears uncomfortable, with the patient who has multi-morbidity preferring to focus on one salient long-term condition and the attempts to smooth out and join up the elements that constitute the single pathway of care. Sectors of care, general practice, hospital specialist, social care and voluntary care in the community, often fail to work effectively together; there is reduplication of effort causing waste of resources, and deficient systems for feedback and learning.[39]

However good the clinical outcomes, integrated care comes with a price tag that is alarming even if it were not subject to inflation. Fortunately there is an easy consensus among population, politicians and professionals: smooth, efficient, seamless clinical and care pathways. This is like apple pie – who can say no?

Financial saving is a major driver of integrated care policies. A virtuous cycle is anticipated whereby more efficient community care will reduce the burden of hospital demand, releasing secondary care savings to further boost the community infrastructure. The mission statement of integrated care might be expressed as: *to improve the quality of the patient's experience through patient-centred care planning that is evidence based, safe and economical.* However, the devils lie in the details, and some of them are demons. For example, how to ensure that hospital savings make their way into the community coffers; how to finance the initial community investment that kick-starts the cycle; how to manage complexity in systems and care pathways when there is more than one serious long-term condition present; is innovative change compatible with shrinking health budgets, and who is in charge? And then there is the major issue of the *commissioning* of integrated care, but more of that later.

If you think that integrated care is like holistic care, taking into account all of the factors and significant conditions that cohabit within so many patients, and trying to manage them all as elegantly, humanely and economically as possible, then you are an idealist (and probably a GP who thinks that this is what we have been about all along). For systems-oriented policymakers, that is a bridge too far, and the ultimate challenge for those who commission care. The current emphasis is on the individual disease pathway, to try to get it right through service redesign and effective commissioning processes. This is challenge enough without addressing the complexities of co-morbidity where several clinical pathways coexist and interact.

To reconcile the single pathway approach with the reality of multi-morbidity, two concepts are promising.

1. *Bundling of services*: an *individualised* care plan that pulls together the elements of disparate clinical pathways and specifies the overall package.
2. *Care pathways*: these are the product of needs assessment and defining patient-centred outcomes to embody *goal orientation* rather than *disease orientation*. Irrespective of the diagnostic labels the goals are defined in functional terms – that is, what the patient needs to be able to achieve in daily life. The *care plan* defines the process of achieving and sustaining this.

CASE EXAMPLE

The 77-year-old widow suffers from type 2 diabetes, arthritis, hypertension and heart failure. Her doctor, mindful of guidelines, defines desirable outcomes as tight diabetic control, normalised blood pressure and reduced use of analgesics to avoid compromising renal and cardiac function. The patient-preferred outcomes include pain relief, less unsteadiness, better mobility and therefore more autonomy. Her preferences carry implications for targets in glucose and blood pressure control, use of ACE inhibitors, beta blockers, and non-steroidal anti-inflammatory medications. Clinical targets may have to be compromised in order to achieve her functional aspirations. Achieving this will adversely affect the clinician's performance in attaining guideline compliance (and, possibly, income). There may have to be reduced reliance on drugs, combined with an increased use of AHPs (for physiotherapy, occupational therapy, dietary guidance and pharmacist support); more intensive surveillance by specialist nurses (in diabetes and cardiac failure); and perhaps the use of telemedicine systems, all coordinated by a named clinician, either the GP or a geriatrician.

Health analysts Chris Ham and Natasha Curry[40] classify forms of integrated care as:

- *Real Integration*, where organisations merge their services
- *Virtual Integration*, in which providers cooperate to work together through networks and alliances
- *Horizontal Integration* refers to providers working together and operating from the same level (e.g. GPs working closely with community social services)
- *Vertical Integration*, where different providers work across different service levels (e.g. GP with hospital specialist, as in shared care and intermediate care)
- *Commissioning based*, where different providers work from a pooled budget
- *Mixed* (the *'make or buy'* model) where, by a combination of commissioning and provision, the budget is used to provide some services but to purchase additional elements from other sources.

The question whether integrated care is disease specific or comprehensive (geared towards a matrix of functional outcomes) may be overcome through enlightened commissioning of care. This will be the key test for the future of CCGs and NHS England.[41] They need to think generic in respect of chronic disease management, to design services around the needs of the person that transcend boundaries between multiple conditions and between sectors of care provision.

There is a variety of terms in use in integrated care that are closely related to the care pathway concept.

Integrated care pathways have been defined as *structured, multidisciplinary care plans that detail essential steps in the care of patients with specific clinical problems.* They have been proposed as a way of encouraging the translation of national guidelines into local protocols and their subsequent application to clinical practice.[42] This introduces a further set of problems into integrated care proposals. Evidence-based practice is considered of vital importance. However, by contrast with tertiary care where, for example, cancer centres work to a tight protocol-led integrated pathway, those in the community tend to be convoluted and trans-sectoral. This confounds much of the clinical evidence base of medical practice and is one of the many recognised problems with getting evidence into practice, as will appear later. Different patients need different plans for integrated care and they are not for everyone.

Care planning is defined, by the Department of Health in 2009, as:

> addressing an individual's full range of needs taking into account their health, personal, economic, educational, mental health, ethnic and cultural background and circumstances. It recognises that there are other issues in addition to medical needs that can affect a person's total health and well-being.[43]

This clunky statement suggests that the Department of Health in England discovered general practice around 2008. Is this not what generalists have always striven to do? However, this places general practice at the hub of chronic disease management, dependent as it is on continuing, holistic case management. Parallel developments in care planning are widespread in other developed health systems.

Case management is a matter of *care coordination*. It aims to reduce duplication of effort and procedures, avoid gaps, and reduce health and social care costs. It is a crucial strand of the UK strategy for chronic disease management. Evidence for the effectiveness of case management is mixed but promising. It sounds a bit like integrated care, but turns the concept into a process.

Linking these ideas together tells us that integrated care is concerned with risk stratification – *identifying* people with complex and long-term conditions, *assessing* their need in a holistic fashion, identifying *desirable outcomes* and specifying the *pathway* of care which informs the *care plan*, and this will be subject to individual *case management*.

Achieving this requires:
- investment and additional resources
- longer consultation times for complex cases
- efficient and compatible systems for sharing patient information
- a multidisciplinary approach
- coordination with other services
- continuity of care.

General practice federations provide a model of the kind of primary care hub that will provide a broad range of integrated services outside the hospital setting.[44] There is widespread opinion that service redesign is necessary to bring about realignment towards community-based care, rather than continuing dependence on hospital-centrism and specialist/disease focus[45,46] – that is, the paradigm shift.

In the UK integrated care is part of the national outcome framework and recommended keys to its successful introduction are:
- share and analyse models of success (not to 'reinvent the wheel')
- lead clinician and lead administrator, to coordinate activity, utilise feedback, act on complaints, rectify problem areas
- promote a fact-managed system, evidence based and responsive to need, managing biometric data
- education to underpin the whole process – better-informed service users, multi-professional learning, initial professional training and continuing learning, overseen by local education and training boards

- goal-oriented approach – encouraging each individual to achieve the highest possible level of health (as defined by the patient)
- participatory patient management – the patient at the centre of the process
- safety-netting to minimise hazards and side effects
- comprehensiveness rather than fragmentation.[47]

Integrated care is further discussed in Chapter 6 along with its implications for health policy. For now, the elements of an infrastructure for integrated care are summarised in Figure 5.3.

- Patient centred, carer sensitive and family-friendly
- Generalist led, multidisciplinary team delivered
- Lead clinician and lead administrator
- Compatible IT systems, data sharing
- Evidence-based, fact-managed protocols that take account of complexity
- Care planning and case management of integrated pathways of care
- Goal-orientation in balance with guideline orientation
- Patient involvement in line with community-oriented primary care
- Specialist nurse key role ('community matron')
- Medical specialist services brought close to the community, shared care, outreach clinics
- Community access to diagnostics, possibly through the so-called Darzi Centre model (polyclinic) or practice federations
- Crisis intervention capacity, prompt hospital access
- Intermediate care processes – virtual ward or 'hospital-at-home'
- Connected health technology – telemedicine, patient-held ('smart card') databases
- Community social services involvement
- Carer support and home care workers
- Supported living facilities, respite care provision
- Voluntary sector involvement, self-management and expert patient programmes
- Task forces for special needs – elderly care, mental disorders, disability support

---

FIGURE 5.3 An overview of integrated care in long-term conditions

A survey of chronic disease management in ten European countries showed that they mostly use a vertical, disease-oriented approach. Evidence suggests that better outcomes arise from an integrated approach to disease within strong primary health care systems.[48]

COMMISSIONING CHRONIC CARE

Healthcare does not just happen. Somebody, somewhere, makes it possible by commissioning it – that is, identifies what is needed, and contractualises how it will be purchased. Otherwise a health service is liable to be chaotic, and this is not uncommon. **Commissioning of care specifies and procures total care required in a given situation.** Consideration in some detail is merited because commissioning is central to healthcare delivery. Furthermore, recent UK health policy is heavily invested in community-oriented commissioning. It may be summed up as *'what, by whom, at what cost?'*

All health economies are beset by funding issues and this is one of the main drivers behind the rapid development of commissioning models. In the United States a model that incorporated citizens' juries was tried during the 1990s in Oregon and invited focus groups to prioritise conditions in rank order of merit in order to prioritise funding. Medicaid went even beyond this earlier Oregon experiment to introduce health insurance by lottery.[49] In the UK the NHS was founded on centralised commissioning, then through serial reforms in 1990, 2003 and 2012 by devolution towards a primary care base. Much of the world struggles on with the chaotic model based on un-coordinated service providers whose message is *'here's what is on offer; come and get it, if you can afford it'*, while governments try to fill the consequent gaps with public health measures and fragmentary programmes of care. In the words of the WHO,

> The great limiting factor on the effectiveness of healthcare is the quality of the vehicle that delivers it to the populace. Where this is based on programmes of reactive disease treatment there are liable to be gaps in provision, health inequalities, escalating costs and poorer population outcomes.[50]

The so-called *'primary care–led NHS'* proposals in the late 1990s in the UK led to the introduction of *local commissioning groups* of clinicians, which then coalesced into larger primary care trusts to achieve economies of scale and risk-sharing that were more broadly based. These failed to break the mould of the earlier regional health authorities and tended to continue their management-led pattern. The Health and Social Care Act 2012 seeks to create CCGs under the leadership of GPs and with two-thirds of the entire health budget for England at their disposal. A new body, NHS England, will develop commissioning outcome frameworks, but it seems likely to exert centralised control.

To base an entire health system on an integrated commissioning model is unique to England. Heavily dependent on GP input, and with participation by service users and lay representatives, these will commission integrated services and packages of care based on identified community needs. That is, if they can persuade the traditionally dominant voices of hospital managers and specialists to harmonise. This is likely to be problematic unless there is widespread adoption of the paradigm shift. Commissioning is hard to do well, since it has exacting requirements that need high-level skills and new methods that include:

- assessing the needs of the population covered
- designing packages of care
- forming an overview of local service provision
- negotiating contracts
- monitoring compliance of contractors
- evaluating what has been delivered
- ensuring cash flow while keeping within budget
- governance and ethics monitoring.[51]

Elements of project management can be contracted out to consultancies, but the cost may be high. In one US programme, administrative support accounted for upwards of 20% of budget, while more generally it is reported that 20%–30% of funding is consumed by firms of providers as overheads and profits.[52] There are fears that competition legislation will force CCGs to put to public tender the majority of proposed services and that this could see the NHS fragmented and opened up to 'privatisation by stealth'.

Commissioners undertake financial and legal risk related to business viability, conflicts of interest, impact on patients and rationing of care.[53] They will find themselves restricting or shutting down aspects of service delivery in order to comply with inevitable cuts in funding. This will be difficult to explain to their patients since local sentiment and opinion always jump to protect existing services. It is not surprising that GPs are wary of entering into these additional responsibilities, possibly liabilities, or that the commercial sector is deeply interested and anticipating substantial profit.

This emphasis on commissioning has been gathering strength for over a decade. But is commissioning part of a GP's role? The Seventh National GP Worklife Survey 2013 found that 13% of GPs have formal involvement and 15% act as commissioning lead within their practice team.[54] This must constitute a substantial proportion of all full-time GPs in England, representing a real diversion of clinical manpower. GPs in the UK have become accustomed to the concept of commissioning, but it has approached a scale that is ambitious. The implications for workload and responsibilities in general practice are considerable. However, in undertaking commissioning they can bring with them the values of primary care, seeing the CCG as the lever on the system that will advance the paradigm shift and further the vision of chronic care in the community. If, on the other hand, they find themselves relieving a bottleneck here or there only to find a logjam elsewhere, or being tasked with solving the crises and problems of hospitals without any other change, then they may find commissioning an onerous exercise in futility. It may be some years before we know. There are valid fears that there may be an underlying agenda to asset-strip the cohesive NHS which is regarded as a national treasure. The democratic mandate would then be replaced with a business model that is accountable only to corporate law and share-holders.[55]

In summary, *commissioning of healthcare is a complex example of clinical management that defines, secures, oversees and evaluates health services*. The UK system of commissioning has become a bold and unique experiment – that of predicating the health services as a whole on community-oriented local commissioning. It is closely related to integrated care, whereby pathways of care are subject to patient-centred, multidisciplinary case management in order to improve the experience of the patient, achieve better outcomes and use resources more cost-effectively. How this will affect the integrity of the NHS, time will tell.

THE QUALITY AGENDA

> If we deny the finest healthcare to any citizen we deny the value of their lives. They become the slaves of unnecessary suffering and disability.
>
> **Senator Ted Kennedy**

Quality is, and always was, an essential ingredient of healthcare. This section could end here, were it not for a few key considerations.

- *There are differing views about what quality means*. It is liable to be interpreted differently by patients (needs or wants?), healthcare workers (more bureaucracy), management (new powers), health systems (better value for money) and society (more control over pushy professionals).
- *Doctors show wide variation in measurements of what they do*, in areas such as consultation rates, prescribing patterns, referrals and admissions. What does this mean and why should it be so?
- *Things go wrong*; adverse events occur and competence is called into question; there must be yardsticks to measure performance.
- *Professional resistance* to quality management is influenced by perceived criticism, professional pride and the association between quality assurance and additional bureaucratic workload.

- *It involves making and receiving judgements*; it raises fears of proceedings or litigation; reflective practitioners may feel that they know their own learning needs and vulnerabilities, and can manage them, but do they?
- *It is easier to validate processes of care than to standardise professionalism*; what we do best may not be measurable (e.g. caring); so do we have to create procedures, protocols and policies for everything?
- *Clinicians are not machines*; things go wrong for them too – in personal health and circumstances. It has been said that only the mediocre are always performing at their best.
- *Bottom line*: the interests of patients have to be protected.

> Society has the right to know if general practice is doing a good and safe job for its citizens.[56]

Quality of practice has always been a core value of professionalism. This is why the Royal College of General Practitioners was founded (in 1952). It campaigned for postgraduate training in general practice and university chairs in primary care, created membership by examination in 1968 and introduced an influential Quality Initiative in 1985. Following these professionally led developments, the UK government has used contractual levers to address and incentivise quality markers. Thus, for over 50 years UK general practice has led, and participated in, a continuous upward trend in quality, with beneficial outcomes. But how is quality of care to be judged? Total quality is an elusive concept and evaluation relies on proxy measures, ones that focus on activity, process, performance indicators, portfolios of continuing education, practice inspections, to name a few. All come at a price in terms of effort, time and expense.

The challenge for professionals is to embrace the *demonstration of quality*, to value the processes involved, to know that the necessary cost to them is worthwhile, and that any judgements resulting are fair and formative rather than inquisitorial and punitive. Pride in one's work, and even enjoyment, should be the motivators, whereas external micromanagement and 'bean-counting' damage morale, undermine self-governance and threaten job satisfaction. And what about those who are found wanting? Quality assurance ought to be more about education than regulation. It is not about uncovering, say, 5% of GPs who are performing badly but addressing that 5% within each of us that could be improved.

The well-known construct 'the Johari Window' has a cell marked 'unknown unknowns'. However good we think we are, there are sectors of performance where we lack insight – we do not know what we are unaware of. Quality process addresses this, bringing it to conscious level so that it is progressively shrunk in size. This is challenging and relies on the trustworthy, humane involvement of external agency.

Quality is not a commodity that can be prescribed. It is a continuous process of safeguarding and improvement through change that is purposeful, measured and evaluated. Rather than regarding it as a criticism of the past, we should see it as an exercise in critical thinking and reflective practice. Smith[57] summarised this agenda for change:

> A deep change in healthcare would be if it became safe, evidence-based, truly patient-centred and concerned with health rather than disease. We've had the rhetoric for years but never the reality.

This statement suggests a convenient framework for further discussion:
- one key issue – does *quality relate to healthcare policy?*
- three planks of quality – *safety, clinical effectiveness* and *the experience of the patient*
- two drivers of change – *management* that moves the rhetoric towards its realisation and puts information into practice so that quality is embedded within the culture of practice; and *governance* – those procedures that demonstrate the implementation of quality-sensitive tools and measures, through creating the audit trail of supporting evidence.

In the UK the Royal College of General Practitioners introduced quality awareness in the 1970s with *practice activity analysis*, recording variables such as consultation rates, hospital referrals, access and waiting times, prescribing of antibiotics or psychotropics, and other indices that reflect what is going on. These can be compared between partners, with peers in neighbouring practices or at locality or regional levels, not for constructing league tables but to interrogate data for meaning, significance and action. Continuous prescribing data analysis and feedback, another significant quality tool, was pioneered in Northern Ireland in the early 1970s, developed by Hugh McGavock as the COMPASS programme, and adopted throughout the UK. It showed individualised practice prescribing rates of a wide range of drugs, their quarterly trend and comparison with mean rates for locality and region. This now informs an annual, external, formative practice review.

Jack Wennberg in the United States first studied variation in performance. He found that some variations were rational, others unwarranted. Practice variability is not, per se, unwelcome or damaging. It reflects a complex of factors that range from the macroscopic ones of health policy and system to the very local and individual.

> To some extent variation can be justified since different doctors care for patients with different preferences and in different social and healthcare contexts but the range of performance is usually wider than can be justified by these

factors; this can contribute to inequity in the delivery of care and potentially also to outcomes.[58]

Ian Kennedy's 2011 report for the King's Fund, *Improving the Quality of Care in General Practice*,[59] found no new ways to measure quality in primary healthcare; he concluded that, in general, care in general practice is good; even where variation exists it is difficult to show that such variances harm patients and variation in prescribing is largely accounted for by case-mix.[60]

One critical review of variance in rates of referral concluded that:

- the phenomenon remains largely unexplained
- there is a lack of consensus on what constitutes an appropriate referral
- patient characteristics accounted for less that 40% of variation
- GP and practice characteristics accounted for less than 10%, perhaps related to the level of tolerance of uncertainty and perception of risk
- the use of guidelines had only limited success in altering referral behaviour.[61]

Just as quality was always at the heart of medical practice and teaching long before anybody invented quality initiatives, it was always part of health policy ever since 1948, when the UK government removed the greatest single obstacle to good services – that of charges for treatment. The past two decades have seen it increasingly formalised in specific areas such as attention to the experience of the patient, patient participation, clinical effectiveness, value for money, safety and governance.

Patient involvement and quality

Our patients are not stupid or hostile. They wish to be involved in decisions and self-management, and they hold GPs and practice nurses in high regard. Few patient complaints or litigations arise from lack of competence or knowledge. The vast majority of them arise from miscommunication, perceived lack of respect for patients' dignity and delays in treatment. They know clinicians are busy and they forgive much provided that they are treated with courtesy and consideration. What patients want is personal communication and humaneness, competence, listening and informing, taking account of their preferences, involvement in decision-making, adequate time and competence.[62] According to the sociologist Hirschman[63] there are three forms of action individuals can take in response to receiving any service:

1. exit – cease to purchase the service
2. voice – express dissatisfaction in the hope of improvement
3. loyalty – continue to support the service.

Patients who *exit* the practice generally do so quietly. In most cases we do not know why and assume it was because they moved house or for convenience. **We could give some more thought to why people quit our practices**, perhaps using an exit questionnaire. With regard to health services, commentators point out that *loyalty* is the most common one, perhaps to an excessive degree (i.e. deference) especially if there is little choice of alternative providers. Each NHS practice is obliged to have a complaints system, and the *voice* of complaint is now well embedded in NHS systems.

Patient participation groups

There is an extensive literature on patient participation groups and how they operate. If they were easy to establish and conduct they would be universal. There appears to be general agreement on their value in principle but less enthusiasm in reality. This is partly due to suspicion on the part of GPs that 'busybodies' and pressure groups would infiltrate their practice decision-making processes with destructive criticism and little care for the costs in time and expense involved in meeting demands that might be made. We fear the 'process issues' more than the principle and it is difficult to achieve balance. Nevertheless, short of a participatory democracy for all our patients there is much that practices can do to gather and respond to the ideas, concerns and expectations of their patients, from suggestion boxes to large-scale surveys. Annual use of a *patient satisfaction survey* is a contractual requirement of GPs in the UK; although these surveys are widely used in research and regulation, there are limits to their value for practices:

- limited ability to capture nuance
- underestimation of the extent of dissatisfaction
- responder bias
- weakness as an outcome measure.[64]

They are also liable to *design bias*, especially when devised by remote authority, they seek answers to questions that are not being posed locally and the practitioners they refer to do not have ownership of the process. So why do we use them? Iliffe *et al.*[65] remind us that

> The ideological reason is that in a democracy service users have rights to influence matters that affect them and that they ultimately pay for. There has been a transformation in healthcare from a providers' market to a consumerist one. The satisfaction of patients' needs should be part of the definition of quality.

Iliffe *et al.* go on to provide further reasons for using surveys: that service users have strong views about whether a service is good or bad, and are the best judges of interpersonal aspects, relating and communication.

In summary, we must ask ourselves what we are doing if not attempting to meet the health needs of our patients. If we don't want to know we shouldn't ask; but if we ask, they will tell us and we ought to listen and respond. There is more to patient satisfaction than groups and surveys. The chief foundation of a listening and responsive practice is a reflective and empathic practice culture, expressing *the four R values* of quality:

1. *relational* – direct dialogue with patients in a spirit of partnership
2. *reflective* – a philosophy of practice that is self-critical within a learning organisation
3. *rational* – distinguish between wants and needs, prioritise them and solve problems
4. *realistic* in scope – setting attainable objectives that are affordable and sensitive to workload implications.

Clinical effectiveness

The remainder of this chapter addresses the broad area of clinical effectiveness, which ramifies into every aspect of clinical practice but is particularly crucial to chronic disease management. There are three main products in general practice:

1. delivery of acute and demand-led interventions
2. preventive, health maintenance and health promoting measures (especially in chronic care)
3. holding work, the continuum of caring, but greatly under-studied.

The first two are eminently measurable and they figure prominently in contracts, quality management and commissioning. How to measure the third one?

Holding work has been defined as:

> establishing and maintaining a trusting, reliable, constant doctor-patient relationship, providing ongoing support without expectation of cure.[66]

The authors of this go on to reflect on its relevance to everyday primary care, particularly in the long-term management of people with complex chronic problems. If substantial value is not accorded to this kind of intensive, rewarding work that patients need, what kind of effectiveness are we measuring? As we have seen, patients attach very great value to the skilfully managed interpersonal encounter. The holding relationship is at risk of becoming an endangered species, the victim of reductionist measurement, perverse incentives and work–time pressure. Time spent 'bean-counting' attracts rewards. The rewarding aspects of therapeutic relationship are under pressure when competing with programmed computer prompts that dominate valuable consultation time. Some values must be regarded as intrinsic to professionalism because of their face validity, irrespective of other requirements or incentives.

Measurement of effectiveness is a thriving industry within health services that ramifies beyond the scope of the individual practice. Commonly used parameters are *outcome* and *cost.*

Outcomes: the three Ms of quality

The earliest outcome measures were simply those of recording and measuring mortality, morbidity and money, but these are not the three Ms in question. There is more to outcomes than measuring what has happened to the patient. The next step is to improve upon observed clinical outcomes and this requires a partnership between patients and their health professionals, with the patient actively involved in self-care.[67] Perhaps the most significant measures of outcome are those that relate to *patient-determined outcome.* Consider, therefore in what way the patient has benefitted, how his or her behaviour has changed and what his or her contribution to the process was. But the starting point is information. Through processes of reflection, analysis, decision-making and action, data can change outcomes, and not just measure them.

This is summed up as the three Ms:

1. *measurement* – the point assessment of variables, defined as outcomes or results of interaction between the patient and the health delivery system
2. *monitoring* – repeated assessments (as in point 1) in a manner that permits causal inferences concerning what produced observed results
3. *management* – the use of information gained from *monitoring* and related sources in the process of clinical decision-making, management of patient care or service delivery to achieve optimal patient outcomes.[68]

In applying these to quality process the levels of measurement are categorised as:
- health status:
  - clinical measurement such as blood pressure, glucose, lung function
  - self-rated health and quality of life, as in disability, pain, fatigue, dyspnoea, psychological well-being
- health behaviours – exercise, cognitive symptom management, adherence
- healthcare use – doctor visits, A&E visits, admissions, length of stay
- self-efficacy – confidence to self-care.[69]

These measures have been developed as research tools for the evaluation of programmes of care in large populations, and these lie beyond the scope of individual GPs or practices since they work from a limited denominator and data set. The more usual practice-based instrument is *audit* (more of this later).

Cost and value for money

In an increasingly cost-conscious environment systems are preoccupied with value for money. It may be difficult enough to measure value (or values!), but the money itself is not simple to measure (otherwise accountants would be redundant). There is a ladder of evaluation levels applied by health economists:

- *cost analysis* measures what is being spent and on what: *crude cost* or price paid for items of service
- *cost–benefit analysis* links financial cost with measured consequences *for the patient*
- *cost-effectiveness* links costs and consequences *for the system*
- *cost–utility analysis* links benefits for *both patient and system* with overall costs.[70]

Prior to *the purchaser–provider split*, brought about by the reforms of 1990 in the UK, NHS managers did not know the price of a cholecystectomy. The tangle of budgetary issues in a system that eschewed direct payment by patients did not easily yield specific data. Cost analysis was a major initial task in establishing the internal market within the NHS, on which commissioning of services was predicated. Much has been learned from the private sector, and one can only hope that the NHS is learning the right lessons.

As for effectiveness of outcomes for patients, this has led to the invention of new units of measurement, such as:

- the quality-adjusted life year (QALY)
- the disability-adjusted life year (DALY)
- healthy life expectancy (HALE).

A consensus on the need to strive continually to drive up quality of care and improve clinical outcomes sits uneasily alongside the imposition of financial savings for health systems. A chief executive of the King's Fund, Appleby,[71] stated somewhat wistfully:

> As the NHS enters a period of little or no growth in funding but incessant demand and cost pressure, the idea that improving quality of services, treatment and care could actually save money is an attractive proposition.

Efficiency savings should be possible through streamlining systems, reducing reduplication of services and improving treatment and these should enhance the health of groups and individuals. However, such benefits are values in their own right and their impact on budgets can only be assessed over a long term. They do not deliver early savings or solve immediate problems. When efficiency economies are called for there is a high risk that simple direct action will be applied, cutting drug budgets, freezing manpower requirements and squeezing service delivery. The quality impact of this is likely to be negative, if not for the patient then certainly for those who staff and deliver services. Appleby concludes:

> Although there is plenty of evidence that poor quality health care and adverse events are costly both for the NHS in financial terms and for the patient in terms of health consequences, there is … a dearth of evidence of the reverse relation, that improving quality leads to lower costs.[72]

Closer to home in the local GP's surgery, there is much that can be done with immediacy and relevance in seeking, collating and reflecting on the views of patients about the processes and outcomes of their treatment pathways. Any resulting audits or significant events analysis should affirm positive outcomes and not merely focus on the negatives. **The full spectrum of quality and outcomes demands our attention.**

Safety and quality

> The trouble with always trying to preserve the health of the body is that it is so difficult to do without destroying the health of the mind.
>
> GK Chesterton

All clinical care involves risk; for example, those probabilities (great and small) that attach to prescribing medicines, their side effects, random and idiosyncratic reactions and unintended consequences in the whole process of care. It is one thing to understand risk as a professional (how many of us do?); it is quite another to convey this to the patient successfully. How much risk is no significant risk? A defined risk, however small, seems greater than an undefined one; ignoring a known risk seems less defensible than ignoring an unknown one.[73] David Misselbrook[74] described practice as being 'about fixing things. Fixing things that go wrong and fixing the risk of things going wrong'.

Risk takes two forms:
1. *general* – as in the at-risk population; what is the attack rate of an outbreak of an infective agent?
2. *specific* – such as the risk of a patient's cancer recurring, or risk difference between alternative procedures.

Risk pervades all clinical encounters; every diagnosis is a statement of probability, to be refined through tests and investigations. In ruling out alternative possibilities we consider (before excluding) rarities that have the worst outcomes before settling on the most probable choice. All our tests entail risk of false results. How much of this do we tell the patient, and how to tell it? We know that truth-telling risks scaring people to death. We tend to adopt a 'final common pathway approach' that is based on an educated instinct and subconscious calculation, erring on the side of safety, and presenting a message that has integrated a series of cumulative, inherent risks. That is all very well until you back the wrong horse, even for good reasons, and then there is an accounting to be faced. This is *risk management*, which may be summed up for the jobbing GP as:

- to anticipate risks and take action to mitigate the worst ones
- safety-net your consultations
- keep good records that show your thinking
- be evidence-based where possible, respect protocols and guidelines, use decision support aids
- discuss dilemmas with somebody good, or seek a second opinion
- seek advice from medical indemnity advisors
- have risk management procedures that are demonstrable such as monitoring hazardous drugs, audit or clinical governance meetings, and active complaints processes
- read all clinical correspondence carefully and fully; watch for 'time-bombs' buried deep within much prose (and the 'PS' over the page)
- foster an open, positive, relationship of trust with patients
- be receptive to patients' ideas, concerns, expectations and feedback
- don't be afraid to say sorry (but do it wisely)
- follow up all your relevant knowledge gaps as you encounter them; document them as a learning diary
- keep portfolios of learning and governance activity that demonstrate a culture of reflective practice
- be nice to your local pharmacists; they stand between you and drug harm.

Medicines management, safety and quality

The sheer volume of patient-related activity and the management of uncertainty mean that adverse events will inevitably occur. Among the commonest are adverse prescribing incidents. Prescribing of medicines is the most salient of GP interventions, with risk to both the patient and the doctor. This is particularly true in chronic care where complex syndromes, multiple pathology, or frail elderly with failing metabolic capacity all contribute to risk and the hazards of polypharmacy. In addition, the universal practice of self-care by patients means that they may be consuming over-the-counter or Internet-sourced medicines without the knowledge of the GP.

Discrepancies creep into the patient's drug list, and issues of adherence compound this. The GP–hospital interface is a major contributor to discrepancy since chronically ill and elderly patients experience frequent hospital admissions. It is well recognised that discrepancies in medicines management processes occur both on admission and discharge from hospitals.[75] In a study, commissioned by the General Medical Council, of prescription errors:

- one item in 550 was associated with a severe error
- one in 20 held an error in prescribing or monitoring
- four in ten patients over 75 had one prescription error in a year.[76]

These figures may suggest a system that is, in fact, functioning remarkably well, bearing in mind that not all errors have critical, or indeed any, consequences. But the existence of error is a problem that requires active management and this report made two recommendations:

1. improve IT systems, including alerts that are rational and reasonable, and reduce 'alert fatigue'
2. improve systems for prescription review and blood test monitoring of medication.

As a key area of risk for all concerned, medicines management demands all care and attention, backed up by robust practice policies and procedures that safeguard especially the interface transitions and take account of patient behaviour. In this the GP has a powerful ally in the community pharmacist, a profession that is becoming increasingly oriented to clinical management and involved in chronic care. With access to clinical measurement equipment, near patient testing and the prescription history of patients, the pharmacist's contribution in monitoring, safety and repeat dispensing is growing. Their expertise is widely imported into the primary care team's skill-mix. They have much to offer – for example, through creating

---

1 Be aware of human factors, training/information needs

2 Have a robust repeat prescribing process/comprehensive protocol

3 Monitor patients on toxic medications

4 Check patient identity before prescribing

5 Verify it is the right drug, correct dosage; beware drugs with similar names when clicking on lists

6 Consider drug interaction and contraindications, especially when over-riding screen prompts

7 Administer drugs correctly

8 Advise the patient of common risks and side effects

9 Develop a clear prescription collection procedure

10 Review uncollected scripts before shredding

FIGURE 5.4 Top 10 tips for safe prescribing (*source*: Medical Protection Society)[77]

practice formularies, performing audits, advising on repeat prescribing and dispensing arrangements, and using their IT to detect potentially serious drug–drug interactions.

The Medical Protection Society provides 10 tips for safe prescribing (*see* Figure 5.4).

To the Medical Protection Society's top 10 tips I would add three more:

1. 'weed' the drug lists (delete, minimise and streamline)
2. pay special attention to the interfaces and transitions (notably hospital attendances)
3. scrutinise all clinical correspondence for drug alteration and reconcile the drug lists, since such changes are not always optimal or clearly identified.

MANAGEMENT AND GOVERNANCE

> The difference between good and bad practice whether in hospital or community is not so much a matter of great knowledge as good management.
>
> **Anonymous conference participant**

Management is not about managers – it is too important to be left to them. Every decision-making team member is involved in management. It is about converting activity into services that are sustainable, robust and effective. Institutions depend on systems and these require coordination, resourcing, motivation and overarching values. The value in this instance is quality: of care provision, the patient's experience of the service, use of available resources and maintenance of the systems that create optimal outcomes.

As a WHO report indicates,[78] quality and effectiveness in healthcare are only as good as the vehicle that delivers services, in this case the practice and how it is managed. As we move from a history of single-handed practices towards large units and federations, the complexity of management increases. For example, in an organisation of **N** people the number of lines (**L**) of communication (possible person-to-person relationships) may be represented as follows:

$$L = (N^2 - N)/2$$

Thus, when $N = 2$, $L = 1$; when $N = 5$, $L = 10$; when $N = 10$, $L = 45$. Where it becomes unrealistic to quality assure each personal action or interaction it is the process and protocols that are the objects of validation.

Management occupies the territory that lies somewhere between policy and administration. It is, perhaps, the enzyme that turns policy into processes that can then be administered, and vice versa. This suggests that policy is cooked up elsewhere, and this is frequently the case. Guidelines and aims that the practice concocts autonomously are like policy *with a small p*, and these may have as much impact and relevance for patient experience as the large-scale, remotely decided (*large P*) Policy of edicts and arrangements. Thus a practice policy on the needs of carers or repeat prescribing may have considerably more impact on quality of someone's care than a national budgetary decision has.

Management principles govern three main areas: people, resources and change. The chief resource in general practice is people – that is, how the team members express the partnership with patients and with one another. The way people relate to their colleagues and perform their own role in an organisation determines how effective they will be. There is always room for improvement. The author W Somerset Maugham, referring to writers, said that only the very mediocre are always performing at their best. Continuous improvement is possible and this is the goal of a well-functioning team. The activities and processes that carry quality improvement into everyday practice for the benefit of patients have come to be known as *clinical governance*.

Clinical governance

> What we are talking about is having in place transparent and failsafe systems for developing and nurturing good practice and identifying and correcting weaknesses and problem areas … In the highly pressurised environment in which we work it is systems that let us down at times, not individuals.[79]

As the first director of clinical governance for the NHS, Halligan promulgated this liberal message, adding that it should not be a punitive process but should aim to emphasise good practice, akin to the educator celebrating an area of ignorance encountered – as a learning opportunity rather than a cause of derision. Continuous improvement based on reflective practice appears to be the core message. The friendly, formative side has been supplemented by the General Medical Council's code, which emphasises that, *'you must protect patients from risk of harm posed by another colleague's conduct, performance or health'*.[80] Clinical governance has been defined as,

> a framework through which NHS organisations are accountable for continuously improving the quality of their services and safeguarding high standards of care by creating an environment in which excellence in clinical care will flourish.[81]

Practices in the NHS are required to appoint *a clinical governance lead*, who is responsible for ensuring that suitable processes are in place, that formal review occurs periodically within the practice and an annual report is submitted to the health trust or commissioning group. This will include an assurance that the doctors have undertaken *annual appraisal* and it will contribute to *3-yearly revalidation* and *recertification*. A menu of activities that constitute clinical governance would include:

- mandatory annual appraisal based on an interview and scrutiny of the portfolio that shows evidence of learning, participation in audit activity, achievement of clinical targets, and regular review of terminal care, mortality and significant event analyses
- regular, minuted meetings for team management and clinical governance
- continuing professional and team development, including annual updating of emergency and resuscitation skills
- a personal learning and development plan for the year ahead
- accumulated portfolios of work carried out, appraisal reports, progress in areas of personal interest, all contribute to recertification at 5-year intervals.

All of this has significant implications for practices and individual clinicians. It can feel onerous in terms of time, effort and resource allocation, and it has the threat of sanctions. As an educative programme it has a distinctly summative bottom line. Those who implement summative assessment procedures have to make provision for remediation. After all, as Abraham Flexner said, '*The power to examine is the power to destroy.*'

A final word about quality in general practice.

There is very little evidence concerning which characteristics of practices correlate with quality outcomes. There is mixed evidence on practice size. Large ones provide greater diversity of services, while small ones demonstrate more continuous, personalised care. One consistent quality indicator is training status. **Approved training practices are rated more highly by patients overall, offer a broader range of services and score lower on ratings of stress and workload for GPs.**[82]

EVIDENCE, GUIDELINES AND AUDIT

Evidence-based practice is the translation of the results of clinical epidemiological studies into daily practice. David Sackett, one of the original advocates of evidence-based medicine (EBM), provides a definition that is accepted by most authorities, including by the Cochrane Collaboration:

> Evidence-based medicine is the conscientious, explicit and judicious use of current best evidence in making decisions about the care of individual patients.[83]

It has been favourably compared with some historical approaches to the sources of knowledge and its application, loosely based on Isaacs and Fitzgerald's[84] satirical summary:

- *vehemence-based medicine* – the advice or opinion delivered by the peers with the loudest voices
- *eminence-based medicine* – the authoritative practices and opinions of our venerated elders
- *reverence-based medicine* – passing on the teachings of a sage
- *avarice-based medicine* – we will do only what we are incentivised to do
- *indolence-based medicine* – taking the line of least resistance and cutting corners
- *elegance-based medicine* – eloquence as a substitute for evidence.

Components and relations of EMB are summarised in Figure 5.5.

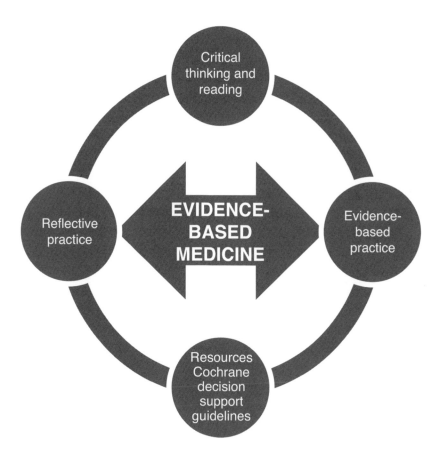

FIGURE 5.5 The components and relationships of evidence-based medicine

Our culture of clinical practice has always sought to be evidence-based; but evidence changes. Indeed, it is only in recent decades that a critical view of quality of evidence has been applied systematically. The writings of the Greats held good for centuries, from Hippocrates and Galen through to Harvey and Koch, with a stately pace of change. The electronic media created a widening of horizons. Where until recently the local medical society or journals were adequate vehicles for promulgating knowledge, we now navigate the global sea of shared information, good and otherwise. Research methodology is now subject to international scrutiny and there has emerged a hierarchical model of evidence, representing degrees of robustness and validity (*see* Figure 5.6). This ranges from received wisdom (medical school, textbooks), through authoritative overviews of current thought (as in journal editorials) to the kind of synthesis represented by international consensus literature of WHO. Serving the global trend, the primary literature of research papers and various grades of trial receive critical analysis; the best are amalgamated as meta-analyses and systematic reviews (*see* Figure 5.7). The generalist is particularly vulnerable in the face of this tide of knowledge, since there are no natural boundaries to his or her discipline. If taken to task and found to have treated a patient with what are currently regarded as suboptimal interventions he or she would be liable to criticism or sanctions. EBM is a double-edged sword, but it is a protective mechanism for doctor and patient. The best-known form it takes is the *guideline*.

---

  1 Common-sense knowledge, face validity
  2 The views of a special interest group (websites, 'cranks' etc.)
  3 Personal experience
  4 Received wisdom
  5 The teaching of a sage
  6 Locally developed guidelines
  7 Peer-reviewed and research-based reports (primary literature)
  8 Case-controlled study
  9 Cohort study
 10 Randomised controlled trial
 11 Meta-analyses of compatible trials
 12 Consensus statements of reputable bodies (e.g. National Institute for Health and Care Excellence; Scottish Intercollegiate Guidelines Network)

FIGURE 5.6 Twelve levels of evidence (note: this is not necessarily a linear progression)

The evolution of EBM is a tribute to the memory of Archie Cochrane, the Scottish epidemiologist. He expressed concerns about the increasing burden due to the

---

- Primary literature: published reports of original research
- Secondary literature: the pulling together of primary data to create an overview (e.g. a leading article in Journal)
- Tertiary literature: consensus statements, reports or policy documents based on the informed and analytic view of a specialised body (such as government, medical college, WHO) and authoritative compilations such as textbooks

---

FIGURE 5.7 A classification of technical literature

explosion of clinical information on physicians in trying to ensure best practice and optimal outcomes. His response was to address the burgeoning, multilingual medical literature, the variable quality of published evidence and the need to streamline clinical decision-making. Through systematising and categorising these he hoped to reduce the clinician's burden. Proponents of his work preserved his name in the structures that codify EBM internationally, the Cochrane Collaboration and the Cochrane Library. The work of Cochrane was promoted by David Sackett of McMaster University, Ontario, who established the Centre for Evidence-Based Medicine at the University of Oxford.

EBM has two main components: evidence-based practice and reflective practice. The former results from critical reading habits and awareness of current guidelines (themselves derived from primary literature evidence) and their appropriate implementation in clinical care. The latter, *reflective practice*, assimilates these within a broadly defined evidence base that includes such subjectivities as the experiences of patients and of the doctor, the clinical outcomes they both experience. It carries this synthesis through into a critical thinking and learning cycle that addresses gaps in information and performance in order to achieve optimal care outcomes.

Guidelines and the management of chronic disease

> The range of guidelines has increased exponentially each year and the evidence to support them has strengthened considerably.[85]

A guideline represents a concise, evidence-based statement, a summary of management decisions relating to a specified condition. It is a form of decision support and it holds the promise of delivering what it describes. But there is a conundrum with guidelines. There are guidelines for everything and loads of reliable evidence, but who can master their quantity and diversity; how valid is this robust body of evidence in the case of the individual clinical decision? If you follow what it says you should achieve an optimal outcome, in accordance with 'best practice'. But is life that simple, even if you have a 'photographic memory'? But first, let's see what a typical guideline might look like.

A guideline begins with a *definition of the target condition*, its *diagnostic criteria*, *subdivisions* of the condition (e.g. variants of epilepsy), its clinical *impact* (or epidemiology), the rationale for the guideline's *derivation* (e.g. the specialism or group of clinicians at whom it is targeted) and its *provenance* (authorship credentials). An essential element of any guideline is a statement about who compiled it, for whose benefit and when, since evidence is protean. This is followed with a decision support paradigm (e.g. a flow chart or decision tree) that indicates action points and thresholds for action, including initiation, termination or alteration in the level of an intervention (e.g. dose of medication), indicative intervals for re-evaluation and indications for exit (e.g. referral elsewhere). Footnotes provide detail – for example, laboratory test ranges, pharmacological options/alternatives. A bibliography of references is an essential final element that locates the guideline in relation to time (they should have a 'sell-by date'), and the current research literature that substantiates the evidence upon which the guideline is founded.

Guidelines are the practical and accessible face of the complex edifice of EBM – specific, targeted and aiming to enshrine and replicate best current practice. A direct but perhaps unintended consequence of EBM is a culture of coercion concerning protocols of practice. When guidelines are assimilated into protocols what becomes of clinical freedom? The twin peaks of medical ethics, '*first do no harm*' and '*beneficence*', are no longer sufficient to keep a clinician safely out of trouble. Adherence to protocol has to be demonstrable in order to be seen to do a good job in the light of current best practice. Thus, guidelines, their construction and implementation, are becoming legally enforceable.

On the other hand, Sackett proposed that guideline creation by individuals and local groups is an excellent educational exercise to be fostered widely. Involvement in guideline creation is an intellectual and skill-building exercise that has the additional virtues of having validity for local application and 'ownership', both of which contribute to adherence. From the educational perspective, any coercive element that creeps in when guidelines are adopted as official policy is regrettable, even if inevitable.

Why should this be a problem? Is not the universal adherence to guidelines of best practice highly desirable? In reality the excellent can become the enemy of the good. There are aspects of guideline use that are problematic. Clinical judgement and circumstances have to have a place, especially in the management of chronic and complex disease when the 'cap just doesn't fit'. Evidence may not automatically translate into best outcomes, for a number of reasons.

1. There is a time delay in creating guidelines from the shifting sands of evidence; no guideline is perfect, or would long remain so.

2. There is a large guideline industry based on special interest groups, commercial and national bodies promoting various product or policy positions of their own; the largest one in the UK is the National Institute for Health and Care Excellence, which has been criticised as a government creation that has to take account of economic factors as well as efficacy, and which moves at a slow pace. Condition-specific groups that have promulgated respected eponymous guidelines include Diabetes UK, the British Thoracic Society and the British Hypertension Society, to name a few.

3. When specialist groups create guidelines that are directed at the territory of other clinicians there are problems of validity, ownership and adherence.

4. Guidelines generally reflect randomised controlled trials carried out on younger, healthier people with a single condition. What do they say about managing the multi-morbid, frail elderly on multiple medications?

5. To be effective, guidelines have to be specific. An individual with multi-organ disease such as diabetes may be subject to several sets of guidelines. In areas of overlap are they all compatible? Creating a protocol based on all is not simple, especially if there are co-morbidities as so often happens in people with long-term conditions.

6. Implementing and monitoring of guidelines is onerous for clinicians, their staff and their patients. Individuals receive multiple 'summonses' to attend the practice for this or that protocol-driven procedure in addition to their other, needs-based attendances. '*Why don't you get your ducks in a row and call me once for all of them?*' would seem to be a fair criticism of our systems.

7. Guidelines may be used by health systems in managerial, governance, regulatory or disciplinary modes. They are a potent lever for change and this can be applied for all kinds of purpose. As one regional manager remarked, '*General Practice is now a target-rich environment, not just a target-driven one.*'

8. One of the key skills in general practice is management of uncertainty; ways have to be devised for teaching and learning this, to supplement the rational use of guidelines.

However well disposed clinicians are towards EBM and the positive value of guidelines, the patient-centred and demand-led culture of general practice is not well adapted for adherence for protocols. This is less true of specialist services. Obstetrics, cancer services, cardiology and diabetology have for many years practised successful, protocol-driven methodologies. GPs, who encompass the full range of specialisms, must grapple with a constellation of guidelines and somehow integrate these into everyday practice. This is complex and GPs are in a transitional state in this regard. No doubt a creative assimilation will emerge in response to this need.

Multimorbidity introduces clinical uncertainty in a way that is unlikely to be resolved by ever more sophisticated guidelines.[86]

Notes on clinical audit

Audit is the basic approach to translating guidelines into practice. The information flow created by the audit cycle demonstrates the use of guidelines and the effects of their implementation. After years when it was professionally led, audit has become a contractual obligation on every doctor in the UK due to the introduction of performance appraisal and clinical governance. The components of audit are now a familiar routine of practice. A substantial team that becomes accustomed to auditing aspects of their work can sustain a wide variety of performance reviews with continuity.

Audit runs into problems when the question posed is too broad or complex. Sustainable audit is simple, direct and focused. It should be possible to carry out an audit in a couple of hours.

Audit questions easily stray into research questions and lead to complexity. Audit asks, 'To what extent, or how well, do we do X?' A research question might ask, 'Why does doing X not provide the expected outcome?' There is a difference in methodology, although they are complementary.

Performing audits opens up the possibility of research in general practice; audit can set a research agenda for the practice by identifying problem areas and posing new questions. Careful audit records should be maintained, otherwise every audit action begins at square one and measures something different, rather than building upon and reinforcing previous effort.

Audit is non-judgemental. It is not a hunt for deficiencies, but an exercise in quality improvement. Thus a low score against the set criteria provokes reflection rather than incurring shame. The use of language should reflect this. High scores prompt the question, are the criteria set too low?

Significant event analysis

Significant event analysis is less formalised than audit, though it often shares in the name audit. It is *reflection in action* in a peer-review setting. It is a method of formative assessment, not a court of inquiry. Its aims are to embed risk management in everyday practice through team-based action reflection on critical incidents such as errors, near misses or adverse outcomes.

It has features in common with audit and may interact with it. To address, in a professional manner, occurrences that have consequences or risk is an exercise in openness, integrity and trust. It is separate from, and additional to, any *complaints procedure* that might also address the same territory and which requires inclusion of the complainant. It may also highlight instances of good practice with beneficial outcomes, not merely focus on negative events.

Audits, significant event analyses and complaints are all matters of record and are logged in the practice clinical governance system for the purposes of appraisal, revalidation and re-certification. These documents are also legally discoverable.

CONCLUSION AND REFLECTION

The only way to summarise this lengthy chapter is in the form of recommendations.

Ten 'Commandments' for general practice chronic care

1. Embrace chronic care – it's what you do
2. Promote patient safety and quality as priorities
3. Manage information actively (or else you will drown in it)
4. Practise patient-centred care (engage, listen, inform, support, respond)
5. Promote patient self-help and involvement (it is their business)
6. Value prevention (in all its modes, including health promotion)
7. Manage clinical pathways of prioritised patients (you have the levers, they do not)
8. Work with health policy, including commissioning, rather than against it (to change it is above your pay grade)
9. Support your team (manage morale, workload, communication, leadership)
10. Teach and train (education is a two-way street, and patients benefit)

POINTS FOR REFLECTION

- Locate the definitions of general practice cited in this chapter; how does general practice in your area or system match up with this? Why not create your own definition?
- In MDT, define (a) leadership and (b) assertiveness.
- What do you understand by continuity of care? In your practice what gets in the way of continuity?
- What are the advantages and disadvantages of practice federations? What barriers might you encounter to any proposal to make your local practices into a federation?
- Keep a record of consultations in which you feel inadequate or perplexed; your feelings may be quite appropriate, but what are they telling you? The issues they raise may indicate significant gaps in your knowledge or skills.

REFERENCES

1. Wagner EH. Chronic disease management: what will it take to improve care in chronic illness? *Eff Clin Pract.* 1998; **1**(1): 2–4.
2. Rogers S. A structured approach for the investigation of clinical incidents in health care: application in the general practice setting. *Br J Gen Pract.* 2002; **52**(Suppl.): S30–2.
3. Van den Hombergh P, Schalk-Soekar S, Kramer A, *et al.* Are family practice trainers and their host practices any better? *BMC Fam Pract.* 2013; **14**: 23.
4. Macdonald JJ. *Primary Health Care: medicine in its place.* London: Earthscan; 2000.
5. Zola I. Cited in: McKinley JB. A case for refocusing upstream: the political economy of illness. In: Conrad P, Kern R, editors. *The Sociology of Health and Illness: critical perspectives.* 2nd ed. New York, NY: St Martin's Press; 1986. pp. 484–98.
6. Macdonald, op. cit.
7. Allen J, Gay B Crebolder H, *et al. The European Definition of General Practice/Family Medicine.* WONCA, Europe; 2005. p. 29.
8. *The European Definition of General Practice / Family Medicine.* WONCA Europe; 2005. Available at: www.woncaeurope.org/sites/default/files/documents/Definition%203rd%20 ed%202011%20with%20revised%20wonca%20tree.pdf (accessed 16 April 2014).
9. American Academy of Family Physicians. *Primary Care.* Available at: www.aafp.org/about/ policies/all/primary-care.html (accessed 22 April 2014).
10. Francis D, Young D. *Improving Work Groups: a practical manual for team building.* Mansfield: University Associates; 1979.
11. McDerment L. *Stress Care.* Surrey: Social Care Association (Education); 1988.
12. Borrill C, Carletta J, Carter A, *et al. The Effectiveness of Health Care Teams in the National Health Service.* A report commissioned by the DOH. Birmingham: Aston University; 2000.
13. Borrill C, West M, Shapiro D, *et al. Team Working and Effectiveness in Health Care.* Available at: homepages.inf.ed.ac.uk/jeanc/DOH/glossy-brochure.pdf (accessed 20 April 2014).
14. Borrill C. Team working and effectiveness in health care: findings from the Health Care Team Effectiveness Project. *Br J Health Care Manage.* 2000; **6**(8): 364–71.
15. National Cancer Action Team. *Characteristics of an Effective Multidisciplinary Team (MDT).* National Cancer Action Team; 2010. Available at: www.ncin.org.uk/view?rid=136 (accessed 20 April 2014).
16. Borrill, Carletta, Carter, *et al.*, op. cit.
17. Ibid.
18. *European Certificate in Essential Palliative Care.* 9th ed. Esher, Surrey: Princess Alice Hospice.
19. Royal College of Physicians, Royal College of General Practitioners, Royal College of Paediatrics and Child Health. *Teams without Walls: the value of medical innovation and leadership.* London: Royal College of Physicians; 2008.
20. Centres for Diseases Control and Prevention. www.cdc.gov/healthliteracy/ (accessed 10 February 2014).
21. Raynor DKT. Health literacy. *BMJ.* 2012; **344**: e2188.
22. McEvoy H. *Health Education – How? Models, methods and programmes* [Thesis]. Londonderry: University of Ulster; 1985.
23. World Health Organization. *The Ottawa Charter for Health Promotion.* Geneva: WHO; 1986.
24. World Health Organization. *Collaborative Project on Identification and Management of Alcohol-Related Problems in Primary Health Care: report on phase IV.* Geneva: WHO; 2006.

25. Smith R. Hamster health care. *BMJ*. 2000; **321**(7276): 1541–2.
26. Ibid.
27. Williams S. Tangled web. In: *UK Case Book*. London: Medical Protection Society; 2009. pp. 8–11.
28. Ibid.
29. Toosey R, Chowdry S. The impact and success of telehealth. *GP*. 2012 Jan 11.
30. Robinson S. Can telehealth ease the GP workload? *GP*. 2010 Nov 26.
31. Lieberman L. Telemedicine. *GP*. 2011 Jun 3.
32. Department of Health. *Research Evidence on the Effectiveness of Self-Care Support: work in progress 2005–2007*. London: Department of Health; 2007.
33. Murray E. Internet-delivered treatment for long-term conditions: strategies, efficiency and cost-effectiveness. *Expert Rev Pharmacoecon Outcomes Res*. 2008; **8**(3): 261–72.
34. Stange KC, Ferrer RL. The paradox of primary care. *Ann Fam Med*. 2009; **7**(4): 293–9.
35. Ibid.
36. Ibid.
37. Gröne O, Garcia-Barbero M. *Trends in Integrated Care: reflections on conceptual issues*. EUR102/5037864. Copenhagen: WHO; 2012.
38. Rickenbach MJ, Wedderburn C. Follow the yellow brick road: integrated care – can we do better? *Br J Gen Pract*. 2012; **60**(601): e587–98.
39. Ibid.
40. Ham C, Curry N. *Integrated Care: does it work; what does it mean for the NHS?* London: The King's Fund; 2011.
41. Mathers N, Thomas M. Integration of care. *Br J Gen Pract*. 2012; **62**(601): 402–3.
42. Campbell H, Hotchkiss R, Bradshaw N, *et al*. Integrated care pathways. *BMJ*. 1998; **316**(7125): 133–7.
43. Department of Health. *Supporting People with Long Term Conditions: commissioning personalised care planning; a guide for commissioners*. London: Department of Health; 2009.
44. Mathers and Thomas, op. cit.
45. World Health Organization. *Innovative Care for Chronic Conditions: building blocks for action; global report*. Geneva: WHO; 2002.
46. Royal College of Physicians, Royal College of General Practitioners and Royal College of Paediatrics and Child Health, op. cit.
47. Rickenbach and Wedderburn, op. cit.
48. De Maeseneer J, Boeckxstaens P. James Mackenzie Lecture 2011: multimorbidity, goal-oriented care, and equity. *Br J Gen Pract*. 2012; **62**(600); e522–4.
49. Finkelstein A, Taubman S, Wright B, *et al*. The Oregon Health Insurance Experiment: evidence from the first year. *Q J Econ*. 2012, **127**(3): 1057–106.
50. World Health Organization, 2002, op. cit.
51. Reynolds L, McKee M. GP commissioning and the NHS reforms: what lies behind the hard sell? *J R Soc Med* 2012; **105**(1): 7–10.
52. Gerada C. From patient advocate to gatekeeper, understanding the effects of NHS reforms. *Br J Gen Pract*. 2011; **61**(592): 655–6.
53. Ibid.
54. Hann M, McDonald J, Checkland K, *et al*. Seventh National Worklife Survey. Manchester: Centre for Health Economics, University of Manchester; 2013. Available at: www.population-health.

manchester.ac.uk/healtheconomics/FinalReportofthe7thNationalGPWorklifeSurvey.pdf (accessed 16 April 2014).

55. Lays C, Player S. *The Plot Against the NHS*. Pontypool. Wales: Merlin Press; 2001.

56. Grol R, Leatherman S. Improving quality in British primary care: seeking the right balance. *Br J Gen Pract*. 2002; **52**(Suppl.): S3–4.

57. Smith R. In: Abbasi K. Change? Yes, we can [Interview]. *J R Soc Med*. 2008; **101**(12): 611–13.

58. Baker R, Roland M. General practice: continuous quality improvement since 1948. *Br J Gen Pract*. 2002; **52**(Suppl.): S2–3.

59. Kennedy I. *Improving the Quality of Care in General Practice*. London: The King's Fund; 2013. Available at: www.kingsfund.org.uk/publications/improving-quality-care-general-practice (accessed 20 April 2014).

60. Hawkes N. Inquiry calls for greater transparency and quality of care in general practice. *BMJ*. 2011; **342**: d1833.

61. O'Donnell CA. Variation in GP referral rates: what can we learn from the literature? *Fam Pract*. 2000; **17**(6): 462–71.

62. Coulter A, Elwyn G. What do patients want from high quality general practice and how do we involve them in improvement? *Br J Gen Pract*. 2002; **52**(Suppl.): S22–6.

63. Hirschman AO. *Exit, Voice and Loyalty*. Cambridge, MA. Harvard University Press; 1970.

64. Iliffe S, Willcock L, Manthorpe J, *et al*. Can clinicians benefit from patient satisfaction surveys? Evaluating the NSF for Older People, 2005–2006. *J R Soc Med*. 2008. **101**(12): 598–604.

65. Ibid.

66. Cocksedge S, Greenfield R, Nugent GK, *et al*. Holding relationships in primary care: a qualitative exploration of doctors' and patients' perceptions. *Br J Gen Pract*. 2011; **61**(589): e484–91.

67. Murray E. Providing information for patients is insufficient on its own to improve clinical outcomes. *BMJ*. 2008; **337**(7665): a280.

68. Davies AR. Patient defined outcomes. *Qual Health Care*. 1994; **3**(Suppl.): 6–9.

69. Foster G, Taylor SJ, Eldridge S, *et al*. Self-management education programmes by lay leaders for people with chronic conditions. *Cochrane Database Syst Rev*. 2009; CD005108.pub2

70. World Health Organization, 2002, op. cit.

71. Appleby J. Does improving quality of care save money? *BMJ*. 2009; **399**: b3678.

72. Ibid.

73. Mackway-Jones K. The rational clinical examination in emergency care. *BMJ*. 2008: **337**: a2374.

74. Misselbrook D. *Thinking About Patients*. Newbury: Petroc Press; 2001.

75. Wilcock M, Lawrence J. Medication at discharge: is enough information provided? *Prescriber*. 2008; **19**(9): 19–22.

76. Avery AJ, Barber N, Ghaleb M, *et al*. *Investigating the Prevalence and Causes of Prescribing Errors in General Practice: the PRACtiCe Study*. London: General Medical Council; 2012.

77. Wilson J. *Your Practice*. 4; Spring 2008. London: Medical Protection Society; 2008. pp. 8–10.

78. World Health Organization, 2002, op. cit.

79. Halligan A. *BMA News Review*. 2000 Mar 11.

80. General Medical Council. *Good Medical Practice*. London: General Medical Council; 2012.

81. Nicholls S, Cullen R, O'Neill S, *et al*. Clinical governance: its origins and foundations. *Clin Perform Qual Health Care*. 2000; **8**(3): 172–8.

82. Van den Hombergh, Schalk-Soekar, Kramer, *et al*., op. cit.

83. Sackett D, Rosenberg WM, Gray JA, *et al*. Evidence based medicine: what it is and what it isn't. *BMJ*. 1996; **312**(7023): 71–2.

84. Isaacs D, Fitzgerald D. Seven alternatives to evidence based medicine. *BMJ*. 1999; **319**: 1618.

85. Smith P. Introduction. In: *Guide to the Primary Care Guidelines*. 4th ed. Oxford: Radcliffe Publishing; 2008. p. vii.

86. Roland M. Better management of patients with multimorbidity. *BMJ*. 2013; **346**: f2510.

CHAPTER 6

A chronic care revolution: service redesign and the policy complex

Contents

CHAPTER OVERVIEW

> Now we want more healthcare for the ageing population and we can't afford the
> more stuff or more kit or more drugs that will provide that.[1]
>
> **Paul Corrigan, former special adviser to Tony Blair**

This chapter examines the main themes of health policy for chronic disease management and explains their rationale in order to make sense of current changes and
developments. It describes the World Health Organization's (WHO's) global analysis,

how certain health systems are responding, notably in the UK and the United States; it will include elementary health economics, explain some building blocks for chronic care policy, and discuss the characteristics of a hypothetical reformed and high-performing health system. It is suitable for all professionals in healthcare and those in training, since it is not specific to any one professional grouping or health system.

I approached this chapter with quiet dread. Policy seems abstract and remote from the home turf of the GP surgery and patient encounters. Much of it lies outside the comfort zone of clinicians. The literature on policy is vast and the scope is global. Yet it affects everything we do. There is much that needs to be explained concerning the current state of thinking about health policy for long-term conditions and it is evolving rapidly. Policies seem to emerge from places that are geographically and culturally far off and be implemented close to home with minimal explanation or field-testing. Policy is important. It dictates the directions of change and specifies the parameters within which we work. Current orthodoxy concerning chronic care could change, but for now there is much in the literature that suggests convergence towards a broad consensus that favours patient-centred, primary care with emphasis on self-help and prevention.

HEALTH POLICY FOR LONG-TERM CONDITIONS: GLOBAL, NATIONAL AND LOCAL

> Healthcare systems in the 21st century need to address the challenges posed by demographic change, technological development and changing public expectations within the context of limited resources. An epidemiological approach to healthcare needs assessment provides a rational framework within which these issues can be tackled.[2]

My medical education and training were devoid of health systems, economics, politics, and anything to do with the organisation of healthcare. The doctor, the patient and the illness were quite enough to be going on with (and the illness appeared, at times, to be paramount). Those were the simpler days of linear thinking and demand-led work practices. We felt ready and eager to enter full-scale practice. Now those who complete training for general practice appear to feel unprepared to enter into full partnership at principal grade directly, despite all the exams, assessments and certification of competencies. This must be related to their late-stage encounters with 'the system of care' and the myriad ways in which this impinges on daily clinical life. Increasingly complex policy frameworks are mirrored by the increasing complexity of procedures, clinical issues and diversity of services that can be provided. One answer to this 'culture-shock' is to increase the length of postgraduate training for general practice and family medicine, but this will only be effective if 'The System' can be reduced to a comprehensible curriculum of learning. Perhaps this knowledge of structure and system should pervade all stages of the curriculum of medical education and training, since any clinical service is only as good as the vehicle that delivers it, and that is what healthcare systems and health policy are all about. All doctors should know about the mechanisms of delivering a health service, just as they need to know about combating disease. If you are unaware of your own healthcare service framework, what are you to make of changes when they occur? And they do occur, with monotonous regularity, at least in the UK. I'm sure the UK is not alone in this. To paraphrase a famous dictum, *the unexamined health service is not worth your commitment.*

Perhaps the greatest driver of development in health services is globalisation – that is, the ease with which influences can travel through physical and virtual networks. This means that countries and leaders can compare what is going on everywhere else and wish things were different back home. These information networks syndicate data on measurements, costs and conclusions, policies and programmes, dreams and disappointments. The data are crunched and distilled by an army of epidemiologists, statisticians and economists. As a result of such external influences there is no purely ideological home-grown, autonomous health system. Consequently, there is close connection between delivery of local service for our patients and developments at global level, those national policies and 'fashion trends' in systems management.

EXAMPLE 1

The St Vincent Declaration emanated from a conference convened in Italy in 1989 by WHO and the International Diabetes Federation. It included representatives of European national health ministries and of patients' representative organisations. It set evidence-based goals and targets for reduction in diabetic complications that influenced national government policy and local provision throughout Europe and beyond. These were taken up in the Americas and Oceania.[3] It noted the rising prevalence of diabetes, predominantly type 2.

It advocated:

- evidence-based policy-making
- adoption of best-practice templates
- a shift in focus from type 1 to type 2 diabetic care
- increased reliance on primary healthcare as the location of the main battle against diabetes
- programmes of care emphasising prevention, early intervention, surveillance and shared care with specialist services.

> It proposed implementation at national level through a rolling programme of reviews and monitored attainment of performance targets, so that nations were morally 'coerced' into adopting community-oriented priorities and appropriate resource allocation, and with improved outcomes.

Thus, this international forum identified a trend of international importance, raised awareness, applied research findings to create a programmed framework of priorities that enabled governments to implement nationwide services that saved lives and improved health on a grand scale. WHO is the leading forum and exponent of this modus operandi. Its global health reports and policy documents are influential in the thinking of health ministries everywhere.

WHO stratifies policy matters into three levels as follows.

1. *Macro level*: national policy, shaped by government and promulgated through fiscal and legal frameworks; it is capable of harnessing *intersectoral action* – that is, cooperation between different departments of government; thus health matters will have components that require departments of education, transport, communications, or the police and justice systems to contribute (e.g. on drugs policy, the control of tobacco use or dealing with environmental toxins). *Intersectoral action is the macro equivalent of multidisciplinary work at micro level.*

2. *Meso level*: the health organisation, especially as it operates at regional or area level; within the reach of local government, municipalities and major third sector organisations; it includes the operational end of the health or social services; for example, the clinical commissioning groups in the UK, or units of the health schemes in the United States, such as within the Veterans Health Administration or Kaiser Permanente Health Plan.

3. *Micro level*: the interpersonal relationships, activities and networks that impinge on the patient – for example, the GP, multidisciplinary practice team or the local patient self-help group.[4]

These strata are not discrete. The boundaries are fuzzy and they influence one another for better or worse. For example, training is a function of the healthcare organisation (meso-level issue) but where it has a direct impact on patient care it may become a micro-level issue. WHO applies this stratified model in its crucial document *Innovative Care for Chronic Conditions*,[5] in which it offers a general critique of current healthcare systems, addressing the following levels.

At the macro level, governments need to make informed and rational decisions, set standards of quality and proper incentives in healthcare, to coordinate and strengthen intersectoral links. There are faults in *legislative frameworks* (they can be cumbersome, restrictive or deficient), in *policy* (reflecting the priorities of yes-teryear), *lack of investment*, perverse or irrational *incentives*, weak *governance* (corruption, chaotic implementation) and poor *intersectoral links*. One example of this is a feeble taxation policy that could, but fails to, reduce consumption of fast food, sweet drinks, alcohol and tobacco (which together contribute to over half of preventable chronic illness risk).

At the meso level, healthcare organisations must streamline services, upgrade the skills of health workers, focus on prevention, establish information-tracking sys-tems and provide planned healthcare; but in general they fail to address chronic conditions (they favour acute care provision and do not give enough emphasis to prevention), equip or train health workers properly (meagre training budgets), or provide appropriate information technology (e.g. for shared e-records, compatible systems).

At the micro level, communication between health workers and patients is para-mount for improving care for chronic conditions; however, there is failure generally to empower people, to value patient interactions, take account of local concerns or give proper recognition to the contribution of primary care.

The WHO document concludes that, 'without change, healthcare systems will con-tinue to grow increasingly inefficient and ineffective as the prevalence of chronic conditions rises'.[6]

Of course WHO is speaking from a global overview of the health services of dif-ferent countries, and these all succeed or fail in their individual ways. It does not regard any nation as standing outside its framework of response to the rise of chronic disease. Since its publication in 2002, the document has already influenced heavily the health ministries of countries across the globe. Most developed health systems show evidence of taking these messages forward in practice, but unevenly. Current health reforms in the UK, Europe, Australasia and North America reflect much of the WHO analysis. It did not appear out of thin air. Therefore a synopsis of the back-ground may provide a point of entry to an area that is increasingly complicated, and illustrate the form and function of health policy matters.

WHO POLICY AND CHRONIC DISEASE MANAGEMENT

Following the formation of the United Nations in the immediate aftermath of the Second World War and with the initiation of its health wing, WHO, there came into being a global opinion forum on health issues. For the first time health matters were not being dictated by colonial administrations, 'mother country' systems or a dominant economic power. All nations had a say, and they began to say it. Armed with the observation that poverty, injustice and ill-health formed a vicious cycle, and with the brand-new Universal Declaration of Human Rights, there began the **global critique of health as a justice issue, and disease as a political/economic one**. This led to the Alma-Ata Declaration of 1979, which asserted healthcare as a right, and participation in healthcare as a duty, of citizenship. It set a deadline, expressed as a mission statement, '*health care for all by the year 2000*'. Most of the world missed it. However, the message was clear and governments heard it, even if it met with a good deal of derision, apathy and misunderstanding at the time. As the saying goes,

> The captain shouts his orders and the crew carry on as before.[7]

WHO provides a very effective laboratory for epidemiologists and number-crunchers. They could do the maths and see the epidemiological time-bomb in the making. It takes longer for political and professional inertia to be overcome, and that is a work in progress. Epidemic HIV/AIDS and tuberculosis in the 1980s helped focus governments on the effectiveness of the epidemiological approach on population health (that is, combining community-level action and the primary care platform for healthcare delivery with evidence-based policy responses). Within a decade these communicable diseases were becoming long-term conditions that are manageable, and even curable. (Of course, fundamental research made a huge contribution to these advances.)

The academic community both informed and benefited from the global forum and international comparative work. An eminent example is what might be termed the 'Starfield Effect'. Barbara Starfield was described in an obituary as:

> perhaps the most influential figure in the primary care research community ... (whose) ... work influenced how policymakers and researchers think about the delivery of health care worldwide.[8]

Her seminal book, *Primary Care: Concept, Evaluation and Policy* (1992), proposed that health systems with a strong foundation in primary care had better health outcomes generally and were more cost-effective than those that are dominated by disease specialists and secondary care. Her strong criticisms of US-style health systems and admiration for the UK's NHS have energised a transatlantic exchange on the provision of healthcare, especially with regard to long-term conditions. This conversation appears to be bringing about a broad measure of agreement on the principles that characterise best practice, as we shall see later. Despite her relative lack of impact within the health system of her native United States, where family practice is still held generally in low regard, much of the thinking around chronic care emanates from this same country. Further examples include:

- *the Chronic Care Model* of Wagner (on which the WHO report *Innovative Care for Chronic Conditions* of 2002 relied heavily)
- *the Stanford Model* of chronic disease self-management (that gave rise to the Expert Patients Programme in the UK)
- *the Trajectory Framework* of Corbin and Strauss (a model of the nursing process in chronic care)
- the models of *integrated managed care* (among them, Kaiser Permanente and the Veterans Health Administration)
- *the medical home*, a US term that equates to the primary care health centre in the UK, and is defined by the US Agency for Healthcare Research and Quality as a model of the organisation of primary care that is *comprehensive, patient-centred, coordinated, accessible, and committed to quality and safety.*[9]

All of these have influenced healthcare thinking throughout the world; all have given us tools and insights that inform the discourse on health that is part of everyday conversation now.

Why the United States? Its health system may not be a beacon of light to the world in terms of equity, access, value for money or population health outcomes, but the United States is the biggest and best-funded population health laboratory anywhere. The US institutes of public health and epidemiology are renowned. Discussion of

---

'OBAMACARE'

Official title: *The Patient Protection and Affordable Care Act*
'Obamacare' was ruled constitutional by the US Supreme Court on 28 June 2012.

Key features:
- by 2014 citizens must possess a health insurance policy that provides at least minimum coverage
- failure to do so incurs a tax penalty payable to the Federal Government ('the individual mandate')
- without this law it is estimated by the Congressional Budget Office that 60 million Americans would remain uninsured
- the Act will reduce this to 27 million, mostly illegal immigrants and those who abstain.

FIGURE 6.1 Features of the healthcare bill, 2012, USA[11]

health policy issues regularly achieves a higher pitch and volume in the United States than anywhere else. A 50-year debate spans the Kennedy/Nixon struggle over healthcare reform, through the abortive Clinton proposals and, more recently, Obamacare (*see* Figure 6.1). The much smaller national 'laboratories' in Europe and Australasia have made their own contributions also. To name a few examples: the British NHS, its welfare state and its serial reforms since 1990; France has been named by WHO as the best-performing health system, probably on account of its chronic care;[10] the Netherlands, Scandinavia, Australia and New Zealand have health systems that resemble that of the UK and substantial programmes of care for long-term conditions. One of the beneficial features of the generic model of chronic disease is that it has attracted and provoked analysis and problem-solving without borders.

UNPACKING HEALTH POLICY

The WHO definition of health policy is our starting point:

> Health policy refers to **decisions, plans and actions** that are undertaken to achieve **specific health care goals** within **a society**. An explicit health policy can achieve several things: it defines a **vision for the future** which in turn helps to establish **targets and points of reference** for the short and medium term. It outlines **priorities** and the **expected roles** of different groups; and it **builds consensus** and **informs people**.[12] (Emphasis added)

What WHO coyly omits from this definition is that health policy is fundamentally about money and how it is spent. However, its definition does indicate the general characteristics of public policy:

- *decisions, plans and actions* – the processes of public administration
- *specific goals, targets, reference points* – processes of management and measurement
- *priorities, within society, defining vision for the future* – context, culture and values
- *roles of different groups, consensus building, and informing people* – the sociology and community work dimension, and local politics – that is, the primary healthcare perspective.

These descriptors indicate the deeply political nature of healthcare and related policy, driven by forces that may be electoral, or with dialectical considerations that may pay scant regard to evidence-based argument. Macroeconomic factors heavily influence health policy, especially since the economic crisis following 2007–08. Health systems throughout the world are facing policy challenges that are similar. They boil down to a core cluster: ***Increasing numbers of people who are ageing,*** *have more long-term conditions, more complex problems and rising expectations, combined with cost inflation, all of which threatens to render high-quality health and social care politically and economically unaffordable.*

EXAMPLE 2

Most health analysts in the United States in the mid 1990s were sure that managed care (whereby purchasers and insurers could control cost and quality by dictating terms to health providers) had become the new paradigm of healthcare, replacing the free-market model. With cost inflation out of control, 50% of health management organisations (HMOs) lost money in 1997–8 in what amounted to a virtual melt-down of the US managed care sector.[13] Since then integrated care organisations appear to be the paradigm most favoured by progressive policy analysts, and are much studied by authorities in the UK.

EXAMPLE 3

About the same time in the UK the NHS was undergoing a transformation from monolithic, centrally funded origins towards a market-based model (albeit an 'internal market'), whereby 'fund-holding' was delegated to the GP practice at local level, and a separation of functions created between the service provider and the body that purchased or commissioned the service (the 'purchaser–provider split'). Details of actual costs of services became quantified and known for the first time; provider organisations were held to budget limits; 'care in the community' policy led to radical reduction in long-stay facilities. These forces led to 'secondary to primary drift' (sometimes referred to as 'left-shift'), and substantial services and sectors becoming contracted out to the commercial sector. Waiting lists for hospital services grew longer and additional money had to be infused into the system. More recent consequences included increased patient and public involvement, and primary care-based commissioning of services.

Changes such as these represent landmarks on the path from the established acute care orientation towards sustainable strategies for tackling long-term problems. The game is changing due to trends that are summed up in Figure 6.2, and these are the more or less universal trends cited by WHO. These factors reflect the acute to chronic, and institutional to community, shift as we have seen in earlier chapters.

Rural lifestyle	Urban, globalised lifestyle
Communicable disease	Non-communicable disease
Maternal/child mortality priorities	Older people morbidity priorities
Single disease focus	Multi-morbidity/co-morbidity
Emphasis on specialist care	Emphasis on primary care
Unregulated health systems	Regulated systems
Health as a commodity	Health as a right of citizenship
Paternalistic care	Participatory care
Better treatment for me	The health of the community/nation

FIGURE 6.2 Global trends in healthcare affecting policy (*source*: based on WHO report *Innovative Care for Chronic Conditions*, 2002).

Cost is the bottom line in policy. Rising costs have generated a decade of moral panic. Given that the game is changing, why are costs such an issue?

- *Human resources* constitute the most expensive single item on the national health bill. An increasingly skilled and specialised body of doctors, nurses, allied health professionals and managers does not come cheap, nor does the constellation of support workers who play vital roles in sustaining large organisations. Regulatory and support frameworks add to this expenditure in terms of transparent recruitment procedures, continuing training, accreditation, governance, restrictive legislation on working practices (hours, health and safety, etc.). Health and social care is a labour-intensive service sector, with very substantial implications for cost management.

- *Capital costs*: our hospital-centred system demands ever more complicated institutions, with more technology built into them and to more exacting specifications. The lead time to commissioning a new hospital is reckoned in decades; the final cost always overruns projections; redesign is routinely demanded and obsolescence inbuilt. These considerations apply also to fitting out and equipping a hospital, not to mention the larger matter of recurring costs in operating it. A hospital is as sophisticated as an aircraft carrier, and equally dependent on auxiliary forces.

- *Costs of drugs and other consumables* – economic analysis of pharmaceutical and biotech industries is beyond description here. A study from the American Association of Retail Pharmacists[14] states that the prices of drugs most widely used by older Americans rose by over 25% between 2005 and 2009 – that is, about twice the inflation rate. The inflation in branded drugs in United States rose by 13.3% in the 12 months from September 2011 against a background inflation rate of 2%.[15] The cost of bringing to market a new drug is only to be contemplated by a multinational corporation; this is estimated in 2011 as $1.3 billion.[16] In the United States cancer researchers are developing more than 800 substances to target specific gene mutations.[17] The cost of those that come to market will be huge, and this will be recouped from sales to health services.

- *Safety and governance*: in the interests of public safety and confidence an elaborate edifice of licensing, regulation, surveillance and auditing measures surrounds all levels of healthcare, and each professional at work. For example, detailed patient-consent requirements reduce the productivity of surgeons. As patients experience treatment regimens of ever-greater complexity, potential hazards multiply along with unintended consequences. 'Saying sorry' is no longer good enough when things go wrong, so restrictive practices and audit trails abound in the name of accountability and transparency. Litigation costs increase faster than inflation. A quarter of the maternity services budget in the UK goes on litigation costs.
- *Commercialism*: consumerism, commoditisation, lifestyle-related aspects of health and commercial influences from the private health sector all exacerbate healthcare cost inflation.

These are the realities of delivering professional services that are evidence-based and state of the art. Guidelines and protocols make their own contribution to cost inflation through over-inclusive testing and monitoring, medicalisation of risk factors, overtreatment and reducing the element of clinical judgement. The issue is not simply one of whether current trends in healthcare cost are affordable. Rather it is how to achieve the best possible health gain for society where there are limits to what level of public expenditure can be negotiated politically. The WHO critique of health economics cites 'five common shortcomings of health-care delivery',[18] which indicate the areas where patterns of service delivery are no longer appropriate and where reform should be directed. These are as follows.

1. *Misdistribution of healthcare.* Julian Tudor Hart's *Inverse Care Law*[19] may be interpreted as the inverse relationship between the need for healthcare and its availability. Thus, those who are least in need of a service are always at the front of the queue when it is being given out and get more than their fair share. Among the aims of any progressive health policy is *equity*. This does not mean even distribution but **ready availability of services and access according to need**. In most countries health professionals cluster within urban areas and around teaching hospitals, to the detriment of rural or less well-endowed areas.

2. *Impoverishing (or impoverished) care.* Chronic illness means catastrophic expenses for many. It is well known that the largest spending health economy in the world is unable to make provision for the health needs of 40% of its population; even for the non-poor developing a chronic condition results in crippling

costs. In most countries too much is expected from too few resources deployed. We think of poor countries in this way, but it is also true of wealthy ones. There are large 'aspiration gaps' between what is promised or expected and what is provided. Where a health budget is based on a percentage of economic productivity (e.g. GDP) and recession occurs there is a shrinking resource base to meet needs, which, in turn, increase further as standards of living are eroded.

3. *Fragmented and fragmentary care.* WHO roundly criticises the dominance of the disease-focused and specialist-led pattern that is such a prevalent feature of all health systems, even those that cannot afford to be so. It calls this 'hospital-centrism', and describes it as 'a disproportionate focus on specialist, tertiary care', providing 'poor value for money', and this has become 'a major source of inefficiency and inequality'.[20] Hospital professionals are channelled into disparate specialist streams, often identified with a disease or bodily system. These have been described as 'silos', and a hospital can be envisaged as a cluster of clinical silos into which patients are labelled and sorted. This kind of structure has a pervasive influence on how professionals are trained, managed, relate and even on how they think. Clinicians become de-skilled in the clinical areas outside their own silo. Individual programmes of care share features of the silo model, for example diabetes care or cancer services. They address defined clinical sectors and create boundaries to care and, while excellent in themselves, consume resources that may have to be diverted from wider purposes. This is especially so in countries where comprehensive services are not affordable, so they invest heavily in specific priority programmes and prestige projects. Silos and programmes have a tendency to grow in complexity and number. They flourish, irrespective of what is appropriate care for the many with complex interacting health and social needs, fuelled by 'the pervasive commercialism of health care in unregulated health systems', and these 'are highly inefficient and costly'.[21] Care is experienced not just as compartmentalised but also as disjointed.

4. *Unsafe care*; paradoxically, hospital-centrism leads to:
   a. *diminished safety*: through poor system design, adverse incidents (such as hospital acquired infection), shrinkage of generalist skills, becoming increasingly remote and inaccessible, expensive and competing with wider priority sectors for a large proportion of health resource, such as provision of proper level of hospital nursing staff and primary care capacity
   b. *the complexity of hospitals* poses problems for management and staffing as shown by adverse reports on several hospital foundation trusts in England in 2013[22]
   c. *silo-based treatment* that is inappropriate for complex and multiple conditions (*undertreatment*) where, for example, a patient in a hospital may receive little attention to his or her other, co-existing conditions

d. *unnecessary medicalisation* (*misdiagnosis*); over-investigation, overtreatment and excessive interventions related to (among other factors) lack of pre-selection or filtering at a pre-hospital stage.

5. *Misdirected care*: the one-at-a-time, single disease approach failing those who have complex needs; preferential resource allocation for costly curative services at the expense of chronic illness, community care, prevention and health promotion; failure to exploit rich sources of health improvement through primary and community care and intersectoral collaboration.

The WHO argument for the radical re-evaluation of health policies concludes with a manifesto of 'eight essential elements for taking action':

1. support the *paradigm shift* (from acute/specialist-oriented to chronic/generalist care)
2. manage the political environment (existing views, practices and values need to change)
3. build integrated healthcare
4. align sectoral policies for health (across government departments)
5. use healthcare personnel more effectively (communication, teamwork and behavioural change; enhanced roles for nurses and allied health professionals)
6. centre care on the patient and family
7. support patients in their communities (support the patients' living and working)
8. emphasise prevention (as a routine component of all health-related encounters).[23]

In launching this broadside against our pervasive and (by many of us) cherished traditions of medical care the WHO is not just a prophet crying in the wilderness. Their analysis is based on, and validated by, leading epidemiologists, policy analysts, by schools and institutes of public health. Most of these are US-based, whence one might expect the contrary view. The political nature of health service reform and redistributive health is illustrated by the prolonged, intermittently explosive debates that are conducted at all levels of US politics since the Kennedy era (as outlined earlier); health is a political issue that ranks, in importance and emotive power, with the economy, gun control and defence. Once again, it is not so much a question of whether we can afford the healthcare that our technology can provide, as, **'What is the best model of healthcare in the light of current projections of needs and resources?'**

The answer? From the available transnational evidence it should be an integrated care model, patient centred and community oriented, based on generalist primary care physicians and their teams, with close specialist support. This sounds to me very much like general practice in the NHS; and Barbara Starfield agrees. This does not make me feel complacent. On the contrary, I feel somewhat alarmed. The UK medical system, its health managers and most doctors are still in thrall to a time-honoured model of hospital-centrism. There is a well-trodden path to cost-saving by simply shifting unmodified hospital activity into primary care. This is not paradigm shift but offloading. Paradigm shift means service reconfiguration with a changed set of parameters, modes of decision-making, resourcing and power base. **Crude secondary-to-primary drift is a trend that threatens to overwhelm general practice as we now know it.**

There is a need for:

- new methods for managing the complex networks that will be necessary for care integration
- new patterns of interprofessional working
- an evidence base of guidelines that are validated for the frail, the elderly who have multi-morbidity, polypharmacy and multiple risk factors and whose care pathways are more like a transmission grid than a pipeline
- service redesign, to render the health expenditure more congruent with renewed health priorities.

It is hard to find good evidence of cost-saving through the incremental reforms since the 1990s in the UK. There are structural costs to implementing change, and the changes envisaged in the chronic care revolution are extensive. Improvements in cost-effectiveness and patient outcomes are being delivered and much of UK health reform reflects WHO thinking. Getting it right in theory is a least something. Whether this means that it will come right in practice, and at lower cost, remains to be seen. It would probably be easier to invent a fully integrated transport system than to achieve the paradigm shift fully. But, if we have the ingenuity to turn an expensive transistor into a cheap multi-gigabyte chip in 30 years, what's to stop us realising integrated clinical and social care pathways that are effective, safe, patient centred, inclusive and affordable?

BUILDING BLOCKS OF THE CHRONIC CARE REVOLUTION
Wagner's Chronic Care Model

> Informed and activated patients interacting with prepared, proactive practice teams reflecting systems-reform.[24]

The chronic care model provides a framework for higher-quality chronic disease management based on Wagner's review of US health policy literature of the 1990s. Throughout the world in the last two decades, attempts to increase the priority and profile of chronic care have invoked this foundational concept. Wagner analysed existing chronic disease management programmes and came up with:

> a functional blueprint or template, as well as a set of organising principles, for basic changes to support care that is evidence-based, population based and patient centred. It defines the broad areas that must be considered but not a specific set of interventions; rather it is a framework in which improvement strategies can be tailored to local conditions.[25]

The six components of *Wagner's Chronic Care Model* are:
1. Self-management support
2. Clinical information systems
3. Delivery service redesign
4. Decision support
5. Healthcare organisation
6. Community resources.

Any similarities between this and WHO's 'eight essential elements' is not accidental. Wagner's model was seminal to the WHO vision. It reflects the emergence, in the literature of the 1990s, of a cluster of core principles:
- patient participation and supported self-help (at all levels of care)
- effective data management (including registry, clinical care, feedback and performance data)
- reconfiguration of existing patterns of service provision (congruent with chronic care priorities)
- acceptance of evidence-based guidelines and protocols as fundamental to decision support, along with specialist advice and provider education; decision support should also be available to the patient to provide prompts and recalls as well as information to assist with making choices and decisions
- improved coordination of care (multidisciplinary, integrated, generalist led, patient centred)
- incorporation of the third sector in care planning (special role in social care and self-care).

These principles may be applied at all levels, (macro, meso and micro) and there is evidence of benefit for patients with long-term conditions when these are integrated into care planning. In building on Wagner's thinking, WHO expanded and reinterpreted the chronic care model for global implementation, placing the emphasis on those dimensions that operate at macro (national and governmental) level that is, on health policy.

Chronic disease self-management programmes

It is now self-evident (but was not always so) that most care is self-care, especially when it comes to long-term conditions. As described in Chapter 4, the fusion of practical self-help and social learning theory, first described in the 1970s by Kate Lorig and Albert Bandura at Stanford University, gave rise to the chronic disease self-management programmes in the United States. This was adapted as the Expert Patients Programme in the UK.[26] Typically it consists of a peer-led 6-week course for sufferers. It has a programmed approach that aims to enhance people's ability to take control in significant areas of self-help. These include symptom management, medicines management, healthy living and lifestyle, use of available resources, and personal growth. Its significance is that it recognises and endorses the principles of participation, self-help in healthcare and the generic model of chronic disease. There seems to be little public debate on the degree to which participation and self-help should penetrate the entire edifice of service provision but it has been assimilated into public policy in health and social care in the UK as a core value.

Integrated care

This is dealt with more fully in Chapter 5. Briefly, the aims of integrated care are to prevent people '*falling between the cracks of care*', between primary and second-ary care, or between health and social care. It is a quest for so-called seamlessness in service delivery and clinical pathways. Again it can be stratified from micro to macro levels, representing the various views of what integrated care is. It may be specific and tailored to provision of coordinated services for individuals and their carers; or aimed at defined groups such as people who suffer the same condition; or at defined populations. While there is as yet mixed evidence for cost-effectiveness of integrated care, there is good evidence of benefit in specific whole populations and in older people.[27]

It may be seen that integrated care is a complex of concepts that range from straightforward local coordinated care right up to the large-scale HMOs that are prominent in the US healthcare scene. Its very variety indicates its flexibility as an idea, and this has considerable appeal for political policy-making. It has been pro-moted as a principle plank of system reform.

Quality and Outcomes Framework

The Quality and Outcomes Framework has been described as the boldest experiment in performance management in Europe. Crucially, it was the result of detailed joint planning between the British Medical Association's General Practice Committee and health managers representing the Department of Health. An essential element of the broad reforms brought in by the 2004 GP Contract in the UK, it ring-fenced approximately one-quarter of a GP's remuneration and subjected this to attainment of performance indicators. Some indicators relate to systems management but the majority of them are matters of chronic care, including prevention. There is provision for locally agreed, enhanced services. There are specified descriptors and measurements, a ladder of performance targets for each and a points system that determines the proportion of target payment gained. The scheme has opt-out and exception clauses; there are regular amendments to the list of descriptors; it is contractually enforceable and requires verification by regulatory visits; submission of detailed statistical returns is required and financial penalties can be imposed. This 'carrot and stick' approach has achieved improvement in standards of clinical care in the areas incentivised, especially where there is social deprivation, it has reduced the 'postcode lottery' effect in healthcare and it has brought about enhanced teamwork in primary care (though it must be said that health indices were improving even before the programme was introduced). It has also helped document the community prevalence of common chronic conditions. However, since it only measures process it has not reduced the inequities in healthcare predicted by the inverse care law, it has greatly increased the amount of administrative work and overall workload for GPs. To the dismay of the government, GPs throughout the UK outperformed their early projections, their average income increased, and the resulting cost overrun caused public criticism of 'money-grubbing doctors'! Public representatives made no attempt to convey to the consciousness of the public the subtleties, objectives or success of this sweeping reform. The political environment was mismanaged. Failure in public perception gives a bitter aftertaste to success, and has been a powerful undermining force that contributes to reform fatigue. This is an example of a perverse incentive. It is difficult to achieve balanced success across all frontal elements in policy change.

Managed care programmes in the United States

A variety of models of managed care have evolved in United States since the 1990s. Managed care means that an organisation contracts to provide total care for a defined sector of need, with a view to controlling costs and improving care for people with long-term conditions. This may be applied to a defined condition or cluster of conditions, or a defined population. There have been many casualties along the evolutionary pathway of HMOs, notably in the 1990s because of failure of business models that were unable to manage health cost inflation. The chronic care model emerged from evaluation studies of these experiments. The organisations that survived are widely seen as templates for the future of US healthcare, and as seminal to what has become known as Obamacare. A number of these HMOs deserve substantial consideration since their names are well known, they are ideas-factories, and they are much studied by UK and European policymakers.

The Veterans Health Administration is an example of real integration. It owns and runs its own hospitals, employs its doctors, manages the full range of care within a budget (derived from the federal government, for the care of former armed services personnel). Following stagnation in the 1990s, it reinvented itself through new leadership and shifted from a model that was centred on its hospitals towards one based on regional networks of integrated care. The new emphasis was on primary and preventive services, and energetic performance management based on clinical quality outcomes and enhanced IT. It shared many features with other integrated medical groups:

- multispecialty medical groups
- aligned financial incentives
- electronic information systems
- use of guidelines
- accountability for performance
- responsibility for defined population
- partnership between doctors and managers
- effective leadership at all levels
- collaborative culture.[28]

Kaiser Permanente, on its website (xnet.kp.org), styles itself as America's leading integrated health plan and the nation's largest non-profit health plan. It was founded in 1945 in California out of a previous workers' contributory health scheme. It is described (Wikipedia) as an integrated managed care system operating in ten states covering nine million members, with over 14 000 physicians. Each regional *Permanente Medical Group* is an autonomous, profit-making professional corporation that is primarily funded through its regional *Kaiser Foundation Plan Center* by claims reimbursements. The *Kaiser Health Plan* hospitals and medical groups are distinct but contractually linked entities. There is a thorough operating plan and governance structure overall. The emphasis is less on its foundation hospitals and more on its primary care groups, which incorporate the following elements:

- family physician or general internist (consultant in general medicine, in UK parlance)
- nursing staff, many of them specialised (advanced primary nurse or nurse practitioner)
- medical assistants
- physiotherapists, health educators, pharmacists, social workers or psychologists
- specialist physicians, easily accessed for opinion or by referral.

The slogan adopted by Kaiser Permanente is '*making the right thing easier to do*'. Their distinctive methodology is risk stratification through *the Kaiser Pyramid* (*see* Figure 6.3). This illustrates population management through focusing on the 20% of their target population who need professional care. The healthy remainder receive any necessary treatment but with emphasis on prevention, screening and health promotion. The 20% that have a significant long-term condition are stratified into three levels:

1. the major portion, 70%–80% of people with chronic conditions, receive *supported self-care*
2. those at high risk receive *active disease management*
3. the smallest portion, deemed to be highly complex patients, receive *case management*.

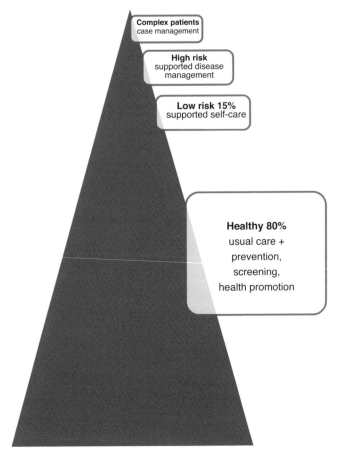

Complex patients
case management

High risk
supported disease management

Low risk 15%
supported self-care

Healthy 80%
usual care +
prevention,
screening,
health promotion

FIGURE 6.3 The Kaiser Pyramid

A unique feature of Kaiser Permanente is that it removes the primary–secondary split for people at all stages of the pyramid of care. It incorporates the chronic care model and integrates organisations and disciplines. Thus doctors from primary and secondary care share the same budget and work within a multidisciplinary centre. Advanced primary nurses carry out case management (like 'community matrons' in the UK). There is great emphasis on measurement of outcomes and feedback. Kaiser Permanente is one of the top-performing and lower-cost systems in the United States and is seen as a model for the rest of the health system. In particular, it has contributed greatly to information-based prescribing quality.* It is considered to be influential in the health policy thinking of the Obama administration.

The term *Obamacare* (*see* Figure 6.1) has been used to denote the controversial reforms introduced in 2012 by the Obama administration that are aimed at opening up healthcare to all citizens through compulsory health insurance, with employers' contributions, backed by state resources. At present, managed care schemes cover a minority of citizens and a limited range of localities. More than 40% of the US population have no health cover at all apart from the accident and emergency department or medical charities. A further influence on Obamacare is *Mass-health*, the well-established programme operating throughout Massachusetts since 2006 (informally dubbed 'Romneycare' for eponymous reasons that, as a Republican, Senator Romney might prefer to forget) that prescribes universal health insurance coverage.

Opponents of managed care systems point to the tight management structures that characterise HMOs, along with the perception by doctors and patients alike that clinical decision-making is distanced from the clinical encounter, thus threatening clinical freedom and reducing personal choice. Also, in the present state of development it is difficult to foresee how universal, comprehensive population provision will prevail, how discrete programmes of managed care will interface and interlock without significant gaps or overlapping (thus leading to exclusion or reduplication) and what will be the outcome of compulsory, occupational healthcare insurance.

Health literature on chronic care in the United States has a different starting point from that of Europe – that everyone should seek to provide for their own needs by purchasing what services they require. The one-to-one, patient-to-doctor, axis has been a cherished value. Services are specialist-delivered; family practice has not been highly valued, highly paid or evenly distributed; there are problems of universal registration; both specialist and family medicine are acute care oriented, nursing has a much higher profile than in Europe and nurses carry out much of the continuing care (it could be said that nurses are the generalists of the US health scene); there is low (but increasing) use of electronic records and data-sharing; barriers to care include deficient out-of-hours provision and front-loaded costs.[29] The developments towards managed care and universal coverage go a long way in overcoming the negatives while preserving the positive features of the US system.

Most European systems, along with, Canada, New Zealand and Australia, show evidence of a chronic care model influencing their health policy,[30] and programmes to improve care for people with long-term conditions are being widely implemented.

---

* McGavock H. Personal communication

As Singh and Ham[31] point out in their international review of systems, the main point of similarity is a move to reorient care from episodic or acute interventions toward a continuum of care which enables better prevention and management in chronic conditions. France, with half of the US health spend, was rated first among 191 countries by WHO, probably on account of its attention to chronic care.

The NHS and the social care long-term conditions model

This UK health policy initiative, published in 2005, incorporates some features of the chronic care model and US-style HMOs, modified to fit the UK culture and the NHS. Singh and Ham[32] summarise its essential features (*see* Figure 6.4):

- a systematic approach that links health, social care, patients and carers
- identifying everyone with a long-term condition
- stratifying people so that they can receive care according to their needs
- focusing on frequent users of secondary care services
- using *community matrons* to provide case management
- developing ways to identify people who may become very high intensity service users
- establishing multidisciplinary teams in primary care, supported by specialist advice
- developing local ways to support self care
- expanding the Expert Patients Programme and other self-management programmes
- using tools and techniques already available to make an impact.

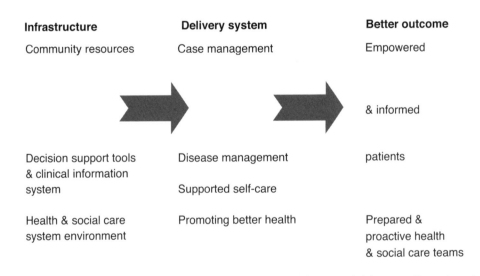

Infrastructure	Delivery system	Better outcome
Community resources	Case management	Empowered
		& informed
Decision support tools & clinical information system	Disease management	patients
	Supported self-care	
Health & social care system environment	Promoting better health	Prepared & proactive health & social care teams

FIGURE 6.4 The NHS and social care long-term conditions model (*source*: Department of Health[33])

SCENARIO: a coffee break

So, our maturing trainee has made a discovery. Accomplished as she is in clinical medicine, half the consultations week after week have little to do with bioscience, pharmacology or clinical reasoning. She had revelled in the challenges she encountered in the hospital training and felt empowered as a result. She is now disorientated and a bit demoralised. General practice is different, and that is her discovery. Not what she had been led to believe. Much of the chat around the hospital had prepared her for 'the frustrations of general practice'; the head colds, tummy upsets and lonely old people who need to talk; solving small problems and referring the rest (appropriately) to the relevant hospital consultant; these were considered to be the essence of what 'a good GP' does. Now, towards the end of the working day she wonders what she has accomplished.

Her problem seems to be that even the regional hospital, with a medical staff of 200–300 spread across a score of departments, does not seem to provide an appropriate clinic for many of the people who present to her. Is that abdominal pain going to go (if anywhere) to gastroenterology, surgery, gynae, or might it be vascular? How can she be sure that it is 'merely irritable bowel syndrome' and, therefore, best treated symptomatically, to avoid 'fixing' the problem through an endless round of unproductive, expensive and bewildering investigations? Investigate! Investigate! says her inner hospital voice. And the patient wants something done. But there are risks involved. Perhaps the worst of these is the risk of somatic fixation in that mysterious realm (is it the amygdala?) where resides chronic anxiety and the obsessional need to medicalise every twinge and pursue the illusion of certainty that it is not cancer. Fear of the unknown – the change in bowel habit, the spot of blood, mild anaemia – any of these might be overlooked at her peril (the doctor's peril, that is), regardless of the predictive value of such symptoms. As she talks I make a mental note to return to the topic of psychosomatic medicine.

But what she means is something less elusive. She is light on psychiatry. She is finding it hard to get to grips with those (30%–40%) consultations that have a significant mental health component. The majority are 'not in the books', or, for those that are, the advice seems impractical. We are harangued about GPs overprescribing antidepressants or tranquillisers but the current mantra, that cognitive behavioural therapy is the answer, has problems: availability; long waiting lists, only to be told 'this patient is not suitable for cognitive behavioural therapy'. Every presentation of anxiety, sleeplessness, stress and sadness becomes a crisis of conscience for her. Can she solve this with a script for a course of this or that, and risk drifting into the horror of being a bad doctor who dopes her patients' awareness of life; or can she find ways of working with them to resolve their angst?

Combining this with painful chronic conditions like migraine, rheumatoid arthritis or inflammatory disease and the decisions become complex and perplexing. Mix in a few family problems like bad relationships or being lone carer for a handicapped child and therapeutic paralysis sets in. She had received the impression that social workers might somehow come to her rescue by sorting out domestic complexity, but few of her concerns fit their criteria for referral.

We suspect, for example, that in the Smith household the total mix of the family's medicine cupboard is being randomly redistributed and that the father with multiple sclerosis is hooked on cannabis supplied by his son who is an ardent user. It's all very difficult, she concludes, as she asks for mental health to be made a learning priority.

Where to start? As her trainer I ought to have a plan of action for this. Even trainees who have rotated through psychiatry find that not a lot of it is transferrable to the general practice setting. So, to first principles: books, case discussions, fieldwork and basic skills training (listening, holding, counselling, etc.). As we sketch out the practicalities she points out that we have nothing under the heading fieldwork.

On the common room notice board there is a flyer announcing a conference on Mental Health in the Community, to be held soon at the university. The content seems helpful: a report on the National Mental Health Review (with responses by service users); updates on suicide prevention, eating disorders and addiction services. The cost is reasonable and it doesn't clash with anything; why not sign up and report back what you learn? Better still, 'come back with a reflective learning diary of its impact on you'.

TEN CHARACTERISTICS OF AN EFFECTIVE HEALTH SERVICE

> Policy-based evidence measures compliance; evidence-based policy introduces measures.[34]
>
> John Seddon, Occupational Psychologist, originator of the
> Vanguard Method of systems thinking

Any high-performing health system must be capable of delivering good chronic care, otherwise it is not performing. The impending challenges presented by the upsurge of demand for chronic healthcare require that health systems must achieve high-level performance without delay. Conveniently, health analyst Chris Ham has provided a short-list of characteristics of a high-performing health service for chronic care.[35] He draws on the chronic care model, HMOs and the WHO paradigm, and integrates these with an extensive review of recent literature on health policy and service management to create a list of ten characteristics, and four strategies for their implementation, which I refer to as 'Ham's Ten–Four'.

The characteristics

1. Ensure universal coverage
2. Care is free at the point of uptake
3. The delivery system should focus on prevention and not just on the treatment of sickness
4. Priority is given to patients to self-manage their condition with support from carers and families
5. Priority is given to primary healthcare
6. Population management is emphasised
7. Care should be integrated to enable primary healthcare teams to access specialist advice and support when needed
8. Need to exploit the potential benefits of IT in improving chronic care
9. Care is effectively coordinated
10. Link these nine characteristics into a coherent whole as part of a strategic approach to change

The strategies

1. Physician leadership
2. Measuring patient outcomes as the lever to drive continuous quality improvement
3. Align incentives in support of strategy
4. Community engagement

The remainder of this chapter will explore the implications of these for general practice and chronic care. To characterise them adequately will necessitate some reiteration of concepts introduced in this and earlier chapters.

1. Ensure universal coverage

Universal coverage is about society and citizenship, and the rights and duties that pertain. The prerequisites for this include:

- civil registration of births and deaths; a comprehensive national register of citizenship
- universal identifiers, a unique personal identity code or number, preferably one that is used across all health, social service or social security transactions
- address code – a postcode or 'zip' that identifies the locality of residence
- a legal framework that makes the privileges of participation enforceable.

For universal inclusion in healthcare, society has to hold some kind of consensus on the principle of *risk-sharing*. This may involve disadvantages for some, as benefits are spread more widely and thinly in order to be inclusive. Three historical examples of different ways of accomplishing this are as follows.

1. The system of occupational health insurance introduced by Bismarck in Germany in the 1880s, elements of which are still prominent in the German health system
2. Soviet systems of total state provision that prevailed in Eastern Europe and much of central and northern Asia through most of the twentieth century, which gives us the *polyclinic* with a one-size-fits-all level of healthcare that was functional but lacked patient centredness
3. The UK national insurance scheme introduced in 1948, founded on universal registration and comprehensive coverage, which delivered the familiar NHS and welfare state

Identity and demographic data that can be coded are fundamental for population medicine, epidemiological studies, measurement of indices and the assessment of need. Without such registry it would be difficult to implement these. What do you think it would be like to run a medical records system without a computer and where surnames or addresses are arbitrary and where there is free choice of physician for any given episode of care?

2. Care is free at the point of uptake

The Alma-Ata Declaration stated that healthcare should be a right of citizenship, hence the slogan 'health for all …'. Not the end of disease, but the beginning of protection for all against the potential ravages of disease. Healthcare, however, is never free. Someone bears the cost, and the price is huge. Worldwide, money is the fundamental barrier to accessing care – in particular, professional, technological care. Where care is a commodity to be purchased or traded for profit, costs are heavy, unpredictable and unaffordable for a large proportion of people. Market forces in healthcare, perhaps paradoxically, appear to drive costs up. Some small, petrodollar-rich states provide free care for all citizens, for the time being. Governments everywhere else struggle to finance and distribute healthcare within budgetary limitations: how much care, at what cost, what is politically sustainable? Most countries have a mixed economy in healthcare; for example, providing population health through public finances and insurance-based state provision for acute care, which may be supplemented by individuals through co-payments or electively through private health insurance. The population health provision often includes health programmes for chronic conditions and other priorities (e.g. cancer services, maternal and child health). Many comprehensive systems require upfront payment, with reimbursement of costs. Frequently reimbursement claims are subject to deductions, excess or co-payment charges and even exclusion of pre-existing conditions.

Very few systems in the world provide open access to unlimited healthcare free of charge. The leading example is the UK's NHS. **The absence of direct charges greatly enhances access to preventive and anticipatory care and health surveillance, and promotes adherence with treatment regimens.** In this regard the NHS is well placed to provide comprehensive chronic illness care. Salient problems include social care provision, access and waiting lists.

3. The delivery system should focus on prevention and not just on the treatment of sickness

Prevention and treatment have always been two sides of the one coin. Where they part company is where health is commoditised, where treatments are priced and sold. It is possible to put a price on a health event that has been prevented, but specific interventions are more marketable. In the commercial sector even prevention is commoditised as, for example, the personal health check-up but without evidence of any benefit to the individual and none for community health.[36] In fact, they may offer unwarranted reassurance, lead to unwarranted tests (and over-investigation) and risk overtreatment (of, for example, mildly raised cholesterol or prostate-specific antigen).

Primordial prevention, addressing the upstream causes of disease, is a matter for collective responsibility at community or state level, where trans-sectoral, coordinated action is crucial. Primary prevention, mostly in the form of immunisation programmes, has transformed the health of children and reduced rates of mortality and disability over three generations. Secondary and tertiary prevention are less directly related to community health although public health medicine would interest itself in reduced recurrence rates of acute events, easing the disease burden and addressing disability. Health education and promotion are essential elements of prevention although cost-effectiveness is difficult to evaluate, despite their face validity. Health benefit is achieved by promoting hygiene and healthy lifestyle, primary and secondary prevention and making the benefits of effective health and social care available to all.

In the UK there are comprehensive preventive services which are based, to a great extent, in the setting of primary care. This minimises the risks of 'preventive overkill'. Aspects of primordial prevention are addressed by the welfare state system and environmental health.

4. Priority is given to patients to self-manage their condition with support from carers and families

As is self-evident from the health pyramid, most healthcare is self-care. Commercial interests would aim to shrink and professionalise self-care as much as possible. The greatest potential for expansion in marketing healthcare is 'downwards', increasing their market share by encroaching into the large self-care zone. The professional health check, alluded to earlier, is an example of an area of professional encroachment into self-care for gain without benefit. Self-care does not exclude professional expertise. There is a real place for competent, informed support for self-care through, for example, ethical screening, risk factor management and 'life coaching', whereby professionals and third sector experts help the patient set and lead the self-care agenda. All health promotion is about change, and successful change management is aimed at adopting, retaining and owning the goals of change. This involves information, support, guidance, motivation and reinforcement towards desired behaviours. The health pyramid has prevention and self-help running right through it from base to apex, contributing to all levels of care (*see* Appendix 3). Among the greatest threats to personal health status are disordered appetites and lifestyles – those addictions, weight disorders and sedentary habits that characterise much of urbanised society. Supported self-management and motivational training are fundamental in the management of these. Another complex behavioural area that strongly influences personal health is *adherence*, and this too requires self-management support.

Ownership, autonomy, participation and self-efficacy all feature on the list of qualities that people with long-term conditions assert as basic values they would wish to see incorporated in their care pathways.[37] These are strongly represented in the third sector organisations and in statutory policies on patient and public involvement. The corollary of this is that any manifestation of *dependency* runs counter to public policy. Residential facilities are being scrapped as if they never had any purpose and every instance of institutional abuse is accorded national headlines. This is conveniently 'on message', since beds are expensive and the money can go elsewhere (but does it?). There is no place like home, and there is unanimity that care should happen in the location of least intensity. But there must be a facility for respite care, for crisis and substitute care or to accommodate people who suffer from extreme disabilities. It is not the acute medical and surgical wards that are closing in the interests of saving money, but mental illness, disability and elderly care units that are easily pruned on ideological grounds. What is to happen to the person with disruptive behaviour due to brain injury or advanced Alzheimer's whose relatives are unable to cope? Self-management is all very well but should there not be limits? Chronic disease self-management programmes are among the policy aims of the NHS.

5. Priority is given to primary healthcare

Not recognition; not equality; but priority. The primary care role has to be brought out of a historical niche of low regard and placed strategically where it belongs, calling the shots on behalf of the patient and orchestrating supporting specialist services. It refers to the totality of primary healthcare, not just primary *medical* services.

> PHC [primary healthcare] is the key to achieving an acceptable level of health throughout the world in the foreseeable future as part of social development and in the spirit of social justice. It is equally valid for all countries from the least to the most developed, though the form it takes will vary according to political, economic, social and cultural patterns.[38]

Chronic care should be person centred, community oriented, generalist physician led and multidisciplinary team delivered. More than that, it should be environmentally aware, trans-sectoral, sensitive and responsive to local priorities, and community-involved. To complete the spectrum of primary care, population health and public health infrastructure should be seen as playing vital roles. The micro, meso and macro perspective renders primary care a much more comprehensive concept than just general practice. This is the basis of health policy endorsed by WHO since the Alma-Ata Declaration. Primary care is indeed GPs, nurses (and allied health professionals) and community physicians, but add to that the full infrastructure of health in the community in all its facets. This applies not just to poor countries where, perhaps, basic primary care is all that is available. It applies to all countries and the wealthy ones, with their status-building centres of excellence, may be the last to realise it. This is where the work of Starfield is prophetic on the international stage. It is not that primary healthcare is all you need, but secondary is secondary; it is the strategic resource backup, not the primary provider. This is not a rationale for dumping additional responsibilities on to GPs through 'mission creep' or contractual coercion, to the point of risking service failure. Most chronic disease management takes place in primary care in most healthcare systems. And those systems that have a strong base of primary care do best.

Primary care must be promoted, reinforced and resourced accordingly to carry forward the battle against chronic disease. **The UK has a resilient primary healthcare system; the public and political rhetoric does not yet reflect this but remains hospital centred**.

6. Population management is emphasised

We have seen that identity and demographic data that can be coded are fundamental for population medicine – that is, epidemiological studies, measurement of indices, prevention and the needs assessment; also that systems of integrated managed care are founded on risk stratification. This means the use of tools to identify people with chronic conditions and to gear support to the level of their risk and needs. The Kaiser Pyramid (*see* Figure 6.3) illustrates this. Integrated information systems create disease registers and identify people who have needs. These facilitate surveillance,

and enable providers to offer services of evaluation and review. The healthy majority receive usual care and health promotion services. The definition of those who
are regarded as being at risk must be done with care. It can appear that the system
is actuarial, aimed at singling out those who are a financial liability to the system,
and this may be stigmatising. Criteria may convey different values and, depending
on the wording, select subtly different populations. Compare *'those who have had
two or more admissions to acute care'* (objective), with *'those who are **most likely to
benefit** from intensive support'* (subjective, possibly discriminating against those
with greatest disability); or, similarly, *'those whose needs assessment shows that **they
are unable** to achieve their self-assessed goals for daily living'*. People with the greatest needs may not be able to achieve much in the way of goals. Pragmatism must be
tempered with justice. The South Yorkshire Strategic Health Authority Model is an
elegant example of development on the Kaiser Pyramid. The 20% at risk are further
subdivided, in increasing order of intensity: level one receives *'standard chronic disease management'*, in level two *'dynamic case management'* and level three, *'proactive
care management'*.[39]

Population management relates also to commissioning of care on a population-
wide basis as created in England by the Health and Social Care Act 2012.
**Comprehensive needs assessment will be the basis for packaging, defining and
contracting for delivery of integrated services.**

7. Care should be integrated to enable primary healthcare teams to access specialist advice and support when needed

Integrated care means a better deal for patients. In principle it reduces waiting that
is due to interface delays and difficulties; it reduces reduplication and waste; it delivers better clinical outcomes and potential cost savings. Some of its complexities
have already been outlined above. Integration should enable primary care teams
to have access to specialist advice and support when needed. This is frequently
lacking. The separation of primary from secondary care means that specialists, by
their very nature, are more remote from the location of usual care. Every specialty
cannot be placed in every local population centre. Legal liability, governance and
professional issues dictate that to maintain high standards and depth of provision,
local hospitals close and district hospitals merge. As one observer remarked, 'if you
live in the dales you live in the dales'. Specialist services retreat into more massive,
remote and specialised 'centres of excellence'. Are we asking specialists to give up
their clinical home in the hospitals, which are increasingly remote and rarefied, to
move into the small townscape of ambulatory centres alongside GPs? It's a big ask,
and maybe that is how it must be. The Darzi Report of 2011 envisaged a polyclinic for
each town or locality in which comprehensive ambulatory clinics would sit alongside diagnostics (radiology, physiology and laboratory).[40] This facility would also

include locality services like physiotherapy, clinical psychology, pharmacy, medical and surgical clinics, with endoscopy and minor surgical facilities; a one-stop shop for most patients. The specialist would then be nearby and easily accessible to the GP for a quick word or an easy referral. The logistic and manpower implications of this are substantial. It would mean GPs relocating also, leaving their 'home' in the neighbourhood surgery, and this too is a retreat from proximity to the patient. Much of the proposed benefits may, alternatively, be derived from the use of intermediate and shared care, provided there are compatible electronic record systems.

Careful use of inpatient secondary and tertiary resources, combined with more robust social care provision, is needed if patients are to be discharged smoothly from hospital wards, leading to reduced back-pressure on the admissions side, and to increased throughput. Pressure on bed occupancy is also eased by developing collateral flow of patients through enhanced community-based services such as ambulatory clinics and diagnostics, day case procedures, intermediate care, enhanced social care and supported living capacity. In summary: **improved access to specialist care, enhanced ambulatory and outpatient care, ease of transition back into the community, intermediate care and rationalised care pathways**. Sounds simple, doesn't it? A bit like treating advanced heart failure – easier in theory than in practice.

In the UK system GPs have been providing levels of integrated care for decades, assimilating patient demand and modulating hospital use – that is, **vertical and horizontal integration**.

8. Need to exploit the potential benefits of IT in improving chronic care

In UK general practice it is easy to take the practice-based applications of electronic media for granted, but GPs in most countries are less fortunate. The NHS has been castigated for a multi-billion pound IT failure (a national integrated clinical information network – the IT Spine – that had to be abandoned),[41] but it supplies every practice with a maintained, networked, multi-user system (for all administrative and clinical functions), an NHS-wide e-mail network, electronic referrals, and electronic links that directly download much laboratory and radiology diagnostics data. It can manage clinic reports and discharge correspondence across the clinical interfaces. This can feel bewildering as one screen after another revolves before the tired gaze. However, it could be worse. In most countries clinicians have to fulfil their own IT needs with little or no support. Many still run on manual or stand-alone systems, even in sophisticated countries in North America (though steps have been taken by the Obama administration to remedy this in primary care).

In Chapter 5 we have already discussed the panoply of gadgets and apps that makes up the world of telemedicine, virtual consultations and connected health, through modems, cell phones, digital cameras, Skype, sensors, transducers, alarms, remote access and Bluetooth, that all can be harnessed to bring the benefits of special skills to the ambulant patient, or to the home and bedside. **Applying proven capability of IT is necessary for effective management of chronic conditions.**

UK health policymakers are investing much optimism in connected health as a large part of the solution to chronic disease management. In the NHS general practice has advanced IT capacity and is virtually paperless, but this is not the case in most hospitals. Integration of IT systems across the interface remains a challenge.

9. Care is effectively coordinated

> The most efficient structure for coordinating care is a system with a strong primary care foundation in which the primary care practice, in partnership with its patients, consciously assumes the responsibility for coordinating care throughout the health care system.[42]

Many of the aforementioned characteristics of chronic care systems contribute also to this one. Chronic care that is not coordinated is fragmentary or fragmented or both (to use the terminology of WHO reports). The role of primary care, the focus on prevention, supported self-management, continuity of care, population management, IT – all of these assume *coordination*. This is particularly crucial for people who are most at risk of frequent referral or admission on account of multi-morbidity and whose needs span both medical and social domains. Shared care, 'hospital-at-home', virtual ward, connected health and the various forms of intermediate care are, by definition, works of coordination and teamwork. This is true also of integrated care, commissioning and multidisciplinary working. This is easy to say but coordination demands procedures, meetings, governance and feedback loops that themselves are demanding in terms of skills, time and support.

In the UK, with its universal free NHS and robust primary healthcare, **the GP is ideally placed to be the coordinator of the diverse services required for chronic care.**

10. Link these nine characteristics into a coherent whole as part of a strategic approach to change

The ten characteristics are not seen as a scoresheet but as the building blocks of an edifice of robust care founded on chronic care principles. This tenth one, like the keystone of a Roman arch, enables the others to fulfil their function. Without it the others are fragments of care that absorb and diffuse resources and do not form a coherent framework. This is the task of leadership, a treatise in itself, but which may be summarised as: setting achievable goals, vision and inspiration, motivating, support, problem-solving and commitment. Leadership is required at all levels – macro, meso and micro. The goals of change need to be defined and understood. Change is a delicate plant and easily subverted. For example, a politician might legitimately define his priorities as the wishes of his voters and constituency interests, and these might be in conflict with the needs of an integrated system of healthcare ('rescue our local hospital!'). The WHO literature would suggest that the guiding principle should be **what society owes to those who suffer long-term conditions and disabilities, including the limitations that reason dictates should be observed**.

Clearly the NHS scores highly in all of the characteristics given here. So why is chronic care still not fully realised? Part of the answer lies with resourcing. However, the systemic stresses incurred in achieving highly on the first nine can compromise achievement of the tenth goal. The overarching one remains elusive.

THE FOUR STRATEGIES

Ham's recommended strategies for *implementing the high performing health service* are worth dwelling on because they are based on authoritative opinion and an extensive literature review. They are (1) physician leadership, (2) improving quality through measuring patient outcomes, (3) aligned incentives and (4) community engagement. They may seem to be heavily influenced by North American thinking; however, as we have seen, much of current thinking originates there and does not necessarily reflect free-market dominance.

1. Physician leadership

Physician leadership is considered to be crucial to any movement to realign health services from acute towards chronic care. Professional inertia can easily subvert any such move and, indeed, has succeeded in doing so in many countries to date. Physicians are critically influential at all levels of a health service, and in both the policy and clinical domains. Their involvement in the process of changing how clinical services are delivered is essential. So also is their commitment to quality improvement. This is not to exclude nursing or other professionals. There is no shortage of examples of nursing leadership in developing and delivering healthcare, and multidisciplinary approaches are axiomatic. There are two particular contributions that practitioners can make in policy matters. One is to influence the political agenda towards **'what society owes to patients'** rather than **'what politicians owe to voters'**. The second is to concretise and **'earth' the musings of management and policy theorists, health economists and analysts to ensure that these are tested against the realities of patient care**.

Much of the thinking around chronic care appears to fall into the trap of spending the same notional health pound several times over. For example, specialist nurses are much valued as case managers for chronic care, for acute primary care triage and specific programmes, as well as in intermediate care. However, they are in limited supply and expensive to train. Very many more will have to be produced if the paradigm change is to be successful. The same applies to the capacity of general practice to absorb all the tasks that 'the primary care revolution' would send their way. Much groundwork will be needed to underpin and define the parameters of physician leadership in the implementation of the new paradigm of care.

2. Measuring patient outcomes as the lever to drive continuous quality improvement

As has been described in Chapter 5, quality management is a fundamental value in clinical care. The kind of quality improvement that is demonstrated in the US integrated care schemes is very managerial indeed. Robust performance management, with targets, protocols and performance-related incentives for the top administrators, have delivered benefits. But that is within the eclectic and vast US health system where physicians and patients have mobility and can exercise exit options. It is by no means certain that tight performance management would function as well in a universal system such as the NHS, which has a near monopoly in provision of services.

The problems of outcome measurement are well known and especially sensitive in professions where the quality of interpersonal relating is fundamental. As Hasler and Schofield[43] said:

> It may be that providing emotional support to both the chronically sick and their family and other carers is one of the most crucial of functions that can be fulfilled in primary care.

Anything that measures this and values it would significantly contribute to driving quality improvement. The Francis Report illustrated how patient care in the UK is adversely affected when an organisation's focus is on managerial goals such as meeting targets and restrictive budgetary requirements without being reflective of human values, 'a culture focused on doing the system's business – not that of the patients'.[44] One of the most notable interfaces in healthcare is that between managers and clinicians. **The successful quality of care agenda is one that is owned by the clinicians and based on professionalism.** The genius of management would be to facilitate where coercion is not essential, to promote a training and educational approach to improve standards, and to free clinicians to do what they do best, rather than burdening them with onerous commissioning tasks, reporting and boxes to be ticked. **Continuous quality improvement should be a matter of continuing professional development** rather than one of continuous management oversight. Is this utopian?

3. Align incentives in support of strategy

> Payment by results becomes payment by activity. Such incentives are often perverse.
>
> **Simon Caulkin (Press columnist)**

Ham observes that organisations that are focused on chronic care have thought through the ways of promoting their aims and objectives. Incentives that are aligned means that they operate in a coherent, collective and mutually reinforcing pattern and avoid the perverse incentive that undermines the ultimate aims. He cites as an example the Quality and Outcomes Framework in the UK, which, as we have seen, attaches payment for GPs to performance indicators that bear on long term conditions. Unfortunately in this case, the financial gain has been eroded through payment cutbacks while the bureaucracy involved has increased. So, despite evidence of health benefits, morale in the workforce has suffered. Aligned incentives can easily slip into perversity. There is more than one kind of incentive, however. **Morale is one of the foremost workforce assets and this should be nurtured** by every possible means.

> What gets measured matters. Measures set up incentives that drive people's behaviour …. What gets measured gets managed – so be sure you have the right measures, because the wrong measures kill.
>
> Simon Caulkin

4. Community engagement

It was Balint[45] who saw the doctor–patient relationship in terms of a mutual investment enterprise that was built up and capitalised through repeated interactions, a capital fund of goodwill that could be drawn upon when tough circumstances required it. It is in this spirit that healthcare structures need to engage with the community health assets. This means intersectoral action at local authority level involving education, leisure departments, and environmental services contributing to the health of the community. In the non-statutory sector, the community development approach is a powerful one for identifying local needs that can be met locally, in collaboration with professional structures. Since healthcare is ultimately self-care, self-help should be central. There is a tough side to this. Equity and realism have to temper aspiration, and community tyranny is like any other tyranny. One of the principles of primary healthcare (as enshrined in the Alma-Ata Declaration) is that **no professional or lay self-interest group has the right to demand a disproportionate level of resourcing**. Furthermore, 'The people have the right and duty to participate individually and collectively in the planning and implementation of their health.'[46] Benefits and priorities of community engagement include: more prevention, contact with hard to reach groups, harnessing the richness of third sector organisations (especially for social care), communications networks for information and education, and conscientising in matters related to health policy so that public perceptions are accurate, in so far as is achievable. Press and media distortion of health policy and its effects is commonplace, and influential. This can perhaps be balanced by community information networks. For example, policy that seeks to incentivise community care by general practice is misrepresented by the press as 'payment to avoid admitting patients to hospital'; payment related to achieving performance indicators is reported as 'bonuses'. One does not seek to harness press freedom but lamentable, partisan and ill-informed editorial stances need to be challenged because they are influential and damaging to healthcare.

All of Ham's four strategies are represented in NHS primary care. However, there is much to be done on them, notably in developing physician leadership within multidisciplinary working arrangements, developing measures of outcome that are manageable but representative of what general practice does, excluding perverse incentives and showing how general practice might move forward with community engagement.

This, then, is health policy. Big, remote, beset with conflicting interests and views and priorities, difficult choices and the ultimate problem of trying to predict the future and plan accordingly with today's money. But it touches systems, influences values and reflects the interests of society. Ultimately policy determines what the people who need help will get and it writes the contract for every healthcare professional.

SOCIAL POLICY AND CHRONIC CARE

This chapter has focused on health policy due to the busyness of the scene and an, admittedly, medical bias. Integration is much talked about and if health policy is not matched by *social policy developments* there is a vital strategic flaw, for at least two reasons. There is a straight and short path from chronic disease to poverty and a reciprocal path from poverty to chronic disease.[47] Second, deficiency at the level of community social care creates problems in hospital throughflow. Among the very reasons for health policy reform is the assertion that hospital usage must be reduced to contain cost and promote the viability of services. One of the prime contributors to pressure of demand for hospital services is the complex of social issues that influence location of care. These include availability of facilities for independent home living, home-based care and family support with respite care, sheltered housing, residences for the elderly, nursing homes and step-down accommodation. Deficiency in any of these results in 'hospital bed blocking' and the overloading of medical services. The recent historical exclusion of long-stay beds from the hospital sector needs to be matched with enhanced social support, community services and strategies for financing these. The Dilnot Commission[48] (*see* Chapter 4) examined ways of mitigating the costs of comprehensive social care for individuals. Among the recommendations was a ceiling on personal liability for care costs through risk-sharing strategies underpinned by public finance. Another novel policy development is the facility for *personal budgets*, which enable the patient to make key decisions about his or her own care needs. On a wider front, the upstream social determinants of health lie, to a great extent, within the realms of social policy. Primordial prevention is therefore a responsibility of government through economic and social policy measures, and intersectoral cooperation.

For fuller discussion of social policy *see* Chapter 4.

A 12-STEP REHABILITATION PROGRAMME FOR HEALTH SYSTEMS

> Every mountain and hill shall be laid low, the crooked straight and the rough places level, to prepare the way …
>
> Isaiah 40:4

1. Support the WHO paradigm shift: from disease and hospital centredness towards patient-centred care in the community; promote partnership and parity of esteem between primary healthcare and the specialist acute sector.
2. Promote education for chronic disease management, based on the chronic disease paradigm, the chronic care model and the disease trajectory model.
3. Emphasise disease prevention and health promotion, with special emphasis on the major preventable risk factors – addictions, obesity, hypertension, lipids, accidents and lack of exercise.
4. Promote public health and intersectoral action for health; tackle inequalities and the other social antecedents of disease.
5. Promote self-help by patients, community involvement, carer-support and social care measures.
6. Address interface issues between sectors of care and between professional groups; align key sectors and tackle roadblocks in access and care pathways.
7. Pursue integration of care pathways and active care management especially for those who are most at risk.
8. Invest in IT for chronic condition management, decision support, information-sharing and connected health, and the skills required for their effective use.
9. Invest in research and development to build the evidence base for rational and realistic guidelines, integration and commissioning of services.

10. Create an aware trained workforce that is fully resourced and well informed on the principles of chronic care and disability support; foster the morale of front-line workers.

11. Apply rational commissioning procedures and optimise resource use especially in manpower and drugs utilisation.

12. Support quality management and make sensible provision for victims of medical accidents.

CONCLUSION AND REFLECTION

Public policy in health and social care affects the lives of everyone. In recent decades the issues posed by long-term conditions have been seen to dominate the policy agenda increasingly. Throughout the world, countries are recognising the necessity to review the principles that underlie their health services and begin to reconfigure them accordingly. WHO has provided leadership in this and has offered a framework for change. The influence of US thinkers is undeniable, far-reaching and diverse. The Starfield Effect, the trajectory model of Corbin and Strauss, Lorig's expert patient and self-management culture, Wagner's Chronic Care Model and the HMO models of integrated managed care have been described. All have been assimilated within the WHO global analysis to produce a framework for robust chronic healthcare planning that is generic. This has not been seriously challenged, although it needs to be interpreted and modified for local application. In the UK adoption of the resulting principles has led to primary care-led clinical commissioning, the quality and outcomes framework, integrated care, intermediate care programmes, the NHS information strategy, patient and public involvement, and the Expert Patients Programme. As with all policy revolutions there are widespread misgivings being expressed: that the clinical commissioning experiment will fail under its own weight; that business model failure will lead to chaos; that specialists will resist any threat to their perceived status; that adopting the influential US models will lead to market exploitation and commoditisation of health; that social care policy will be the Achilles' heel of health reform. An understanding of policy is crucial, however distant and legalistic it may appear, since it should be influenced by all levels of decision-making including at the levels of the practitioner, the patient and the community. Policy is also about money; the payment for health services; making sure that the expenditure is rational and productive; commissioning decisions that govern the quantity and direction of spending; the assurance that services purchased are of sufficient quality and fit for purpose. Health policies must match up to the realities of what patients need, what professionals can realistically deliver and what is politically affordable.

Times are turbulent in the NHS. They are turbulent in healthcare everywhere. Our lives, whether as clinicians or patients, are being shaken up. At the root of policy issues lies the question: how are we going to manage the challenge of chronic disease now and in coming decades? The healthcare workforce, especially in NHS primary care, which is so crucial for building the proposed edifice of chronic disease management, has not been sold the vision. Rather they feel reproached for problems that arise in implementation, and harangued to do more and better. The consequent morale problem reflects a failure in strategic leadership on the part of policymakers and government, and this may be the real Achilles' heel of the entire venture. The solution may lie with an educative approach, along with reinforcement of primary care manpower, so that they can ease back on the treadmill sufficiently to be receptive to the vision for chronic illness care, and that is the object of the next chapter.

POINTS FOR REFLECTION

- How familiar do you think you are with the structure and workings of your health system? How might you improve on your knowledge?
- Primary healthcare team members are far from the levers of power, but not as far as they might think: what channels of communication and representation are open to you? (Colleges, unions, local politicians, non-governmental organisations, etc.).
- Can you participate in these, or attend meetings as an observer?

REFERENCES

1. Corrigan P. *GP*. 8 December 2012.
2. Stevens A, Raftery J, Mant J. *Healthcare Needs Assessment*. 2nd ed. Vol. 1. Oxford: Radcliffe Publishing; 2004.
3. King H. WHO and the International Diabetes Federation: regional partners. *Bulletin of the WHO*. 1999; **77**(12): 954.
4. World Health Organization. *Innovative Care for Chronic Conditions: building blocks for action*. Geneva: WHO; 2002.
5. Ibid.
6. Ibid.
7. Klein R. Cited in: Iliffe S. *The New Politics of the NHS*. 3rd ed. London: Longman; 1995. p. 191.
8. Roland M. Barbara Starfield: an appreciation. *Br J Gen Pract*. 2011; **61**(589): 523.
9. US Agency for Healthcare Research and Quality. Defining the PCMH. Available at: www.ahrq.gov/page/defining-pcmh (accessed 21 April 2014).
10. Singh D, Ham C. *Improving Care for People with Long-Term Conditions: a review of UK and international frameworks*. London: NHS Institute for Innovation and Improvement; 2006.
11. 111th United States Congress. The Patient Protection and Affordable Care Act. Available

at: www.gpo.gov/fdsys/pkg/BILLS-111hr3590enr/pdf/BILLS-111hr3590enr.pdf (accessed 24 April 2014).

12. World Health Organization. *Health Policy.* Available at: www.who.int/topics/health_policy/en/ (accessed 21 April 2014).

13. Bodenheimer T, Grumbach K. *Understanding Health Policy: a clinical approach.* San Francisco, CA: Lange; 2005.

14. American Association of Retail Pharmacists. Press report. *New York Times,* 6 March 2012.

15. Available at: www.reuters.com/article2012/11/28/us-expressscripts (accessed 17 April 2014).

16. Economic Intelligence Unit. *The Future of Health Care in Europe 2011.* Available at: www.janssen-emea.com/future-of-health-care-in-europe (accessed 21 April 2014).

17. Saporito B. The new cancer dream teams. *Time.* 2013; **181**(12): 20–7.

18. World Health Organization. *The World Health Report 2008: primary health care now more than ever.* Geneva: WHO; 2008.

19. Hart JT. The inverse care law. *Lancet.* 1971; **297**: 405–12.

20. World Health Organization, 2008, op. cit.

21. Ibid.

22. *The Mid Staffordshire NHS Foundation Trust Public Inquiry; the Francis Report.* The Mid Staffordshire NHS Foundation Trust Public Inquiry; 2013. Available at: www.midstaffs publicinquiry.com/report (accessed 17 April 2014).

23. World Health Organization, 2002, op. cit.

24. Bodenheimer T, Wagner EH, Grumbach K. Improving primary care for patients with chronic illness. *JAMA.* 2002. **288**(14): 1775–9.

25. Glasgow R, Orleans T, Wagner E, *et al.* Does the chronic care model serve also as a template for improving prevention? *Milbank Q.* 2001; **79**(4): 570–612.

26. Department of Health. *The NHS Expert Patients' Programme: self-management of long-term conditions; a handbook for people with chronic diseases.* London: HMSO; 2002.

27. Ham C, Curry N. *Integrated Care: What is it? Does it work? What does it mean for the NHS?* London: The King's Fund; 2011.

28. Ibid.

29. Schoen C, Osborn R, Doty MM, *et al.* A survey of primary care physicians in eleven countries, 2009: perspectives on care, costs, and experiences. *Health Aff (Millwood).* 2009; **28**(6): w1171–83.

30. Singh D, Ham C. 2006, op. cit.

31. Ibid.

32. Ibid.

33. Department of Health. *Supporting People with Long Term Conditions: an NHS and social care model to support local innovation and integration.* London: The Stationery Office; 2005.

34. Seddon J. Interview, BBC Radio4, 9 February 2012.

35. Ham C. The ten characteristics of the high-performing chronic care system. *Health Econ Policy Law.* 2010; **5**(Pt. 1): 71–90.

36. MacAuley D. The value of conducting periodic health checks. *BMJ.* 2012; **345**: e7775.

37. McEvoy PJ. Patients with long-term conditions, their carers, and advocates. *Br J Gen Pract.* 2013; **63**(608): 148–9.

38. World Health Organization. *Primary Health Care: report of the International Conference on Primary Health Care, Alma-Ata, USSR, 6–12 September 1978.* Available at: www.who.int/publications/almaata_declaration_en.pdf (accessed 6 December 2013).

39. South Yorkshire SHA model. Cited in: Singh D, Ham C. 2006. Op. cit. p. 23.

40. Department of Health. *High Quality Care for All: the NHS next stage review; final report (the Darzi Report)*. London: Department of Health; 2008.

41. BCS, the Chartered Institute for IT. *The NHS Information Strategy: 'add health informatics'.* August 2012. Available at: www.bcs.org/content/conWebDoc/47069 (accessed 7 December 2013).

42. Bodenheimer T. Coordinating care: a perilous journey through the health care system. *N Engl J Med.* 2008; **358**(10): 1064–71.

43. Hasler J, Schofield T, editors. *Continuing Care: the management of chronic disease*. Oxford: Oxford Medical Publication; 1990.

44. Report of the Mid Staffordshire NHS Foundation Trust Public Inquiry, op. cit.

45. Balint M. *The Doctor, his Patient and the Illness*. London: Churchill Livingstone; 1957.

46. World Health Organization, 1978, op. cit.

47. World Health Organization, 2002, op. cit.

48. Dilnot Commission. *Fairer Care Funding: the report of the Commission on Funding of Care and Support*. (The Dilnot Report). London: The Stationery Office; 2011.

CHAPTER 7

The learning and teaching complex through the chronic disease paradigm

Contents

CHAPTER OVERVIEW

In this chapter all the elements of the story, the full chronic disease paradigm, are brought together. The image that comes to mind is Hercule Poirot, gathering all the suspects and retelling the story, with highlights or action replay. Here, we review our understanding of the issues concerning long-term conditions, to reflect on what we know, and how this might be communicated to students, trainees and through in-service training. An educational model is described that points to the main domains of knowledge and practice. While the reference point is general practice, UK-style, the majority of concepts and issues have their counterparts in the health systems of other countries and have relevance to other clinical specialties, although some translation of terms may be required. This section will not dwell on the nuts and bolts of medical education but on the curriculum of needs throughout the learning continuum. It begins with a brief account of training for general practice in the UK.

> Current and future trainees should be trained in integrating care.[1]

MEDICAL EDUCATION IN PRIMARY CARE: A UK PROFILE

> Training capacity is required not only for the increasingly complex clinical work of primary care, as comorbidity becomes the norm and the focus shifts more and more from the out-patient clinic to the surgery, but for the new roles – needs assessment, service design, commissioning and quality assurance, among others – that the 'new' NHS will demand.[2]
>
> Roger Jones, former editor of the *British Journal of General Practice*

Familiarity with chronic care is not an optional bolt-on to medical education but a keystone. Learning about primary care is fundamental to this. Education and training are essential arms of creating and maintaining a functioning and professional healthcare system for the benefit of patients, if it is to serve them well. A survey of the views of 100 academic deans on the curriculum content of medical schools, carried out in the United States in 1997, produced a 'wish list' of the top 12 topics.[3] Nine of them relate directly to chronic care: ambulatory care, prevention and health promotion, primary care, use of electronic information systems, care of the elderly, interdisciplinary teamwork, psychosocial care, community social problems and patients as partners in healthcare. The remaining three are highly relevant to it: the doctor–patient relationship, professional values and ethics. It is difficult to imagine a platform for conveying these coherently other than community-based teaching about chronic care – that is, in general practice or by general practitioners.

General practice, in the UK at least, has been in the vanguard of medical education for 50 years, pioneering methods in learner centredness, individual and small group teaching, and formative and summative assessment.[4] Primary care has become a key educational resource for the whole medical system by providing a broadly based delivery platform for much of undergraduate clinical teaching, foundation training and specialist training for that 50% of the whole profession who will become GPs. Accordingly, GP teachers are the best-trained, and the most widely dispersed, medical teaching force in the UK. This has been achieved with minimal resourcing:

- no additional premises or personnel allocation
- remuneration levels that barely cover the cost of clinical time substitution
- instructor training that is minimal and undertaken largely at their own expense

- no allowance for preparation and supporting activity, not to mention research and development (R&D).

There is, according to a report by the heads of the five London medical schools, good research evidence of positive effects of undergraduate teaching for students in the community that benefits the students, the practices, health professionals and patients.[5] It is well established that training practices score more highly than average in quality assessments. Community-based teaching accounts for 15% of the curriculum of London medical schools (and probably more elsewhere).[6] Students become familiar with primary care methodology and a case-mix that reflects community prevalence; they see a full system at work and an overview of the health service, by contrast with the single specialty teaching hospital departments; they receive one-to-one tuition and personal attention; they experience the professional lifestyle of the majority of doctors, the locus of over 90% of clinical encounters and management of the full range of illnesses in their ecological setting; and they gain an alternative view of hospitals – from the outside.

At graduate level much has changed in the UK in this century:
- some exposure to general practice during foundation training
- selection for the 4-year graduate training is carried out by GPs
- the training programme is based in general practice with a GP educational supervisor
- approved training posts in hospitals have to have some community relevance
- a day-release group programme during the hospital attachments
- two separate placements in general practice over 18 months with day release throughout
- a radically reconstructed professional qualification, MRCGP (Membership of the Royal College of General Practitioners) examination
- a national curriculum, revised in 2013, that tabulates the range of learning objectives that constitute the UK model of practice
- grounded on workplace-based and e-portfolio-based learning, clinical skills assessment and a clinical knowledge written test.

Chronic care subsists within the national curriculum but it is not highlighted as a coherent framework per se. In order to make a disparate body of knowledge accessible, there should be an emphasis on core generalisable knowledge, transferrable skills and problem-solving from first principles. Trainees often end up feeling insecure in their state of knowledge, despite having acquired a great wealth of it in the 10 years since embarking as students. It needs to be systematised, cross-linked and experienced in context to make sense of the galaxy of learning tasks they encounter. One way of integrating diverse fields of knowledge is through problem-based learning. Another is by selecting major cross-curricular themes, such as chronic illness care. Any proposed curriculum of chronic illness care should not compete with the established training curriculum. It should supplement and inform it, guiding background reading and identifying issues for discussion. The chronic disease paradigm is proposed for use in teaching and training in order to:

- emphasise the experience of patients, their involvement and their contribution to self-care
- present the community perspective as the default setting of clinical care
- introduce new descriptors such as the chronic care model, the trajectory model, the World Health Organization (WHO) paradigm shift and integrated care
- facilitate a critical evaluation of healthcare policies
- point towards the evidence base that underlies these
- link these with their existing knowledge of basic clinical sciences, including the social sciences
- locate procedures, such as those of the quality and outcomes framework (QOF) which may be construed as serving mainly administrative purposes, within a composite philosophy of chronic care.

Current and future trainees should be trained in integrating care.[7]

HOW IS CHRONIC CARE TAUGHT?

The apprenticeship model, within a validated training practice, is fundamental to providing an individual, mentored, workplace-based experience in a protected learning environment.

- Through immersion in primary care they learn experientially; the full menu of chronic illness care is encountered through the regular round of practice activity as they build up their e-portfolio and reflective learning diary
- Encounter multidisciplinary teamwork in the various practice-based clinics, case management discussions and team meetings, and through the governance procedures
- Take medical care to patients in their homes and care facilities, in addition to office-based encounters
- Follow through the clinical pathway of those admitted to hospital and participate in intermediate care plans, as well as other methods for bridging the interfaces of care settings
- Become intimate with an integrated practice information management system, its uses and abuses

Regular personal tutorials with the trainer build on these experiences; much of their content may be mapped against the chronic disease paradigm, as trainees currently do to the national curriculum.

Over 15 years of using this teaching tool has shown it to be easily applied. Each domain (complex) may be regarded as a mini-programme that is expanded in the fashion of a 'drop-down menu'. The same holds for *the disease trajectory framework*; by drawing attention to the evolving, longitudinal nature of the patient's journey with chronic disease, stages may be analysed, trends discerned, impending crises identified and preventive perspectives reinforced. Discrete, point observations may be converted into a map that has predictive value, raising questions about the patient's health and functional status such as:

'What is changing in his social environment that accounts for this deterioration?'

'Do we envisage him dying within the next few months?'

'We seem to be stuck in a rut. Are there other services or clinical resources from other sectors of care that might be of additional use?'

'What can she not do now compared with a month ago?'

'These data appear to be unchanged from last month; is she really stable or is she fluctuating?'

Similar approaches apply to parametric data, where graphing the discrete measurements turns observations into predictive trends. The archetype of this is the infant developmental weight chart, where loss of predicted trajectory heralds a problem even before actual weight loss is evident, prompting heightened alertness or proactive intervention.

Modelling is a classic mode of teaching in medicine. Actions and attitudes speak louder than words. It can be tempting to regard the chronic sick, those with disabilities, the mentally ill, the addict, the frail elderly, the patient with complex needs or the non-complying person as 'heartsink patients', but a practice team that approaches these as positive challenges to clinical management skills will teach much of lasting worth. Equally important learning takes place through the downtime chatter in the common room. Here colleagues are free to regress – have a 'moaning coffee break', abreact, recover and prepare to 'return to battle'. We have to be real. The important thing is what the students or trainees learn from such times.

Personal self-care is a vital area of learning for chronic illness care. The essence of burnout is a loss of a sense of meaning in what you do. The chronic disease paradigm provides a cognitive framework which can make sense of the tide of repetitive, dull, minute, precise tasks, and the five (or more) hours daily spent communing with the computer screen. It demonstrates why this may contribute as much to chronic care as do the face-to-face consultation sessions. There is, of course, a wider agenda in relation to self-care, as will become clear later.

A salient task of trainers is to help the student or trainee learn how to learn. This involves building confidence and self-reliance through affirming the student or trainee's strengths and turning weakness to advantage. The area of ignorance can be redefined as a learning opportunity, that quest for knowledge gaps that shrinks the zones of unawareness (as in the Johari window concept) as a discovery that is to be celebrated – and filled. It has been said of those in training that they come to the job overburdened with information but underequipped with perspective.[8] In responding to this, it is important to affirm what they know, to keep putting them in touch with the wealth of knowledge they already possess and to help them to spend it wisely by systematising and applying it. Almost certainly, their most undervalued memory stock will be of epidemiology, social medicine and psychology, all hovering below the threshold of recall. Like computer hard drives, much may have been corrupted or deleted but everything can be de-fragmented and reconstructed at the hands of an expert. Chronic illness care draws on these as the basic sciences of patient centredness. If this is regarded as *an attitude*, then it is a challenging thing to teach. It is simpler to teach patient centredness as a *social construct* that includes family and caregivers within a community context. The attitude will follow if it is well modelled also by the practice teacher and team.

There are two main approaches to teaching a new subject area: by immersion or incrementally. Both can be effective, but this poses the demon dentist question: '*Would you prefer one minute of agony or 10 minutes of suffering?*' The first one, plunging learners directly into complexity, can lead to bewilderment and negativity. This is hazardous unless it is thoughtfully based on the principle of *cognitive dissonance*, which deliberately confronts the learner's preconceptions to bring about change.[9] Cognitive dissonance is illustrated in the second scenario, 'Tutorial time', in Chapter 1, where the bright new trainee is put in charge of a complicated family illness situation. The second, gradualist, approach uses building blocks to work sequentially towards the desired goal. Linear clinical pathways are practised before allowing responsibility for clinical complexity or high levels of multi-morbidity. A family case study may be instructive, as in the first scenario, 'A case study', in Chapter 3 – like peeling the layers off an onion.

Both approaches have merits. The gradual approach keeps to firmer ground but risks being tedious. I recommend trying the former one with the trainee who is resistive, sceptical or dismissive of what is being offered, or for the high-flyer who thrives on challenge. Monitoring and safety-netting apply, naturally. As Festinger[10] (the thinker behind cognitive dissonance) observed, 'Humans are not a rational animal but a rationalising one.'

Teaching is frequently at its best when both trainer and trainee are exploring ideas and discovering connections together. You don't have to know everything to be a great teacher. The process of learning is often of more value than the product, as long as you have some vision concerning what the desired product is. **The chronic disease paradigm is an aid to learning, not a goal of learning.** Unpacking and repackaging it is the learning process. Suitable outcomes may include creating a personal set of general guidelines that crystallise the management of chronic conditions, to try to improve upon the paradigm and personalise it.

If management of chronic disease in its fullness is now the essence of general practice, then learning to manage long-term conditions in the community setting is fundamental to the curriculum of training. Rather than being diffused across the range of different diseases, the course of training should centre on principles, generalisable knowledge and transferrable skills that may be applied widely. Disease-specific areas may then be highlighted as they are encountered. This approach is particularly recommended for programme directors who run the day-release group schemes. Small group work, round-table discussions and problem-based learning are the natural milieu for debating dilemmas, developing ideas and promoting conceptual growth.

As for undergraduate teaching, my own experience is limited to individual and small group tutoring. The technicalities involved in university curricula I must leave to academics and faculties. However, an outline for a special study unit is included below (*see* 'A special study unit for students'), for use as a small group elective module. Also included is an outline curriculum for trainees (*see* 'The curriculum of chronic illness care'), which can be adapted to continuing professional and team development, and, in the final chapter, clusters of headings that relate to chronic illness care.

A WHO report calls for 'a transformation of healthcare workforce training to better meet the needs of patients with chronic conditions'.[11] It goes as far as stating: 'A workforce for the 21st century must emphasize management over cure and long term care over episodic care.'[11]

THE CHRONIC DISEASE PARADIGM

> You in your small corner and I in mine …
>
> **Susan Warner, from a popular Victorian hymn**

Clinicians can be forgiven for having a limited, niche-bound view of the broad field of chronic disease management. This has to be expanded if the daily round of work is to be sustainably meaningful. A simple form of the paradigm is shown in Appendix 1 and involves, as we have seen, four basic domains that surround and interact with that of the patient. These are the disease, the clinical, the community and the policy complexes. Education is the theme that constitutes the sixth domain and this has been named the learning and teaching complex. It does not appear within the paradigm model because it is like wallpaper that runs right across it. Research and development might be seen as an extension of this, having relevance to all of the complexes (but that would merit another book). These domains will be unpacked in the following pages.

What is the meaning of the chronic disease paradigm?

The chronic disease paradigm is a conceptual framework to embody and promote teaching of the full 'life cycle' of chronic illness within its total environment:

- its consequences for patients
- the emerging challenges it poses for societies and health systems
- its implications for organisation at macro, meso and micro levels
- how policy and evidence are changing the direction of healthcare priorities
- the consequent need to train and retrain professionals appropriately for changing roles.

By filling in the context of developments in policy and work practices this fulfils the following functions:

- makes sense of what individual clinicians do as cogs in the big wheel of healthcare
- sustains morale in the face of reform fatigue: much box-ticking, hoop-jumping and keyboard-tapping is dispiriting unless there is perspective and meaning
- provides a platform of teaching-learning
- indicates and validates the centrality of general practice, and why **all clinicians ought to have exposure to primary care in the course of their formation**.

In short, **chronic illness care has all the attributes of a specialism in its own right**. It encompasses depth and breadth of knowledge, skills and method; there is a corpus of evidence and literature that is growing rapidly and points to R&D needs attuned to the community context. As a specialism it is not the property of any one professional group and should not be constrained into a new specialist box. By definition, **chronic care is multi-professional and it should find a place in the curricula for all professions that contribute to the care of the chronic sick**. Clearly, it lies at the core of general practice and there are few activities in general practice that do not in some way fall within the scope of chronic illness care. Even the demand-led, acute aspects, out-of-hours services and pre-hospital resuscitation can be subsumed within chronic care, since chronic diseases often have an acute beginning and manifest crises along the trajectory as features of their natural history. So, while the emphasis may be on the GP, the chronic disease paradigm deserves a strong representation in basic medical education, foundation training and general professional training for all specialisms. The same should apply to general nursing training, with appropriate modification, and to all allied health professions in the community, especially physiotherapy and occupational therapy (where chronic care is already represented), pharmacy and social work courses. **Multidisciplinary training is a growth area that is not yet well codified or much represented in medical training programmes.** As long ago as 1997 in the United States a survey of academic deans concluded:

> Changes in health care delivery and an increasing generalist orientation are influencing academic deans' perspectives on needed curriculum changes, and there appears to be considerable support for medical school curricula that will foster a broader, more humanistic role for physicians.[12]

The six components of the chronic disease paradigm will be reviewed in the form of notes for teaching and discussion, drawing together the salient features of each, as described more fully in the previous chapters, although changing the sequence. As a tool for clinical education it ought to start with the patient and family's experience of living with long-term conditions.

THE CHRONIC DISEASE PARADIGM UNPACKED
Domain 1: the patient complex
The participants
- The person who suffers from one or more significant continuing conditions that cause impairment, disability or oppressive symptoms that require professional interventions
- His or her family and informal carers

Dynamics
- Addresses the micro level (i.e. the individual patient and those intimately involved); most healthcare is self-care; most patients wish to be autonomous and own their condition and take responsibility for it.
- This has implications for their participation, involvement in their own treatment, their capacities to influence service provision at all levels, assisted by organisations and expert patients, self-management programmes, mediation and advocacy.
- Self-help capacities have to be supported with timely diagnosis, interventions, information, materials and services; functional capacity and the activities of daily

living are crucial to well-being and offer valid goals for care management; valid clinical goals may have to be revised.

- Patients should receive care in the setting of least intensity.
- Multi-morbidity, polypharmacy and complex clinical pathways are common features of chronic illness; so are relapses, deterioration and death.
- The household participates in the social attributes of the person who suffers disease: deprivation, loss, stigma, limitations and relationship stress, in addition to any immediate roles as informal carers.
- Carers are at risk; frequently it is the old and sick who look after the old and sick; some carers are underage and they have special needs; support for carers is part of chronic condition management; on request a carer assessment may be carried out by social services.

Issues

- The role and responsibilities of being a patient raise issues of self-efficacy and agency, capabilities, mental capacity, confidentiality and adherence.
- The norm of self-care breaks down easily through individual factors such as physical and mental capacity, isolation, motivation and adherence; what, if any, are the limits of participation and involvement; how to manage problems in expectations, dependency and adherence, resolve conflicts of interest and instances of unreasonable demand?
- Where there is social disintegration, or in an impersonal and urbanised society, what substitutes for family and neighbourhood care?
- Who is the 'next of kin', the principal carer, the key-role person? Frequently these do not coincide. Who can act on behalf of the patient? Who is entitled to know what, and how much?
- Relationship complexity: loss of intimacy, 'personality change' and role reversal, risk management; prevention of domestic violence, abuse of elder and dependent persons; breakdown in caregiving.
- Normalisation: how to assimilate illness and disability into a new lifestyle that may be stable?
- How might clinical pathways be rendered minimally disruptive?

Key messages

- Trajectory awareness: to promote continuity and anticipatory care; chronic conditions are like the unwelcome, disruptive guest in the home of the patient; doctors meet them only episodically.
- Self-care is crucial and needs reinforcement.
- Breakdown of family care jeopardises chronic care at its very root.

Key professionals
- GP, social worker, district nurse

Basic science
- Sociology, social psychology

Domain 2: the clinical complex

The participants
- The GP and the primary healthcare team, clinical and technical specialists, allied health professionals, service managers

Dynamics
- Micro and meso level (i.e. the personal physician, the multidisciplinary team, the service systems required for patient support); patients are managed at the level of least intensity with preventive approaches, early minimal interventions and at the lowest appropriate level of specialisation.
- Patient-centredness means respecting the ideas, concerns, expectations and needs of the patient, assimilating these into plans of treatment and reinforcing the patient's self-care capacity.
- The GP is the point of first contact and is the key professional; the GP filters and formulates initial responses, actively seeks out early disease manifestations; acts preventively; coordinates any further clinical course that may include hospital referral or admission; involves the appropriate supportive services and resources; has key roles in health promotion, and risk factor management.
- Specialists provide high-skill backup to primary care; their technical knowledge and specialised equipment serve the clinical pathway of the patient; they may undertake longer-term roles through inpatient or outpatient (ambulatory) follow-up and outreach modalities.
- Hospital care is expensive, disruptive, distant and alien to the patient; its use should be focused on selected patients and based on assessed needs.
- Minimising hospital usage ought to release resources for enhanced services more convenient to the patient and under generalist continuing care.
- Clinical interfaces are bridged by intermediate, connected and shared care, specialist nurse services, step-down facilities and community social care.
- Continuing management by generalists in the community reduces risks of over- or underdiagnosis, loss to follow-up, conflicting care plans, reduplication of clinical effort, needless polypharmacy and systems failure.
- Efficient use of clinical communication systems facilitates record-keeping and coordination of care; effective electronic systems play a key role in chronic illness care.

- General practice is a key medical training facility.

Issues

- Managing the interfaces between locations of care, transition point handover, integration of clinical and social care pathways, and multidisciplinary care are all areas that require service-based R&D.
- The 'medical model' of (conventional) care, and current professional specialities, derive from historical institutions in response to acute care imperatives; can this successful model be transformed to meet fresh challenges in continuing care (the paradigm shift)?
- Good chronic care is consistent with good acute care; can the converse work?
- Professional role boundaries, inertia and rigid line-management practices create barriers to realising integrated care for chronic conditions; what are the implications of the paradigm shift on medical identities?
- Waiting lists for services and choke points in systems create problems of accessibility, linked with problems in hospital throughflow; these are toxic to integrated care.
- Gaps in skill-mix and manpower require creation of new roles and expanded capacity: more general physicians ('hospitalists'), community-based physicians' assistants or biometric technicians, more career GPs (to balance the part-time or sessional doctor trend); improved entry of nurses into primary and community care and nurse specialist grades.
- Despite adventurous and often enlightened public policy, the downstream administration is frequently oppressive, heavy-handed and micromanagerial; heavy emphasis on regulation, procedures, and paperwork interfere with service delivery and use up resources.

Key messages

- Minimally disruptive patient pathways, longitudinal trajectory view, asking: *'What is this person's daily life like and how can its quality be improved?'*
- Advocate, navigate and signpost for the patient pathway.
- You are not alone out there – think team and resource people; what additional skills are required?
- Manage resources prudently, especially the expensive, specialised ones; support team morale and protect the services you provide from exploitation and abuse from any quarter.
- Know the job description of all key players – who does what?
- Teach and train.

Key professionals
- GP and team, specialist nurses and allied health professionals
- Clinical specialists and technical and diagnostic services
- Service managers

Basic science
- Chronic illness care, education, service management

Domain 3: the community (or social) complex
The participants
- Social worker, social care team and care workers
- The third sector: non-governmental organisations (NGOs), voluntary and charitable organisations and institutions, local networks for self-management and health support

Dynamics
- Micro and meso level: the vital local community relationships that surround the patient complex; kindly neighbours who 'pop in'; faith-based communities, workplace, social clubs or sports and leisure amenities.
- Third sector organisations, many disease-specific, offer resources of information, group support, advocacy, volunteer visiting, self-management programmes; many provide services such as day centres, specialist nursing or physiotherapy services; welfare rights advice is a key service (Citizens Advice Bureau).
- The community grows micro-organisations like a wood grows trees; self-organisation is one of the attributes of a community; community development is the praxis of finding local solutions to local problems; community structures are vital in complementing formal care services at low cost; they know where the stress points of society are showing locally.
- More formally, the social services provide specialised teams with powers of intervention (elderly, disability, learning disability, child protection, etc.); they are responsible for administering social care provisions and care packages.
- The social security system of welfare allowances is a vital social service.

Issues
- Society's lost legion of workers inhabit community groups, voluntary bodies and NGOs – underpaid (if paid at all), with insecure contractual conditions; yet flexible, creative, busy and responsive to needs; many NGOs have sophisticated operational plans, service delivery, R&D and networks of influence right up to national level and beyond.

- Self-help organisations offer support, socialisation, self-management and poverty support; funding is mostly charitable, insecure or short-term; many employees tend to experience minimal wages, poor conditions and contractual insecurity.
- Regulation of community organisations is essential but this risks stifling small-scale operations and initiatives, since they rely heavily on volunteers, retirees in search of a useful role, and low-paid workers.
- They need professional support; do they deserve your 'pro bono' contribution (management committee, training and so forth)?
- Formal social care is controversial; its funding requirements are escalating; clients are liable for costs.
- Deficient supply of domestic support, 'step-down' provision and residential social care leads to back-pressure on hospital services and perverse incentives towards hospital dependency.
- A shrinking base of family and neighbourhood-supported care through demographic changes, urbanisation and social fragmentation reduces the 'village network' of support and casts the issues of need into the public services.
- Community caring is not the cheap and easy solution that governments desire; 'care in the community' policies easily descend into 'care by the community' realities.
- 'Secondary to primary drift' does not appear to apply to funding.

Key messages
- Know what is 'out there' in your locality and find out how to access their services.
- Support voluntary sector activities and NGOs; they need your skills and they will be useful to you and your patients.
- Explore gaps in local services and lobby for, or organise, a remedy.
- In commissioning activity, take opportunities to promote the community care perspective; primary care, local initiatives, skill-base, and organisations.
- Take multidisciplinary case conferences seriously and attend where possible.

Key professionals
- Social worker, social care workers
- NGOs and third sector workers: specialist nurses, counsellors and other therapists
- Community workers

Basic science
- Sociology, social science of community development

Domain 4: the healthcare policy complex

The participants

- Government and elected representatives; international bodies; civil service and other public administration personnel
- Health service senior management, academics; researchers; health economists
- Public and environmental health officers; professional associations and unions
- (Perhaps also the press and broadcast media)

Dynamics

- Macro-level (mostly): governments legislate, determine public policy and administer macro systems; health and social care systems are political; they are the biggest spenders of public money; they express the public consensus on underlying values such as market-based or risk-sharing philosophy, spending priorities and intersectoral coordination.
- The healthcare system expresses policy, converting it into service priorities.
- Public and environmental health bridge the gap between health policy and local service sectors through statistical analysis, emergency planning, public safety, hygiene, health promotion, and addressing the social antecedents of disease through intersectoral action and epidemiological surveillance.
- Public policy in most countries concerning chronic disease is generic and has high priority; related policy positions include community care, participation, equity and combating health inequalities, governance, quality and workforce training.

Issues

- Being political, public policy is influenced by public opinion, pressure groups, media, fashion, short-term electoral considerations, economics and transnational factors. Its strategies may be value-driven, inherited, dialectical and not always evidence based. (To quote a campaign slogan by a medical organisation some years ago: Q. *'What do you call a man who will not take medical advice?'* A. *'The health minister!'*).
- Benefits of chronic care require long-term perspective but heavy short-term investment, and this is a political conundrum.
- There is never enough money for the health and social systems; they are the biggest employers and they compete with other national priorities; they have to demonstrate valid achievement; this is problematic since the spending, especially in chronic care, is seldom geared to the needs of those who are paying the taxes, who tend to be younger and acute care oriented.
- Alignment of diverse interests is rare; rationing is unpopular, government needs to save money, professionals want to improve and innovate, consumers want

more choice and less waiting, the press wants lurid stories; there can be conflicts of interest.

- Inertia is passive opposition to change: all the players demonstrate inertia, not always in proportion to the magnitude of a proposed change.
- The inverse care law observes that those least in need of a service are the ones most likely to take advantage of it; areas of deprivation merit preferential programmes and may require task forces of special provision; can health inequalities be overcome?

Key messages

- All practitioners should seek to comprehend the big picture, the full chronic disease paradigm, and the part they play in it.
- Policies, like governments, come and go; the triad of doctor, patient and illness is constant.
- Analyse macro-policy and derive micro-solutions; SWOT analysis (strengths, weaknesses, opportunities and threats); participate in collective action to shape policy; work on policy rather than against it – policies may be massaged and managed to suit local circumstances.

Key professionals

- Public representatives, elected and appointed office-holders (at macro level)
- Directors of trusts, clinical commissioning groups and social services, health system managers, consultants in public health (meso)
- The workforce that delivers services (micro level)

Basic science

- Epidemiology, social policy, health economics

Domain 5: the disease complex

Key participants

- The 'Dragon', which personifies all the chronic conditions as a collective force; the Dragon's ecosystem
- The whole health service, notably primary care

Dynamics

- Macro, meso and micro levels are all involved in combating the Dragon.
- International health policy consensus regards chronic disease as collective; WHO recommends coherent responses through adopting the chronic care model and paradigm shift, and countering the environmental and social antecedents of disease.

- Prevalence of chronic disease is increasing in line with demographics and improving survival through crises, but with impaired living and increased multi-morbidity.
- Consequently, patients experience years of living with impairment, and the effects of ageing compound the accumulation of conditions.
- Chronic disease is not randomly distributed but correlates with deprivation, age, adverse genetic factors, and impaired access to services.
- Additional hazards from chronic disease include co-morbidity, complex treatment regimens, polypharmacy and iatrogenic factors.
- People live longer with good medical and social care; chronic illness is treatable and, to a degree, preventable.
- A small number of risk factors underlie the bulk of chronic disease; prevention is crucial and it runs right across the disease trajectory.

Issues

- Countering chronic disease is impeded by reliance on systems designed for acute disease management that are disease centred, specialist dominated, capital intensive and hospital based.
- Prevalence of chronic disease is increased through emphasis on acute care systems; this is not a criticism; acute episodic care is a necessary, though not sufficient, response to disease.
- The trajectory model of chronic disease should guide responses and working practices: continuing and anticipatory care, monitoring, prevention and care management.
- Expectations to demonstrate quick and measurable outcomes are inconsistent with the nature of chronic conditions.
- The disease wins through attrition, demoralising everybody; how to persevere through repetitive tasks, routines of protocol and torrential data flow with constant vigilance and ensured quality of service?
- Morale, purpose and meaning are crucial to the functioning of a chronic care workforce; how are these managed?
- Intense scrutiny, managerialism and punitive criticism intensify workforce burnout and undermine professionalism.
- Attention to the upstream causes of disease requires intersectoral action on social and environmental factors; these lie beyond medical control.
- Have medical education and professional training adjusted to the challenges posed by the chronic care model?

Key message

- Chronic disease is a big challenge and a burden, but it is a 'normal' experience and creative responses can promote normalisation of life.
- It is never defeated; know your enemy; managed coexistence means that even with good care, people will deteriorate, relapses and crises will happen, and every system is imperfect; things go wrong.
- Quality in care safeguards professionals as well as patients; embrace it; patient centredness maintains focus on the aims of work when the processes of work are tedious or onerous.
- Leadership is the maintenance of team morale, vision and purpose.
- Think trajectory: prevention, trends, care pathways, integration, partnerships of caring.
- Teach and train, especially around chronic disease management.

Key professionals

- Everyone! GP and primary care team, in partnership with the patient and the full clinical and social care services, each playing their part within the policy framework.

Basic science

- Epidemiology, service management, chronic illness care theory

Domain 6: the learning and teaching complex

Key participants

- All clinical students, and practitioners in training and throughout their careers
- Colleges, faculty, trainers, clinical tutors and educationalists

Dynamics

- Learning and teaching are two sides of the one coin; continuing learners make the best teachers and teaching is a powerful learning activity.
- Teaching is one of the characteristics of a professional and an obligation on doctors back as far as Imhotep, Hippocrates and Maimonides; the honorific title 'doctor' means teacher.
- Modelling is a key teaching strategy; people watch each other and draw conclusions from what they observe, even non-verbally.
- In clinical work, teaching skills are essential to motivating, informing, reforming, bringing about change, health promotion, negotiation, mediation, advocacy, dealing with risk and risk factors, management and leadership.
- Professionals may do this well or badly, but they 'cannot *not* teach'; hone your skills.

- Medical training should emphasise methodology in learning: questioning, reflectiveness, problem-solving, accessing sources of information, critical appraisal of evidence, self-help – learning how to learn and become autonomous learners.
- A key aim of training is to supplement linear thinking with lateral thinking as cognitive styles – to both analyse and synthesise; they are synergistic, not antagonistic.
- Chronic illness care is not a new science, but an emerging discipline; it has the characteristics of a specialism – that is, an identifiable area of practice that requires mastery of a body of knowledge and skills, is transmissible, draws on and creates a technical literature and evidence base, and identifies R&D priorities.
- The root meaning of the word *discipline* is '*adhering to a body of teaching*' (root derivation: *disciple*); motivation is required, not coercion or oppression.
- Teaching and learning chronic illness care as a coherent model contributes to professional well-being, especially in those sectors most intimately involved – notably, general practice. It puts forward a philosophy of praxis and a meaningful context that makes sense of disparate and, in themselves, unspectacular but essential activities.
- Working and learning together contributes to multidisciplinary team development; continuing professional development for chronic care must include the team dimension.

Issues

- Chronic illness management is interdisciplinary; training for it involves all clinical professions, but does it do so in reality?
- Multidisciplinary learning is in its infancy; it should be a growth area.
- Specialisms, historically, have generated specialties, specialists and institutional superstructure; these have attracted status, power and command of resources; this results in 'disease-centrism', the 'silo-based' nature of teaching hospitals, and the medical profession has been influenced by these.
- Is chronic illness care a specialism?
- Generalism has been eclipsed in hospitals and undervalued in society; consequently it is poorly esteemed in the political sphere and in media portrayals.
- Development of community-oriented primary care has been greatly outstripped by growth and investment in secondary and tertiary care; community-based continuing care, managing multi-morbidity and population medicine (needs assessment, managing risk and prevention) require a different paradigm, one that already exists in general practice.
- Shifting the paradigm is a challenge that is fundamentally one of education and training.

Key message

- Chronic illness care should be treated as a specialism; professional education, training and continuing learning should reflect this and contribute to the R&D agenda.
- Multidisciplinary education is taking place, but there is more to it than attending lectures together.
- The chronic disease paradigm, the chronic care model and the trajectory model are basic building blocks of a curriculum for teaching and training.
- Chronic illness care training should begin in medical school, inform all graduate training, form the core of generalist training and continue throughout career; other disciplines involved in chronic care should adopt this, especially nursing and social work.

Key professional:

- Educationalists at all levels; all clinicians as autonomous learners

Basic science:

- Educational theory and practice; chronic illness care

CHRONIC ILLNESS CARE: A SUMMARY FOR STUDENTS AND TRAINEES

In Chapter 1 there is a section entitled chronic disease management in a nutshell. The ideas set out there have been developed through subsequent chapters. Here they are re-reworked to provide the background for the educational framework.

Chronic disease is a hot topic. It is in everyone's interest to optimise chronic illness care. The press and broadcast media are full of chronic disease controversy. Governments everywhere are wringing their hands over the ways and means of tackling it and paying for it. Serial changes in contracts, regulations and requirement are symptomatic of this struggle. New challenges arising from a 'climate change' in healthcare and the rising tide of disease prevalence challenge all clinical professionals to meet the legitimate needs of our patients in new and creative ways. Embrace chronic care. It is not boring and it will not go away. It will shape the future of most clinical jobs.

Chronic disease is generic, despite its great biodiversity, and its ecosystem can be defined and managed. The chronic diseases (also referred to as non-communicable diseases, long-term conditions) thrive on a limited number of widespread and preventable risk factors, and a common range of management strategies may be applied; people with long-term conditions experience a large core of shared challenges. There is an international health policy consensus around the generic model of chronic disease and that it is primarily the province of community-based generalists. In the

NHS the GP is the only clinician who has a direct input across the spectrum of conditions and specialised areas. This makes it an exciting career, like the conductor of an orchestra rather than as a concert pianist.

Chronic illness care pervades the medical curriculum and general practice training should revolve around it. What aspects of primary care do not fall within the chronic care perspective? The filtering of all undifferentiated presentations is the platform for risk assessment, early diagnosis, prevention and health promotion; managing acute illness aims at rescue from immediate threat so that longer-term interventions may be put in place, converting a crisis into a safeguarding process; this also applies to emergency and pre-hospital care; family medicine promotes self-management and patient autonomy, and supports the care environment. The public health functions of primary care address risk factors, primary prevention, secondary prevention, evidence-based medicine and quality. Practice management ensures the effectiveness of the delivery vehicle – a team base, information systems, and procedures for quality assurance and patient safety.

The family home is where chronic disease resides. Chronic diseases impinge on family life, the activities of daily living and capacity of families to support the patient's self-care. Family carers carry the disease burden and share in the resulting disabilities. They experience the same social determinants of health, genetic issues and risk factors as the index patient. Situational crises and social breakdown may herald the onset of disease or may result from it. Frequently it is the vulnerable, the very young or the old and sick who care for the vulnerable, the old and the sick.

Chronic disease is dynamic. The trajectory model illustrates the typical phases of its extended timeline. The need to respond to trends rather than point observations prompts prognostic, proactive and preventive measures; discrete data become parametric, turning tables to graphs. The natural history of chronic disease predicts that relapse, crisis and progression will occur; it demands continuity, responsiveness and anticipatory care, and redefines 'therapeutic failure', as distinct from 'therapeutic deficit', within this perspective. Chronic illness is the sum of all concurrent chronic conditions, plus any intercurrent events that contribute to impairment. People with long-term conditions can get sick too, and pre-existing conditions can mask the onset of new illness. Good chronic care presumes good acute care and people with chronic diseases should not get stuck in a 'chronic sick pigeonhole'. Other things happen too.

Chronic diseases are not randomly distributed – they tend to cluster and predispose to further misfortunes. The trajectories of all concurrent conditions, acute and chronic, synergise and interact as multiple clinical pathways mesh. Major risk factors also tend to be interdependent, synergistic and correlate with personal and family lifestyle, and living conditions. Complexes of need, multiple interventions, polypharmacy and iatrogenic adverse events are frequent hazards. Those most at risk of chronic disease are frequently among the least equipped for self-management. This is where professional input is most needed. Remember the inverse care law.

Chronic disease management is multidisciplinary. All the clinical disciplines, medical and allied health professionals, have evolved in their present form for good reasons. The ranges of their skills, knowledge and toolkit are complementary, and are reinforced through coordination. Accelerated evolution of these will be required in order to meet new patterns of multidisciplinary working in an integrated way. Interfaces between services give rise to loss of continuity, delays and patients getting 'lost to, or lost in, the system'. Multidisciplinary teamwork promotes integration of care and discovery of innovative services.

Risk stratification identifies priorities. By definition, priorities have to be selective. There are scoring systems that inform needs assessment based on variables such as functional capacity, age, frailty, organ impairment, social support needs and pressing symptoms. Intensive interventions should be reserved for the 5% or so who are highlighted as having complex needs. It is these who will benefit most from individualised case management.

Managed care has been intensively developed, mostly in the United States. It is a model that may translate well into UK general practice as coordinated, responsive and proactive care-planning, concentrating resources on the most needy and invoking specific specialty contributions. Nurse practitioners ('advanced primary nurse' in the United States) oversee continuity of process and, with medical backup, act as the key worker or manager of the care plan. Optimal care aims would include individualised, minimally disruptive care pathways for patients, in the setting of least intensity, with integration of processes of service delivery. 'Holding work' is a term for active professional presence that is supportive in an otherwise unchanging situation and is additional to any clinical intervention. It is an aspect of chronic illness care that is highly valued by patients, if not rewarded by systems.

Prevention is not just about stopping things happening. Modes of prevention are classified as primordial, primary, secondary and tertiary. Health education, health promotion, surveillance, screening and risk factor modification are all modes of prevention, along with immunisation and attention to social functioning. Prevention runs right through the chronic disease trajectory. It is very dependent on systems of teamwork and information management. Terminal care is a special zone of preventive action, being based on anticipatory care planning. Preventive work is often repetitive and unglamorous but, where cure is improbable, it is a mainstay of continuing care. The existing model of palliative and terminal care ought to point the way to improving the management approach for earlier trajectory stages in all serious chronic diseases.

Quality of care is an essential concern, not a bolt-on activity. Total quality is not about 100% scoring but about 100% commitment to professionalism, the craftsman's pride in his work. Nevertheless, it has to be demonstrable to create quality assurance for both patients and the healthcare system. While it is not practicable to quality assess every activity, quality assurance of each professional, process and policy is feasible and manageable. Thus, people management is crucial. This combination, backed up with appropriate performance indicators and informed by rational guidelines, forms the spine of clinical governance. Guidelines are tricky things and need reflective application. Leadership and modelling high standards of practice complement quality management. Quality and governance should serve, rather than dominate, chronic illness care.

The health system expresses public policy. Professional roles are socially determined, defined, validated and rewarded. Healthcare is political and does not exist in isolation; otherwise it is arbitrary or chaotic. Somebody somewhere commissions health services. Clinicians ought to make their voices heard; to work on the system rather than against it; to get to know it and focus on the positives; to analyse policies critically (SWOT analysis means appraisal of strengths, weakness, opportunities, threats); to convert threats into opportunities; to guard basic professional values; examine macro-systems to derive micro-solutions. Individual professionals need a collective voice to speak to power. This is done through professional associations and colleges.

Personal and public involvement is an imperative of democratic societies. The medical model approach casts the patient in a passive role. By contrast, the chronic illness model of care defines the patient as the key player. This is in keeping with the WHO model of primary care, within which primary medical care is but one contributor. Self-care is fundamental and needs to be validated and enhanced. This has given rise to the concept of the expert patient and self-management programmes, as promoted by third sector organisations. Patient centredness implies eliciting and responding to the ideas, concerns and expectations of people. This is served by processes such as commissioning, service-development, integration and quality. Patient-determined outcomes, functional ones such as mobility, independence or symptom-relief, may trump clinically prescribed ones (such as guideline adherence). Doctor and patient become partners in care. Partners, however, can fall out, and the relationship needs tending by both parties. Patient participation, like democracy, is a great principle but a hard taskmaster, and 'the devil lies in the detail'.

CHRONIC ILLNESS CARE: A NEW SPECIALISM

To regard clinical chronic care as a specialism does not mean transplanting the silo model of hospital specialist into the community, thereby fragmenting the generalism of the general practitioner. It is rather to formulate a philosophy of praxis that enlivens a broadly based body of knowledge, fosters research and development, defines goals to be achieved and promotes the dignity of the professionals who practise it. General practitioners may take pride in numbering chronic illness care among the specialisms that constitute their expertise. As we move towards the realities of integrated care pathways and community-oriented commissioning of care the applied discipline of chronic illness care should be defined as a core module of the curriculum for medical schools, basic and specialist training, and continuing professional development.

A generic curriculum outline and a module for students are shown below.

THE CURRICULUM OF CHRONIC ILLNESS CARE

This outline curriculum may be applied to the various stages of career path, with modification to take account of level of experience and learning needs.

Theory and knowledge content
- Characteristics of chronic disease; the impact of long-term conditions on public health and society; disability as a long-term condition
- Models of disease and the natural history of chronic disease based on the trajectory model of disease (the disease complex)
- The patient, the family and informal carers in chronic illness or disability (the patient complex)
- Community and society support through chronic illness: professionals, voluntary sector services, NGOs and institutions; formal carers; the problem of social care (the community complex)
- Bringing healthcare to the community setting: the nature of primary healthcare; location of clinical care and interface issues; hospitals and specialist resources (the clinical complex)
- Politics, policies and funding for health and social care; the WHO paradigm shift and Wagner's Chronic Care Model (the policy complex)
- Issues in chronic care: commissioning, integrated care pathways; evidence-based and critical thinking; the quality agenda and governance
- The chronic disease paradigm – pulling together the essentials.

Practice-based learning
- Case studies in chronic illness, to illustrate application of the chronic disease paradigm
- Reflective diary of learning episodes; for example: from a clinical seminar on a long-term condition, a review of guidelines on a particular condition, a clinical dilemma encountered

- Produce a practice policy in a particular area of chronic disease management
- Quality assurance reporting: a practice team meeting; audit selected chronic care issues and processes; discuss a significant event; analyse complaints received
- Fieldwork: placements, attachments and visits to various settings related to chronic and continuing care (e.g. a hospice, a cancer unit, a rehabilitation unit, social security office or Citizens Advice Bureau)
- Multidisciplinary working and learning; reflective diary on a case conference in social services or community paediatrics
- Team-based discussion of special issues in chronic care: multi-morbidity, polypharmacy, risk factor management, access to services and promoting patient self-help

Practice-based research
Investigate, document and reflect on practice activity analysis and audit-related activity based on questions such as the following.
- What is the rate of hospital admission in people with multiple diagnoses?
- What are the circumstances and rate of readmission within 1 month of discharge?
- What is the use of accident and emergency department and out-of hours services by chronic disease sufferers?
- What is the best balance of time allocation between open available appointments, dedicated clinic sessions and follow-on slots for chronic care?

Assessment activities
- Self-assessment: PUNs (patient's unmet needs) and DENs (doctor's educational needs); personal learning plan and portfolio of learning undertaken
- Periodic reporting on work done on the framework outlined above
- Peer assessment of case reports; team evaluation
- Appraisal and revalidation procedures; these scrutinise quality of long-term care and the learning portfolio
- Examinations: for students, their qualification examinations; for trainees, the Membership of the Royal College of General Practitioners examination; for lifelong learners, a new diploma in chronic illness care

A SPECIAL STUDY UNIT FOR STUDENTS

These are sometimes called curriculum enrichment or electives.

Aims of module
- Understand the significance of chronic disease
- The generic approach to chronic disease and its management
- Apply the chronic disease paradigm

Concept
- Envisaged as a 2 or 3 week attachment for a group of six to eight senior students; each student assigned to a teaching practice; a hub and spoke arrangement; in partnership with a general hospital; local GP tutor coordinates the practice programme, seminars and the hospital-based aspects; individual tutors assigned

Method
- Mornings – attend clinical sessions; afternoons, a group seminar with tutor
- Problem-based approach with case-based and action learning, audits and directed reading; individual fieldwork includes visit to the hospital laboratory, imaging departments, clinics (e.g. diabetic, oncology or rheumatology), residential and day centres, a hospice, the Citizens Advice Bureau, with reporting back
- Students rotate across practice clinics and appropriate hospital locations
- Selected patients' pathways and carers' experience: identify, interview and report back

Theory and knowledge content
- Represented by seminar topics: definition and meaning of chronic disease; impact on the patient, family and society; the chronic disease paradigm; epidemiology update; what sociology contributes; family medicine and community care; how health services work; developments in chronic illness care

Assessments
- By individual and group tutor reports; performance of assignments and presentations; terminal assessment exercise (marked assignment, e.g. learning diary, reflective diary or extended case study)

Evaluation
- By medical school lead and participants

SCENARIO: Reflections of a trainer – learning through chronic disease

By the end of her trainee programme, with 18 months of it spent in general practice, what do I hope our, now not-so-new, trainee will have learned?

I would wish her to be enthused by her experience of learning primary healthcare, and particularly about dealing with chronic disease. There is a steep learning curve experienced by all trainees when they encounter the reality of professional practice. The progression from basic qualification, through hospital-based graduate training and into the community is challenging, disorientating and subject to overload. In addition to the cognitive overload of new knowledge there is the perplexity that comes with beginning to 'manage messes', as Schön expressed it, and to work alongside a myriad of related professions. Junior doctors in general practice are especially prone to this overload as they adjust to the new setting, systems, rhythm of work and the immense diversity of problems that present to them. Supportive, protected, graduated exposure with frequent opportunities for reflection are essential in fostering the positivity, relish of challenge and thirst for knowledge that are every professional's best defence against burnout and drop-out.

At the same time she should have learned to respect herself, her accomplishments, the fund of knowledge and skills she has mastered, her role and her discipline. She represents the peak of a huge, complex and expensive pyramid of training founded on her hard-won accumulation of knowledge, skills and values (the ethos that is her heritage). She is the product of a great investment by society and it is her responsibility to ensure that she, in turn, constitutes an asset to that society. She should realise that at the end of formal training, whoever the patient and however perplexing his or her presenting problem, she has a mass of knowledge and skills to draw upon. She will know something about everything or, if not, how to find out.

Without proper self-respect, high morale and confidence in the worth of her discipline her efforts will be frustrated, blunted and pose the risk of damage to vulnerable patients. This confidence must be balanced with realism about her own limitations, fallibility and dependence on others in every aspect of professional life. Collegiality, the valuing of the discipline and those who share in it, is an important component of this self-worth and, therefore, of performance.

More particularly, I hope she will have discovered that by focusing on the needs of the chronic sick, and learning about chronic disease management in general, she has covered the broad curriculum of training for general practice (she was already conversant with much 'obs and gynae', clinical medicine, etc., from a sound hospital training). Experience gained through managing acute episodes, relapses and crises renders her well equipped to deal with acute illness and cope with emergencies. Familiarity with the complexities of repeat prescribing takes her into pharmacology across a very broad range of therapeutic substances and awareness of the necessary hazards of polypharmacy. The emotional roller coaster of relapse–remission, breaking bad news or managing anticipatory grief will provide opportunities for developing the range of interpersonal skills that underlie every kind of consultation. She has had to practice the counselling approach to emotional problems, relationship difficulties and conflict management. Health education skills and motivational interviewing are frequently called upon in working with people who have chronic conditions. Palliative care skills are as essential to managing advanced chronic disease as they are for cancers and especially in the terminal phases of both.

As to the management and administrative side of training, she will have become familiar with all the systems operated within the practice. She will have learned that chronic disease management is very systems dependent. Any practice that delivers well in the areas of asthma, diabetes and cardiovascular disease has the management capacity that will make it effective in dealing with all other clinical demands. The IT systems that operate well for chronic disease are more than capable of high quality clinical recording, prescribing management, interfacing with hospital departments and lab/radiology links. The call and recall function for screening and surveillance is equally applicable to chronic disease as it is to cancer prevention, child health surveillance or maternity care.

In mastering these procedures she will have learned to value the management team that operates them. She has attended and observed in operation the various team meetings for information exchange, problem solving, administration, palliative and terminal care, clinical governance and the monthly clinical topic evening. By making a special study of chronic disease in general she is acquiring transferrable knowledge, generalisable skills and, I trust, the fundamental attitudes of professionalism.

In addition to this list of clinical management aspirations I should hope that she has got close to those who bear the suffering of chronic illness, and to their carers. If she has not achieved this then most of the above is technical training that might equally well take place in a skills lab. Essential as technical competence is, at the end of training this should almost be something to be assumed. Where the real learning takes place is through serial and continuing encounters with people who bring to the clinical encounter their vulnerability, their fears, struggles, defeats and resilience. If we lose sight of the person within whom the disease resides, we have lost touch with our own humanity. When the magnificent waves of scientific intervention have spent themselves on the rocky shores of progressive disease it is the human qualities of the clinician that are put to the test. Patients value practitioners who excel in this above all and they will forgive such a practitioner much incidental shortcoming. As the old saying goes, 'If you treat patients well you will always be remembered; if badly, you will never be forgotten.'

Not uncommonly doctors and nurses have found their vocation through their own experience of illness, in themselves or in their immediate family. We are humanised and sensitised through such experiences. I would not wish a profound illness experience on our young trainee. However, she has been encouraged to enter into the experience by proxy. That means the continuing exposure to ill people, not just in the consulting room, but in their homes, for that is the address where the disease also resides. A patient's illness exists for the doctor during the 10 minutes or so of the consultation before we are on to the next task. The illness goes home with him or her, and continues through the dark of night and the light of day. With the passage of time the trainee has seen the ups and downs, the trajectory, of a selection of such diseases. Unless she has encountered the other members of the household and kinship circle she has little grasp of the full impact of the particular disease. When serious acute illness occurs, its impact on the family can be dramatically obvious. In the case of chronic and degenerative disease it is less dramatic but no less profound. It may not be an exaggeration to propose that the majority of carers live lives of quiet desperation, modulated by the vagaries of the patient's fluctuating state. In some cases they themselves are the presenting symptom. I well recall my first domiciliary encounter with a patient with Alzheimer's. I was called out to a situation of uproar that had spread through a cluster of relatives and neighbours who were at their wits' end as to how to cope with the florid behaviour of an old man who, by the time I arrived, was sitting quietly in the corner of his neighbour's living room, with nothing on, in a state of total indifference, smiling. What I remember most clearly are the feelings of helplessness, loneliness and anxiety that paralysed any analytical and interpersonal skills I might have possessed. With hindsight, I was internalising and mimicking the feelings that the group of carers were experiencing. In that moment we were experiencing the disease together. This is the voice of the illness making itself heard and we must learn to tune in to it, otherwise we learn little that is of value about the management of chronic disease that could not have been conveyed by a pathologist or epidemiologist, by distance learning or out of some book.

What I am getting at is really quite simple. Our emotions and feelings in a clinical setting are our antennae that detect what is going on around and within the patient. They are a diagnostic tool. It takes practice, through repeated exposure, to recognise and accept that this is so, to step back, evaluate the experience and value it as holding the keys to a considered, positive response, even where no curative or pharmacological one is evident. Thus, I hope that through occasional exposure to the loneliness of standing by the patient's bedside feeling professionally naked, she will have made discoveries about herself that will be of lasting value to her.

So, I hope that she will have learned through our reflections on chronic disease management that the patient is the epicentre of it all, but that those who are in the immediate circle of relationship are also afflicted with the disease and share in the suffering. Which just illustrates an old truism in family medicine: it is not always clear who is the patient.

A few more matters I should like to think she has grasped.

She came face to face with the economic impact of the chronic disease complex while filling out a detailed life assurance medical report and finding herself saying, 'Why does this person bother applying for life assurance?' Perhaps he needed a loan, a mortgage, had a family business problem … On discussion, the wider message was not lost on her. Loss of working capacity for the patient; losing out in career development on the part of key family care givers or even difficulty for them retaining their jobs; additional expenses in buying in extra care support; the additional costs of turning up the heating or having heavy laundry needs; loss of credit-worthiness … There are so many impacts that it is not surprising that half of those with disability live at or below the poverty line. All this may be offset by payments from social security. However, I recall our trainee's look of shock after she was sent on some computer-based fieldwork, to list the commonly available allowances and she had discovered that they were all substantially less than £100 per week (some of them taxable). I think this modified her attitude to those who depend on benefits and bring in bulky forms to be completed.

I think she is beginning to quite enjoy attending multidisciplinary case conferences with social services. She remarked on the absence of preconceived animosities between the various professional groupings represented around the table, the skilled chairmanship, and the egalitarian procedures that accorded involvement to the patient and their advocate. Each contributes their piece of the jigsaw puzzle that facilitates decisions about the extent of the care package that is put in place and periodically reviewed. The resulting minuted document provides a detailed pen-picture of the case, an overview that enriches our practice-held file and renews our interest. She finds such meetings valuable opportunities for networking, which is useful in further cases. When she goes to work elsewhere she will carry the memory of this as a template for exploring the local services available.

I know she will similarly network with the pharmacists in her new locality, valuing their skills in enabling patients to self-manage their medication, and their tactful phone calls when one of her prescriptions seems not quite right. Perhaps she will also contract with a pharmacist for periodic sessions of advice on auditing aspects of prescribing and revising the practice drug formulary.

I do not know if she will find much time to visit her patients when they are admitted to hospital, but I hope she will make opportunities to do so. The concept of continuity of care is under threat from changing work practices, but such visits carry a strong message to the patient that she is still their doctor. It also enlists the goodwill of the hospital staff and enhances the flow of information and cooperation. Of course time is a scarce resource but it can be well invested in networking with local hospital staff, showing an interest in what the local facilities are and who the various specialists are.

The same applies to the myriad voluntary community and self-help groups that exist in every area. They represent, serve, inform and advocate the interests of their constituencies, and are often hungry for support from health professionals. The reputable majority will not seek to manipulate and exploit the doctor, and her willingness to attend an AGM or speak at an information evening will show support and add to her networking. A young doctor in a new practice area has much to gain from such exploration. Health education and presentation skills can be practised and this builds the portfolio of evidence of professional development that is part of annual performance appraisal.

Her professional development activities might lead her to explore the area of 'medical politics', those professional bodies that represent the views of the profession and its interests in relation to the 'employers' – the health trust, or whatever they happen to be called now (it keeps changing). She will have observed that one of our training partners serves on the local commissioning team, helping to negotiate and reconcile local priorities in health and social need with the resources available. She has seen the benefits such wider involvement brings to the practice in terms of information and perspective. In due course she will make a first-class trainer.

To sum up, I hope that at the end of her training she has benefited and derived satisfaction from deepening her understanding of the nature and behaviour of chronic disease (particular ones as well as the generic awareness that has been emphasised), and that our emphasis on the natural history and trajectory of disease has provided a window on the fascinating fields of clinical epidemiology and evidence-based practice. This perspective will enhance her ability to approach the initial management of even a rare or unfamiliar disease from first principles, this to be backed up by more leisurely homework on its details through the usual resources (texts, library, Internet, etc.). However, she might consider developing a special interest in a couple of major chronic diseases. Having a particular grasp of one or two in depth provides a firm footing of methodology, which is transferrable much more widely. Becoming 'a rheumatology buff, an addiction addict, a diabetes sweetie, a respiratory breeze'; it is amazing how frequently she will find any of these throwing light on her general run of consultations. In the UK the 'GP with Special Interest' is a significant development as a career enrichment feature, and such posts are generally related to the care of one or other of the chronic diseases. I hope she will have grasped the fundamental message that life for a generalist is all about that persistent mantra that has not changed in over two millennia, from Hippocrates to Balint and beyond, the triangle of medicine – the doctor, the patient and the disease.

There is one final wish. It is that she will also have a life, somehow! But time is on her side. She will have other personal priorities that need to be realised. She may need career breaks or part-time working patterns for a while, but I trust that what she has learned through our reflections on chronic disease will stand the test of time.

CONCLUSION AND REFLECTION

- Learning and teaching are two sides of the one coin. The root word for *doctor* means *teacher*. All professionals are career-long learners. All need to work on learning skills.
- Clinical teaching skills overlap with those of consultation, counselling, motivational interviewing, imparting information to patients and health education. All need to learn how to teach.
- Multidisciplinary teamwork requires group skills; this ought to mean interdisciplinary and group-based learning.
- Encourage trainees to get involved in action learning – through committees, case conferences, audits, adopt and follow-up a chronic patient, attend practice clinics, go to a Balint group …
- Teach and train.

REFERENCES

1. Royal College of Physicians, Royal College of General Practitioners, Royal College of Paediatrics and Child Health. *Teams Without Walls*. London: Royal College of Physicians; 2008.
2. Jones R. November Focus. *Br J Gen Pract.* 2012; **69**(580): 794.
3. Graber DR, Bellack JP, Musham C, *et al.* Academic deans' views on curriculum content in medical schools. *Acad Med.* 1997; **72**(10): 901–7.
4. McEvoy PJ. *Educating the Future GP: the course organiser's handbook.* 2nd ed. Oxford: Radcliffe Medical Press; 1998.
5. Rosenthal J, Stephenson A. General practice: the future teaching environment – a report on undergraduate primary care education in London. *Br J Gen Pract.* 2010; **60**(571): 144.
6. Ibid.
7. Royal College of Physicians, Royal College of General Practitioners, Royal College of Paediatrics and Child Health, op. cit.

8. Samuel O. *Towards a Curriculum for General Practice Training.* Occasional Paper 44. London: Royal College of General Practitioners; 1990.

9. Festinger L. Cognitive dissonance. *Sci Am.* 1962; **207**: 93–107.

10. Wikipedia. *Cognitive Dissonance.* Available at: http://en.wikipedia.org/wiki/Cognitive_dissonance (accessed 21 April 2014).

11. World Health Organization. *Preparing a Health Care Workforce for the 21st Century: the challenge of chronic conditions.* Geneva: WHO; 2005.

12. Graber DR, Bellack JP, Musham C, *et al.*, op. cit.

CHAPTER 8

Meeting the challenges of chronic care

Contents

CHAPTER OVERVIEW

In this final chapter the salient messages will be re-worked with particular reference to the GP as a team leader, looking at some problem areas and practicalities, followed by a concluding summary. The processes of general medical practice, according to the UK model within the NHS, will be trawled for areas of pressure, conundrum and challenge. This may be of some interest to practitioners elsewhere since, ultimately, GPs everywhere show remarkable convergence in their daily concerns. What emerge are lists, hints, opinion and speculative answers that may have scant reference to any evidence base. Brainstorming has validity as a process tool even while lacking strict prioritisation or even feasibility. Each of us, in our small corner, has to SWOT analyse (strengths, weaknesses, opportunities and threats) the circumstances of practice in order to refine our systems and discover new responses. GPs tend to be creative about how they work. They have contributed greatly to the success of the NHS to date and, no doubt, they will continue to rise to the challenges.

WE HAVE A PROBLEM ON OUR HANDS!

> We trained hard, but it seemed that every time we were beginning to form up into teams, we would be reorganised. I was to learn in later life that we tend to meet any new situation by reorganising and a wonderful method it can be for creating the illusion of progress while producing confusion, inefficiency and demoralisation.
>
> **Gaius Petronius (66 AD, attributed)**

In the UK, and elsewhere as we have seen, chronic disease is increasing in prevalence, complexity and impact. But this is only part of the problem. Paradoxically, it is the consistency and loyalty of medical professionals that pose equally substantial challenges. We are slow to let go of a tradition of medicine that is institutionally centred. We run the risk of failing the paradigm change test, refusing to budge, or adopting grudgingly and minimally the precepts of community-oriented primary healthcare as the chief locus of chronic care.

As professionals we had been cast in a mould at an early stage. For doctors it began with the alma mater; the university and teaching hospital, the stately morning teaching rounds, 'my old chief' in this or that specialty; the pathology professor who addressed us in Greek on our first day and traversed our orbit again some years later to dissect the secrets of disease and the final solution of obscure riddles laid out on a slab or a slide; all preparing us to tread the wards feeling like young gods with newfound powers, sealed against the inroads of fatigue and observed anguish. It took years of inner-city practice to dent my armour. At some level the glamour persists with its hold over our identity. This is reinforced by the well-informed society that is stirred by news of breakthroughs; the 'tomorrow's world' of manipulating the elements of life, of inheritance, of microorganisms micrographed and slain; the defeat of cancer; of imaging at molecular level; and the ultimately alluring concept of the centre of excellence.

And yet, in 2013 we learn that all is not well in the health service, even in general practice. The Seventh National GP Worklife Survey, commissioned from the University of Manchester by the Department of Health, reports the lowest levels of job satisfaction since 2004, the highest levels of stress since 1996 and rising numbers preparing to pull out of clinical practice.[1] A British Medical Association survey of 500 GPs in 2012 reported that 46% were emotionally exhausted, 42% experienced depersonalisation and 34% felt they were not achieving much.[2] Patients struggle to get an appointment at the entry points of the health system; they may lie overnight on a trolley in accident and emergency (A&E) because there is 'no room in the inn'; despite all our IT capacity there is confusion about their prescriptions; and granny's care home is being closed down because the government says there is no more money. In fact £5.8 billion have been squeezed out of an already low cost NHS in 2012, which prompted the Chair of the BMA Council to suggest that if the NHS were a country it would barely have a credit rating.[3] While community services are creaking there is a growing load of morbidity that defies the august structures of our palaces of treatment. We still believe in the household gods of progress and venerate the temples of science but our faith in their power to heal has been shaken. This calls for a reformation. Not one that would destroy major institutions, but a review of our value systems that would lead to reformulating our expectations, adopting a humbler approach – that health must be husbanded from the bottom up rather than being bestowed from the top down. Such a reformation is a challenging process. It makes demands: that the ill become involved in shaping the course of their illness; that the well actively guard their wellness and make demands that are reasonable; that communities and societies assume responsibilities towards the vulnerable; that professionals find their proper place in the quest for health; and that policymakers find the structures that promote the health of the people.

This problem is crystallised by the rise of chronic disease. The increasing weight of the numbers that chart the disease burden is apparent in all societies as people live longer, accumulate more diagnoses, and are rescued from the causes of premature death only to face additional and often tougher challenges. We cannot just rely on increasing wealth to buy more treatments, as the treatments become dearer and more hazardous while wealth, and the means of generating it, slips beyond our ability to control it. The trajectories of co-morbid disease reveal the limitations of the highly differentiated structures we have inherited. The locus of disease has shifted from the clinical setting to the domestic but the ethos of our training still reflects former priorities. Our reliance on technological medicine, validated by past triumphs, now risks losing the war on chronic disease by its reluctance to serve rather than dispense healthcare. Have our health service priorities been the pursuit of disease science at the expense of their honorific title – the two words Health and Service?

There is a framework to address this. It is called the paradigm shift and it is clearly expressed by the World Health Organization (WHO). It appeals to reason, justice and pragmatism. It calls for a fundamental attitude change that applies to all societies and at every level for a quiet revolution rather than a violent coup. I see it as embodying the humble approach. The word 'humble' comes directly from the Latin root *humus*, which is the soil of the earth, the low ground from which springs organic growth of great diversity, from mosses to trees. What we reap from it depends on the quality of the *humus*, what we plant and how we tend it.

To reiterate, the elements of the WHO paradigm shift:

- support the paradigm shift
- build integrated healthcare
- align sectoral policies for health
- use healthcare personnel more effectively
- centre care on the patient and family
- support patients in their communities
- emphasise prevention.[4]

This is a statement of agreed principles, not detailed enough to constitute a blueprint as it stands. At first glance it appears to be a top-down model, placing politics and policy at the head of the list. However, the first clause is not an instruction to government level; it is *a broadcast call for support* that will make it possible for the other clauses to become political and policy realities. It democratises the manifesto. It challenges all to internalise it, and that includes all doctors and health professionals. It specifies patient-centred, family-focused, community-located preventive action. In medical terms that means primary care.

This makes it incumbent on GPs to rise to the challenge and all other specialised physicians to lend their support, willingly and unreservedly, as a matter of principle. It invites GPs to provide services that are outward-looking, in solidarity with the community to serve the needs of patients and their immediate carers. The preventive perspective is comprehensive, embracing the total trajectory of the disease process from primordial to palliative. This is the primary care paradigm shift and it has to be enshrined in medical training. All those in training have to be educated in the values and meaning of generalism and continuing community care before some go on to specialise their skills. Other clinical professions must reflect this in their training programmes, in accordance with their particular methodology. Yet there is in the UK a widespread failure to grasp this. Hence, in general practice there are problems in morale, recruitment and retention. Primary healthcare and chronic illness care have to be at the heart of the curriculum of training for medicine and allied health professions.

THE NATIONAL HEALTH SERVICE IS WELL PLACED

The NHS that has evolved in the UK since the 1940s will be the location of the remainder of this section. It is the archetype of a health and welfare system that is based on distributive justice and it has been the template for many other countries. Despite the background noise of criticism and signs of internal stress, authoritative analysts at home and abroad regard the NHS as leading the world in fairness, accessibility and quality. It scores highly against 'Ham's Ten–Four' analysis, as we have seen. In funding and operation it is accountable to democratic control; it is free of charge to patients, technically advanced and quality controlled; it expresses values of patient centredness and public involvement, it promotes prevention and self-care, and it has a strong foundation in primary care. The popularity of the NHS is beyond doubt. Nigel Lawson (former UK Chancellor of the Exchequer) once described it as the nearest thing the English have to a religion. Since its inception it has been subjected to reform by successive governments, both of left and right. Despite this continuing moulding its fundamental characteristics have remained firmly rooted in public ownership, comprehensiveness and accountability to society. It has been endorsed by generations of voters and by accumulating evidence of performance. It would follow from this that the UK should not be seeking a new model of healthcare delivery. The NHS ought to be exempted from party political conflict. Having got the broad framework right in conceptual terms, there should be a cross-party consensus around its overall form. It should be regarded as akin to a nature reserve, to be managed according to sound, objective evidence related to best practice. Developmental investment to strengthen primary care further would predict more rational and economic use of precious hospital and specialist care resources, and enhanced overall care. Who could say no to that?

However, there are threats. Commoditising services and piecemeal privatisation, it is feared, will fragment the cohesive NHS model; overloading GPs with conflicting priorities diffuses their energies; micromanagement results in reform fatigue and declining morale; diversifying the GP identity will blur the concept and further damage recruitment. In terms of cost, international comparisons cluster close to 10% of GDP (with the exception of the USA). Society should demand evidence to show why this is deemed to be unaffordable. There must be yet some room for spending in order to save, and to safeguard life, especially in the interests of improved performance through application of the principles of the chronic care model. A further consideration is that the NHS depends on recruitment from abroad for about one-third of its medical workforce, the majority of these reaped from the health services of poorer nations and different systems of training. The UK undertrains for the requirement of its system, and this must be addressed if there is to be a cadre of doctors who are trained according to the priorities and values of the UK system. Asset-stripping poorer nations and less-developed systems makes a mockery of progressive development of UK medical curricula.

IS GENERAL PRACTICE MEETING THE CHALLENGE OF CHRONIC DISEASE?

In the UK, as everywhere, there is an insatiable growth in demand for health and social care services. This results in overload in the acute medical sector capacity

– hospital wards, A&E units and organisations that provide out-of-hours services. There is a tendency for officials to ruminate in the public media and wonder why GPs are not solving these problems, why they are not open all hours for immediate access, why they are admitting too many patients, why they are failing in proactive management and why they are allowing crises to occur. Many years ago, on returning from working in rural Africa, I was tempted to ask how many doctors a health service needs. There was no satisfactory answer then and there is certainly not one now. Whatever the perceptions, uses and abuses that apply, there has to be a public conversation about what is expected from primary care. Hospital bed capacity is shrinking and A&E units are being closed on safety grounds related to staff shortages, insufficient 'cover', patient safety or budgetary reasons, and 'normal clinical services' are expected to operate even outside conventional hours to improve access.

Unlimited availability on such a basis is not compatible with an expanding role in chronic illness care in the community, within the present levels of resourcing in UK general practice. We must guard against stretching too thinly the finite capacity of primary healthcare. When medical services are free of charge at the point of uptake, they face unlimited expectation and demand. Excessive demands on GPs lead to diminishing returns, whereby 'effective interventions are not feasible and feasible ones are not effective.'[5] Not surprisingly, people want the archetype of the avuncular and paternalistic 'Dr Cameron and Dr Finlay' (of AJ Cronin's novels) who will hold them through their crises; they also desire at the same time to have the fast-response technological efficiency of a clinical rescue machine, and all non-urgent (although important) normal care services to be available at times when the stockbroker is not broking his stock. Is the ideal partnership between doctor and patient, then, unrealisable? Partnership is mutual, and has to be worked at by all the participants. People are entitled to assert their right to a voice and to demand to be treated as partners in caring, especially when they suffer chronic illnesses. However, can partnership be nurtured, or indeed survive, in an atmosphere of criticism, threat of litigation, disappointed or conflicting expectations and not infrequently, misuse of services?

Allied to this conundrum is the unprecedented North Atlantic failure in financial and banking governance that has robbed 500 million people in Europe of resource reserve, not to mention growth. It is variously called recession and austerity. The difference between these terms is that whereas recession *hurts*, austerity *kills*. Health outcomes will suffer, service development will stall and high expectations of quality of care across all sectors will be disappointed. Governments always find themselves poorly placed to confront societal expectations and behaviour with respect to healthcare utilisation, but especially when they have to attempt to impose austerity measures. They seem tempted to mount an appearance of response through projecting blame for local service failure, increasing regulation and the micromanagement of health professionals. This is where workforce enthusiasm, morale, recruitment and productivity become casualties of circumstances. In times of austerity social conditions deteriorate and demands on healthcare intensify. It is then that the NHS needs greater resources, not less.

Nevertheless, ideals should be guarded and nurtured otherwise we lose the future. If we admit defeat in every sector of the chronic disease paradigm, the only victor will be the disease complex: the Dragon wins. Whatever else is lost through times of crisis, core professional values should be preserved. It is in this spirit that I commit the results of personal brainstorming to paper, as a challenge to others to pick away at the problems we all face and to create more authentic models for the way forward.

There is an undoubted conflict between the GP's roles as first-contact physician and continuity manager of chronic illness care. Equilibrium is elusive for the time being but local solutions will no doubt play a significant role in finding shortcuts and viable compromises, if not grand solutions. Attention to time management skills, honing routines and protocols to leaner dimensions, reducing reduplication of effort and economising: these are basic and constant concerns of practice management. It is worth noting here that one positive meaning of the word *austerity* is an *absence of frills* and a *positive regard for unadorned essentials.* In clinical services people ought to be satisfied with good plain fare rather than expect a champagne breakfast.

The enemies GPs face are disease, the fear of disease, fear of possible litigation or other medico-legal sanctions arising from adverse outcomes – not the general public or the other divisions of the caring services. Indeed, patients are our greatest fans, and GPs consistently receive a huge vote of confidence in public opinion polls. It is my experience that the old and the chronic sick are the least complaining and most appreciative of patients. Where conflicts of expectation occur, they tend to arise in the acute sector of primary care, at the open end of our high-volume filter. However open-ended or capacious, it is liable to become clogged and exhibit turbulent flow. As Schön said, we manage messes. If chronic illness care is to increase substantially, the problem of primary care access for acute ailments must be addressed and this will require national, service-wide strategies to back up local solutions. For example, the nurse-led 'drop-in centre' is an innovation that has been greatly valued by the public, especially young parents.

So, the message is, dump the fears of persecution, work diligently, keep good records and pay your indemnity dues so that you can focus on doing battle with disease, shoulder to shoulder with your comrades and patients. GPs in the NHS are already well placed to do so.

A MENU OF TACTICAL RESPONSES

> For every complex problem there is a solution that is simple, neat and wrong.[6]
>
> **HL Mencken ('the Sage of Baltimore')**

Managing the full trajectory of chronic disease should be entirely congruent with general practice. Who else is in a position to do it? The responsibility is ours. It has gradually worked its way into our portfolio of responsibilities and it will increase further its impact in primary care. For GPs, the 'crock of gold at the end of the rainbow' would contain treasures such as:

- ease of access for patients in accordance with their need
- longer, uninterrupted consultation times
- protected time for the various categories of essential practice activity – clinical, management and training
- afford to have a personal assistant each
- workload substitution – delegating or leaving down some existing activity when the need arises to assume new tasks
- less administration
- more space to accommodate the various services that might be offered
- to be allowed to get on with what we do best – seeing our patients
- a bit of appreciation now and again from government.

In other words, to be able to provide a comprehensive service that is, as one Ulster GP put it, '*handy, cheap and good*' (i.e. user-friendly, cost-effective and competent). However, as with the circus ringmaster's whip, when you tweak one end the other end cracks. It is perfectly possible to achieve these points, but not necessarily all at the same time. Nevertheless, it is a fair start when you draw up your wish list and examine each item individually for possibilities – to be debated, piloted, evaluated and implemented. Envisage solutions that can be prioritised into a plan of action. Every plan is a composite of small solutions. Practice management is partly about chipping away at the blocks – examining macro-problems for micro-solutions. Recognise that you cannot change the NHS systems or society's expectations of them; you can only change yourself and, perhaps, your team, and there are limits. Also, solutions cost money or its proxies (time, effort, personnel, meetings, equipment or space). Do not scorn micro-solutions or easy changes (that is, those ones you have already thought of or implemented). Everybody, from you up to WHO, is struggling against the rising tide of demography and disease burden. Even maintaining the status quo may be counted as success when the river of events is in spate and the tide is flowing against you.

Expansion in the chronic illness management aspects of general practice ought to mean that existing aspects of practice will move over or go away to accommodate them. This is improbable, but try to envisage how slimming and trimming might be processed, to reduce the 'weight' of procedure and to abate 'noise', that background of distracting trivia, the meaningless messages that demand attention and interfere with priority signals. Inappropriate use of top-level skills slows down the whole system. Not everyone needs doctor time. If this can be safely freed up at the acute, front end it will contribute to an increase in chronic illness care capacity. The looming workforce crisis in UK primary care relates to problems in recruitment and retention, early retirements and the increasing popularity of part-time jobs and 'portfolio careers' in general practice. Sessional doctors provide valuable services, and are perhaps most usefully deployed at the acute end of practice. There may have to be a 'quasi-consultant' grade of GP who carries strategic and executive functions. A joint report from The King's Fund and Nuffield Trust recommended that clinical commissioning groups provide funding to free some GPs for one day a week to focus on personalised care planning and strategic planning for their practice.[7]

TAKING STOCK OF UK PRIMARY CARE

'Ham's Ten–Four' model for a high-performing health service was introduced and discussed in Chapter 6.[8] Once again, it provides a convenient framework, for stock-taking, suitably redirected at the GP and the primary care setting.

1. *Universal coverage.* As a GP in the NHS you are an essential cog in the machine that is committed to providing comprehensive healthcare for all. Your NHS is endorsed by the UK population mandate since the 1940s. You have inherited a remarkable system of healthcare. You know who your patients are, and they know you. Do you know the community prevalence of the salient chronic conditions in your locality – who has what in terms of long-term conditions and disabilities in your practice population?

2. *Care is free at the point of uptake.* As a GP you have no defensive barriers against the patient. At times you may *wish* you had, but it is good for the people. You have no direct profit incentive to skew your decision responses to patients' needs. This may limit your income but it keeps you honest and keeps down costly and wasteful overtreatment. How can you manage *low-risk demand* so as to protect the service priorities of healthcare provision?

3. *Focus on prevention, not just treatment of sickness.* General practice in the NHS is a true health service. You have already assimilated much population medicine within your remit – immunisation and child developmental surveillance, the secondary prevention of the big non-communicable diseases, and much tertiary prevention in palliative and terminal care. How do you delegate and responsibility-share the routines of preventive work?

4. *Priority for patient self-management and carer support.* You are a family doctor with access to patients' homes, where chronic disease subsists. Is there more you can do to promote self-management, promote patient involvement or support the role of carers?

5. *Priority is given to primary care.* As a GP in the NHS you participate in the leading primary medical care system, yet you still inhabit a system that retains a hospital-centred culture. Can you be more assertive of the unique value of primary care? Can you prevail on hospitals to more closely support your work and be responsive to your needs?

6. *Population management is emphasised.* In your average-sized practice you manage healthcare for around 10 000 persons, coordinating open-ended, continuing, preventive and responsive care. You serve a local community and know its stress points and strengths. You are well placed to involve and invoke the local amenities, non-governmental organisations and social services. How might you carry out community needs assessment, risk-stratify your patients or inventorise local community services and health resources?

7. *Care should be integrated.* With your primary care team you have been developing, amid many distractions and with rudimentary support, ways of coordinating the vertical and horizontal axes of needs and resources. You already provide continuing and personalised care for the long-term sick and those with disabilities. What do you need from specialists and institutions to better achieve integration? What do you do to improve joined-up, minimally disruptive care for your chronic sick?

8. *Need to exploit IT to improve chronic illness care.* You are the best-equipped, most IT-literate and e-connected part of the health service, and you are world leaders in this regard. How do you manage and adapt current systems to serve more elegantly your needs, to economise your IT interface time and reduce screen fatigue?

9. *Care is coordinated.* GPs in the UK are familiar with the interface issues of hospital admission and discharge, managing the total medication load of each individual patient, working with a team of nurses and allied health professionals, and liaising with family carers. New challenges arise in extending integrated care, intermediate care, multidisciplinary working and commissioning of care. You are well placed to take on coordination – you are doing it already. What factors limit your effectiveness as a coordinator of care? What skill deficits and what obstacles do you encounter?

10. *Linking the nine characteristics in a coherent strategy for change.* But what change? Are we not sick of change? Why more change? Let me suggest that the nine characteristics are, in fact, processes and that change is inherent in each; further, that much of the implied change is already accomplished. You

have much experience of managing change and growth. So the tenth characteristic means refining the processes and applying them gradually to strengthen
the coherent strategy. All of the process characteristics are highly relevant to
chronic illness care. Taken collectively, they reflect the entire primary care
chronic illness programme.

As a GP you are delivering a great deal of this at micro and meso levels; you should
hope that further up the line, at macro level, others are doing half as well. But each
of the ten headings has raised questions for general practice:
- How well do we do this?
- How might we do it better, leaner and more effectively?

These are the stock questions of quality management that form the basis for clinical
audit. The well-worn audit path might usefully be applied to these as a measure of
the quality of chronic illness care. However, it is vital to remember that you do not
have to undertake all of this personally. You have a team of skilled people to share
the responsibilities.

Ham, of course also proposed four strategies: (1) physician leadership, (2) outcome
measures of quality, (3) alignment of incentives and (4) community engagement.
These were conceived with health services of every kind in mind. In the NHS we
might hope that the others 'upstairs' are forging ahead with these. For example,
when we are going to see any aligned incentives? Questions for GPs include how
good are we at measuring outcomes and how deep are our present levels of community engagement.

In summary, within the NHS we are fortunate to have both the structural vehicle for high-performance chronic care and the skilled professionals who are well
equipped to drive forward programmes of chronic care. This happy conclusion validates the present, and lends optimism about the future. It is not simply an exercise
in complacency but it has become increasingly clear as I worked around the chronic
disease paradigm and its appendages. I believe that **GPs in the UK are not sufficiently aware of the validity of what they do**. They are aware of the treadmill they
labour upon and the chorus of voices telling them it is not good enough and that
they ought to try harder and they have to do more. Commentators have described
this as 'hamster care'. It is fully possible that more can be achieved, not by treading
harder but by moulding, trimming and adapting the present state so that capacity
and effectiveness in chronic illness care are enhanced.

It is to be hoped that this is not also a self-satisfied UK manifesto that relegates
workers in other systems and jurisdictions to inferior status, with a future of mala-
dapted work patterns. Doctors, nurses, social workers and allied health professionals
tend to be conscientious people who enter the caring professions for intelligent

reasons, many of them altruistic and idealistic. None are responsible for the system or ethos they enter, since each of us stands on inherited ground. Professions and health systems have great inertia and there is frequently little the individual can do to influence the developments or directions of change or policy. What individuals anywhere can do is to inform themselves about the principles of chronic care and the full chronic disease paradigm, and to **incorporate these into personal modes of practice – especially in their teaching** and training activities as the foundation of future progress.

SLIMMING PRACTICE, WEIGHT REDUCTION AND NOISE ABATEMENT

The items that follow might not immediately reduce your workload. However, as a checklist it may help you identify areas to address or select for inclusion in a practice development plan. An early model of business management emphasised four facets: (1) plant (premises), (2) personnel, (3) equipment and (4) product. These are considered in turn, with hints on how efficacy for chronic illness care might be addressed without entirely losing sight of feasibility and resource implications.

1. Plant

The plant is the fixed asset – premises and usable space.

- Identify **choke points** related to premises – adequacy of waiting room, treatment rooms, reception and issues that affect through-flow; also disability access, health and safety, and an emergency response plan; maximise and diversify treatment room areas for nursing procedures and nurse-led clinics.
- Value-added **use of public spaces** to advertise services, health-related messages, information on self-health using light displays, DVD presentations, posters, leaflets – *delegated but actively managed.*
- Optimise use of space throughout **hours of opening**; expand as needed by renting space in nearby buildings for back-office activities, meetings or training space; think about a Portakabin if extension is not realistic; federate with other practices to improve space utilisation.
- **Excess computer** terminals and ports for opportunistic use with laptops (caution with security issues in use of Wi-Fi).
- **Co-location of services** means accommodating specific skills or providers within the GP premises even though they are not core team, e.g. counsellor or addiction adviser.

2. Personnel

Personnel are all those directly employed and attached clinical staff, and the administrative team.

- **Nursing team**: consolidate it, through direct employment and co-location where possible; enhance and optimise the skill-mix; maintain home-nursing capacity; promote and train to nurse practitioner level for enhanced decision-making, telephone triage and specialised nursing services; expand and support nurses' autonomy; reserve the highest-skilled nurses as key workers for clinics (diabetic, vascular, respiratory, etc.) and programmes such as bio-monitoring hazardous drugs including warfarin; the nurse and health visitor may cooperate to run a *well-being clinic (for risk factor and lifestyle management)*; spare nursing time through minimising nursing bureaucracy and devolving routine tasks to nursing assistant or phlebotomist, or introduce a 'biometric technician' who can take responsibility for collection of samples and lab transit, carry out electrocardiograms and non-invasive biometrics (e.g. weight and blood pressure); nurses may assist in telephone follow-up of patients, especially the housebound.
- **Employ a pharmacist** for sessions devoted to enhancing quality of prescribing, systems for managing repeat and indirect prescribing, maintaining the practice drug formulary, performing audits, and overseeing red/amber list drug safety with minimal reduplication of monitoring and testing; use repeat dispensing to minimise re-ordering.
- **Expand the team** with sessions by a physiotherapist (back pain clinic) or counsellor (relationship and family problems, bereavement support and other personal crisis); other allied health professionals?
- Create **desk officers**, posts of special responsibility that extend the reach of existing staff; for example, for IT support, create and manage a website; filter, triage or redirect incoming mail or e-mail; oversee and administer the screening system.
- Create **task forces** and **leads for key areas** such as clinical governance, prevention, commissioning.
- **Promote team members** to the point of their competence (underemployment is wasteful and dispiriting); reward initiative and volunteering for responsibilities; train, appraise and affirm; nurture team morale (I know, it all costs money!)

3. Equipment

Equipment mainly covers diagnostic, communications and data processing.

Diagnostics

- **In-house and locality-shared access** to imaging, endoscopy, cardiology screening tests, tissue sampling for cytology, biopsy and clinical chemistry; direct access to these eases choke points and minimises referral and waiting lists, and it reduces frustrations for patients by accelerating clinical pathways.
- **Near-patient and self-test** devices for diabetes, lipids, warfarin, oximetry, simple biometrics.

- **Connected care** systems for monitoring less ambulant patients.
- **Maintenance** of equipment and **user skills** (especially resuscitation skills and apparatus).

Patient access systems

- Optimise user-friendly **phone-in capacity**; spare incoming phone line capacity by using mobile phones and e-mail for outward communication; employ electronic access for patients prudently (it creates expectations of instant response and other hazards); use 'return call' processes for enquiries, nurse triage, phone consultation and to filter requests for services.
- Have a **'quick-sick'** stream to assess patients' urgent, but not necessarily serious, needs that might not need doctor time.
- **Auto-check-in** systems can reduce reception queues (if properly used).
- **Information and guidance** for patients, using in-house and electronic facilities, signposting to online resources via a website platform that can carry multiple kinds of links for supported self-care and information support.

Informatics

- **Nurture the clinical record**: ensure that diagnostics and data-download systems mesh with the practice computer network to avoid reduplicating input effort; ensure consistency of recording – that all clinical users are trained to input, edit and delete data responsibly and accountably. The clinical database spares time and trouble if it is well tended. It is 'organic' – it grows, and grows wild, unless tended, pruned, shaped and fed the right stuff; it is easily infected and parasitised with unwanted material; exclude unnecessary inputting and 'scanning-in'.
- Use **online information** resources and **decision support** to minimise library or reference work; also a web-based information database for patient use or to generate educative handout leaflets.
- Employ a **data-desk** manager, IT technician, website manager.
- Integrate the system with laboratory and hospital services by on-line electronic linkage.
- Use an electronic diary and daybook; to syndicate to team all relevant 'news' and patient events.
- Software development takes place further upstream but can be influenced through a **software users' group**: to declutter and prioritise screen presentation, minimise flags and drop-downs, and combat 'alert fatigue'.

4. Product

In general practice, product means systems and services.

Systems

- **Teach and train** – this embeds systematic thinking and reflective practice, and promotes quality of care.
- **Fix choke points** and work on access issues.
- **Responsibility sharing**: create desks to oversee, for example, reliable call and recall; the system of screening and surveillance; internal network desk to filter and redirect accurately all incoming messages, including e-mail.
- Care-planning to **share out responsibilities**; risk-stratify to focus care management.
- Integrate and **bundle diverse services**, customised to suit the individuals with complex needs.
- Review less: **redirect** holding work, stress management and relationship problems to a counsellor and risk factor management to the well-being clinic; use phone-review for the house-bound.
- Use **virtual ward** concept to manage selected patients through crises; make sure it has a 'revolving door' so that capacity for high-level care is protected.
- Automate recurring prescribing; minimise complexity of drug lists through **periodic review**; what is appropriate, essential and safe?
- Use a **practice formulary** actively to simplify and safeguard prescribing decisions.
- Turn discrete data into analogue form, graphs rather than tables, to highlight **trajectory trends** where possible.
- Turn areas of chronic care into onscreen protocols or guideline-type documents to streamline decision-making (**decision support**).
- Liaise with hospitals, trusts and clinical commissioning groups about reformatting the communications they send you – for example, letters that are recurrently excessive, over-inclusive, anonymous, misdirected or *serve their purposes rather than yours*; that contain action points hidden in voluminous prose and which are not highlighted; to reduce and compact letters and documents to screen-friendly format that can be speed-read – for example, a functional, informative letterhead with an identifying subject and source tag at the top for ease of reference, classification and recall; (we don't need to know that our hospital is a non-smoking hospital with community commitment and a fancy logo); this is **essential risk management**.
- Confront **waiting lists** – they waste everybody's time and the work doesn't go away, it accumulates; you are the advocate for the patient; 'downstream obstruction creates flooding upstream', with heightened risks for both patient and GP; find collateral channels around fixed obstructions to flow.
- Pool management functions, skills and back-office tasks with **neighbouring practices** (perhaps through federation).

Services

- Prioritise **self-management** by patients; engage, inform, involve and signpost to further services; people who are ill are not always at their best; the sickest may be least well placed to self-manage; remember the inverse care law.
- Minimise **doctor dependency** and work on adherence issues.
- Manage **frequent attendees** actively and non-judgementally; remember that they occupy higher risk status.
- Examine **inappropriate use of services**; confront if necessary (but responsibly); some will be attention-seeking, but can their needs be met?
- Review less (but safety-net): extend intervals and use the phone; rationalise and bundle tests ('we'll get your diabetic bloods done while you are in for your lithium check') and **minimise duplication** of effort; task-share or redirect follow-up tasks where possible.
- Do not replicate specialist clinics; supplement them; **shared care** means meshing services.
- Manage **interface issues** actively; transitional and handover points entail additional risks for the patient.
- Confront delays and waiting lists, but **safety-net** patients (until they are progressed onwards through the system).
- Share extended services with neighbouring practices; consider formal **federation**.

For the sake of completeness, a checklist for self-care by the clinician

- Recall the big five risk factor list for chronic disease – obesity, lipids, addictions, lack of exercise, hypertension; they apply to you too!
- You are of little use to others if you have serious unmet issues.
- You are a danger to all (yourself included) if you have untreated illness (e.g. depression, addiction or stress disorders).
- Sick people are often not at their best, and neither are you – make allowances; avoidable conflict squanders time and emotional energy; chronic illness is painful for all concerned and you share in it.
- Develop an area of special interest in, say, a clinical, educational or representational role; or become a GP with a Special Interest (a sub-specialist).
- Develop reflective practice habits – for examples, a learning diary, a portfolio of achievement, and enjoy continuing professional development events.
- The quality agenda is not about finding a proportion of doctors who are underperforming but searching out that proportion within each of us that could improve.
- Evaluate your work; receiving feedback is important but you are more likely to perceive and internalise criticism; direct patient feedback is not the sum

total of your worth, though it is worth listening to; there are other means of self-evaluation.

- Audit is non-judgemental and formative; it reveals areas where you could do better.
- Resolve complexity by breaking it into bite-sized chunks; analyse macro problems to find micro-solutions.
- Therapeutic failure, relapse and crises are intrinsic to the trajectory of chronic disease; you may be blamed for much but it is not all your fault.
- Identify a colleague whom you trust as a mentor, as a reference person to confide in.
- Know when to take a break and practise stress-busting tactics.
- Protect your home from carried-over negativity; tend your work–life balance and **significant relationships**; get a hobby and get a life.
- Engage with your team, foster morale and mutual support, identify burnout in others; create fun team events.
- Have 'moaning coffee' time without guilt, but don't overindulge; constant moaning breeds alienation.
- Remember Maslow's hierarchy of basic needs: optimise your working conditions; a pleasant consulting room is a boon to your patients as well as to yourself.

CHRONIC CARE GUIDELINES FOR THE GENERAL PRACTITIONER

This final section is a checklist of issues for GPs, to help them to create their own solutions to their own problems. Given that much of the chronic care paradigm change is well advanced in the NHS and especially in general practice, what are the priorities now?

1. To assert that chronic illness care has at least equal value to that of acute treatment services. Good chronic care provision assimilates the skills of good acute care, while the reverse does not hold. In educational and skills training chronic care deserves high priority.

    Unsolved problem: the medical and lay cultures remain hospital and disease oriented.

2. Recognising that our default position in the past has relied on episodic, reactive care on the medical model, to move beyond that and prioritise continuous care, based on the trajectory model of the illness process. When illness is chronic we need to convert episodes, encounters and observations into trends, pattern recognition, prognosis and preventive action (anticipatory care). There is a need to retrain ourselves in this and to model it to our trainees.

    Unsolved problems include how to process this task of longitudinal surveillance without objectifying people, but with early minimum interventions and minimal disruption; also we need reliable software that will shortcut tedious data entry by converting discrete data into continuous data, preferably in graphic form that reveals trends and intervention thresholds.

3. Medical leadership in multidisciplinary teams implies expanding our clinical reach to take account of the full chronic disease paradigm. Primary *medical* care should ensure:
    i. that good management addresses the patient and family's self-help and support needs
    ii. inclusion of the social complex that links the patient complex with community services
    iii. that the policy complex both informs and enhances service development
    iv. that the learning and teaching complex delivers training for chronic care as a routine of practice, in order to address comprehensively the needs of patients.

    Unsolved problem areas here include interdisciplinary group working and learning. Our trainees need to be instructed on this.

4. Personalised, managed care of multi-morbidity in prioritised patients is the main aim of integrated care. This is routine in general practice for the terminal care trajectory phase. Such an approach would be highly desirable if it were generalised through the disease trajectory for those who would benefit from it, especially the non-ambulant or those with heavy symptom burden. This is beginning to be seen in practices, and hospices are extending their remit beyond cancer care. The Patient's Passport, a new and promising tool being developed by RCGP Northern Ireland, is a patient-held record for use in advanced chronic and terminal disease.[9] Training in palliative and terminal care skills is a good preparation for extending this kind of teamwork practice beyond cancer care, to encompass chronic heart failure, respiratory failure, degenerative neurological disorders and severe disability.

    Unsolved problem: how to manage the consequent patterns of work sustainably.

5. Teach and train as part of routine practice; assimilate this into the routines of practice life. Chronic illness care begins with medical school and involves the whole team.

    Unsolved problems: the lack of a chronic illness care curriculum; clinical teaching tends to be restricted to accredited practice teachers; there is historical deprivation of practice teaching facilities and resources for training in educational techniques.

6. Marathon training. Morale, resilience, peer support and commitment are frequent casualties in primary care. As the load of chronic disease management

accumulates these need to be sustained. Current trends exacerbate this problem area.

Unsolved problem: we lack structures and skills and methods to respond effectively to the morale crisis. There is probably another book on this yet to be written by someone.

CONCLUSION

Writing about chronic disease is like trying to photograph a multidimensional and fast-moving target; and, as with the Rubik Cube puzzle, it is difficult to align all the variables as a neat solution. I am conscious of the limitations inherent in telling this story. Attempting to describe the issues and components of chronic disease has required straying widely around our principal concern, that is, the wellbeing of our patients. It is impossible to avoid writing from a particular perspective or point of reference. I have spent my professional life as a GP and teacher within the National Health Service of the UK, and these form the only framework that I can adopt authentically. I am not in a position to prescribe for other countries and health systems, nor to tell specialists how to be special, managers how to manage or policy-makers to legislate. I cannot even advise GPs how to do their job since every practice is a unique microcosm within the NHS galaxy. However, two particular constituencies are being addressed directly: (1) the primary healthcare team, and (2) students, trainees and lifelong learners in health-related professions, with some optimism that readers from other backgrounds will benefit through carrying out their own translations around the universal concepts presented.

Regretfully, at the close of this account of chronic disease, I am unable to declare the death of the Dragon. However, if you recall the fable from Chapter 2, the well-aimed sword thrust by St George saved the life of the Princess Sabra and the resulting axillary injury disabled the Dragon to the point where it could be confined. Victory over the Dragon only took place when the people of the Kingdom of Lasia mended their ways through righteous living. No doubt this included healthy exercise, the avoidance of empty calories, eating up their vegetables and going 'cold turkey'. Their health services inevitably played a part in this and reflected the benefits.

So, what lessons does the story hold for us in terms of policy and practice?
- Tackle the well-known risk factors and emphasise prevention.
- Address the social determinants of health and disease, and confront health inequalities.
- Adopt the paradigm change to endorse the key role of primary care.
- Adjust the current emphasis on increasingly rarefied episodic care towards chronic care.
- Enhance research on the big chronic diseases with the emphasis on delivery of

appropriate services and integrating clinical pathways; this is needed especially in chronic mental illness, Alzheimer's and other neurological syndromes, multiple disability, vascular disease, diabetes, addictions and cancers.

- Develop community social service care pathways.
- Nurture a healthcare workforce that is adequate in numbers and thoroughly trained from the start in the principles of chronic care.
- Preserve the cohesive model of healthcare based on universal free access, risk-sharing, comprehensive personal and population medicine, and incentives that are aligned towards patient-centred outcomes rather than profit-taking.

The UK is fortunate in having such a vehicle that has stood the test of time and electoral endorsement for over 60 years; it has delivered sustained progress at individual and electoral levels. To fragment it in favour of managerially-led and for-profit programmes would be both unnecessary and retrogressive. The vehicle works and only needs to be up-graded and re-tuned to the challenging terrain that lies ahead, and that is sufficient challenge.

The elements of this story point to an NHS-style model with realigned priorities that endorse the GP and primary care team, and re-invigorate them with vision and a new sense of purpose. If general practice is appropriately staffed and resourced and has the backing of the specialist sector the impending threats will become manageable. The challenges lie in priority-setting, political leadership, finding the financial resources in difficult times, and provision of relevant training for the healthcare workforce.

These chapters have mapped out and explored a wide territory that is characterised by growing controversy, complexity and bemusement. There is much in the recent developments around chronic disease that mystifies and alarms clinical front-line workers. One aim of this book has been to summarise and demystify the clouds of terminology in the policies and practice of healthcare that are accumulating over the territory of chronic disease. A further aim has been to highlight three new concepts that transcend systems of care.

1. That chronic diseases, in their bewildering diversity, may usefully be thought of as *a single genus*; the natural history and ecological analysis has pointed to generic measures that indicate the possibility of managed coexistence with this growing threat.
2. *The chronic disease paradigm* provides a constant reminder of the full context of chronic disease management as the vehicle for effective chronic illness care. It locates all the stakeholders within a comprehensive framework that recognises and values the contribution of all of them. It may help define areas in need of research and development.
3. The *disease trajectory model* stands as a challenge to a clinical mindset that relies

on episodic and fragmentary approaches to patient care; it prompts physicians especially to adopt the chronic care approach – a preventive, prospective and patient-centred awareness.

This triad provides the basis for an *educational* approach to chronic care, as *distinct from a regulatory, micromanaged* one. It is applicable at all stage of clinical career and offers a teaching aid for all involved in training. All clinicians have a calling to teach and train. Educational skills are closely related to the skills of communicating effectively with patients. People are hungry for information, interpretation and guidance. What we individually might do differently, therefore, is to reorient our consciousness around these four coordinates: the generic model, the paradigm, the trajectory and the educational mission.

Will this change the way we think and act? Will it change the way we organise our working practices? Will it change the way we teach and train? Will patients benefit from all of this? Whatever the answers to these questions, we will not go far wrong if as individual practitioners, irrespective of our nationality, system or specialty, we hold the patient and family at the core of our concerns; coordinate best practice to smooth the pathway of their experience; attempt to minimise any necessary disruption to their lives; hold and support them through their rough times; continually strive to improve the ways we deliver services; and pass on this mission in breadth and depth through example and educational commitment.

It all begins and ends with the patient and family, for it is they who carry the burden of chronic disease.

REFERENCES

1. www.population-health.manchester.ac.uk/healtheconomics/research/FinalReportofthe 7thNationalGPWorklifeSurvey.pdf (accessed 18 April 2014).
2. Davies M. Revealed: half of GPs at high risk of burnout. *Pulse*. 4 June 2013. www.pulse today.co.uk/home/battling-burnout/revealed-half-of-gps-at-high-risk-of-burnout/ 20003157.article#.Uy085xzUR21 (accessed 18 April 2014).
3. Porter M. New Year Message from the Chair of BMA Council. 30 Dec 2013, #6483333.
4. World Health Organization. *Innovative Care for Chronic Conditions: building blocks for action*. Geneva: WHO; 2002. pp. 4–5.
5. Sun Xin, Guyatt GH. Interventions to enhance self-management support. *Brit Med J*. 2013; **346**: f3949.
6. Mencken HL. www.brainyquote.com/quotes/authors/h/h_l_mencken.html (accessed 21 April 2014).
7. Iacobucci G. Government must act to ease strain on GPs, say Nuffield Trust and King's Fund. *Brit Med J*. 2013; **347**: f4612.
8. Ham C. The ten characteristics of the high-performing chronic care system. *Health economics, policy and law*. 2009; **5**: 71–90.

9. Abbott A. *Communication and Continuity in Progressive Life-limiting Illness. A report by the Royal College of General Practitioners Northern Ireland.* Belfast RCGPNI. [Publication Pending.].

A simple integrated chronic disease management paradigm

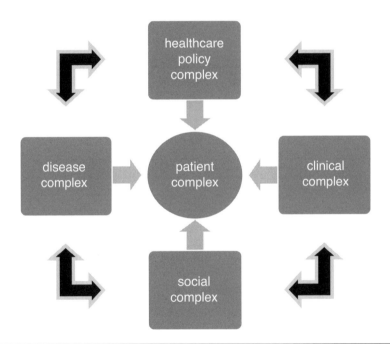

NOTES

The *patient complex* represents the person who has the chronic condition[s], the immediate family carers and social circle of those affected.

The *disease complex* represents all matters related to the pathological condition and the disease consequences.

The *clinical complex* represents the total response of all clinicians and allied professions in primary, secondary and tertiary care.

The *healthcare policy complex* represents the health system, those institutions and policies that constitute the framework of health delivery.

The *social complex* represents the response of society, statutory and voluntary services and welfare system.

The *learning–teaching complex* subsists throughout all domains.

The trajectory model of chronic disease

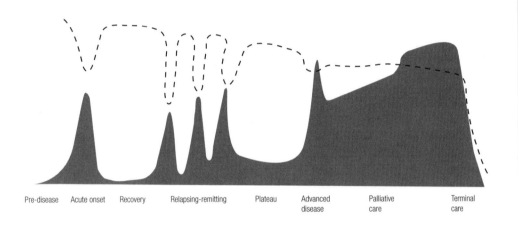

Pre-disease | Acute onset | Recovery | Relapsing-remitting | Plateau | Advanced disease | Palliative care | Terminal care

A timeline of progression in disease activity, phases of change, and (dotted line) corresponding loss of functional capacity

Modified pyramid of levels of care

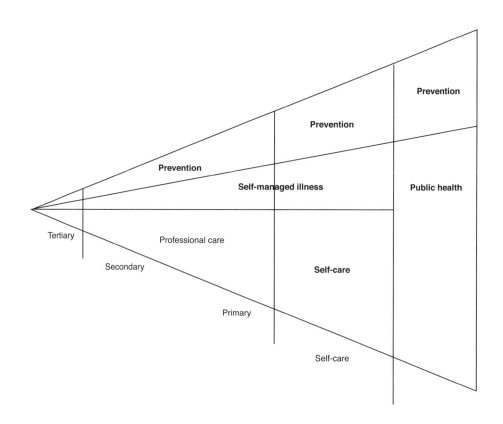

Index

CPD with Radcliffe

You can now use a selection of our books to achieve CPD (Continuing Professional Development) points through directed reading.

We provide a free online form and downloadable certificate for your appraisal portfolio. Look for the CPD logo and register with us at: www.radcliffehealth.com/cpd

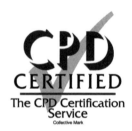